25,000+
Baby Names

25,000+
Baby Names

Bruce Lansky

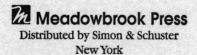

Meadowbrook Press
Distributed by Simon & Schuster
New York

Library of Congress Cataloging-in-Publication Data

Lansky, Bruce.

25,000+ baby names / by Bruce Lansky.
   p. cm.
   Summary: "Includes more than 25,000 popular and unique names, complete with origins, meanings, variant spellings, and notable facts and namesakes"--Provided by publisher.
   ISBN 0-88166-491-X (Meadowbrook Press) ISBN 0-684-03450-6 (Simon & Schuster)
   1. Names, Personal--Dictionaries. I. Title: Twenty-five thousand plus baby names. II. Title.
   CS2377.L348 2005
   929.4'4'03--dc22   2005003741

Coordinating Editor: Angela Wiechmann
Proofreader: Megan McGinnis
Production Manager: Paul Woods
Graphic Design Manager: Tamara Peterson
Cover Photograph: Jim Cummins

Published by Meadowbrook Press, 5451 Smetana Drive, Minnetonka, Minnesota 55343

www.meadowbrookpress.com

BOOK TRADE DISTRIBUTION by Simon and Schuster, a division of Simon and Schuster, Inc., 1230 Avenue of the Americas, New York, New York 10020

10 09 08 07   11 10 9 8 7 6 5

Printed in the United States of America

Contents

Introduction

When you think about names for your baby, you'll find yourself daydreaming about what he or she may look like and be like. And you'll find yourself thinking about your hopes and dreams for the newest member of your family.

You'll put first, middle, and last names together and say them out loud. Someone watching you may think you're talking to yourself.

You'll also find yourself fascinated by all the names you read in the birth announcements; names in your local child care center, school, church; names in the news, in books, in movies, on television, on your favorite team, or on the Internet.

Don't be surprised to discover that you've developed a "fashion sense" about which names are currently "in" and which names are currently "out." As a result, you may find yourself considering:

- names from other countries and ethnic groups;
- names that have been recently created (perhaps a name you've made up yourself);
- names that feature new spellings of familiar names;
- names for a girl that once were more often used for boys, and vice versa;
- names that are traditional surnames.

You'll probably consider some names your parents never did. Interesting, unusual names from all around the world surround you. Pick up the sports section and you'll read about Shaquille, Kobe, Andre, and Lleyton. Turn on the radio and you'll hear Shania, Beyoncé, and Alanis perform. Go to the movies and you'll see Uma, Charlize, and Angelina.

This book was designed to open up the whole world of names to you. I scoured the world for popular and unusual names that just might work for your child.

I created this book to give you the choice of a lifetime—interesting and unusual names from all around the world are right at your fingertips.

Happy hunting,

Bruce Lansky

Ten Factors to Consider When Naming Your Baby

If you have a name you like, you already know how pleasant it is going through life with a name that "fits" or "feels right." If you don't, you know how unpleasant it is to go through life with a name that, for whatever reason, doesn't work for you.

It may help to test each name you're considering against a list of factors that could affect the way a name will work for your child. This will help make the subjective process of selecting a name more objective for you.

Using the chart below, give each name you're considering two points for a positive rating on any criterion, one point for a medium rating, and zero points for a negative rating.

I realize that this scoring system has a built-in bias toward names that are relatively common and familiar—and therefore easy to spell and pronounce. However, you're free to give extra weight to any factor you like. If, for example, you love exotic names that are unfamiliar (and potentially hard to spell and pronounce), you might want to double the weight of the "uniqueness" and/or "sound/rhythm" factors. I hope this process helps you find a name that works both for you and your child.

Factors	Positive	Medium	Negative
1. Spelling	❏ easy	❏ medium	❏ hard
2. Pronunciation	❏ easy	❏ medium	❏ hard
3. Gender ID	❏ clear	❏ neutral	❏ confusing
4. Stereotypes	❏ positive	❏ okay	❏ negative
5. Sound/Rhythm	❏ pleasing	❏ okay	❏ unpleasant
6. Nicknames	❏ appealing	❏ okay	❏ unappealing
7. Meaning	❏ positive	❏ okay	❏ negative
8. Popularity	❏ *not* too popular	❏ popular	❏ too popular
9. Uniqueness	❏ *not* too unique	❏ unique	❏ too unique
10. Initials	❏ pleasing	❏ okay	❏ unpleasant

The 100 Most Popular Girls' Names in 2005

2005 Rank	Name	2004 Rank	Rank Change	2005 Rank	Name	2004 Rank	Rank Change
1	Emily	1	—	26	Hailey	24	−2
2	Emma	2	—	27	Jessica	21	−6
3	Madison	3	—	28	Victoria	28	—
4	Abigail	6	+2	29	Jasmine	26	−3
5	Olivia	4	−1	30	Sydney	27	−3
6	Isabella	7	+1	31	Julia	32	+1
7	Hannah	5	−2	32	Destiny	39	+7
8	Samantha	9	+1	33	Morgan	31	−2
9	Ava	25	+16	34	Kaitlyn	33	−1
10	Ashley	8	−2	35	Savannah	41	+6
11	Sophia	15	+4	36	Katherine	35	−1
12	Elizabeth	10	−2	37	Alexandra	37	—
13	Alexis	11	−2	38	Rachel	34	−4
14	Grace	13	−1	39	Lily	52	+13
15	Sarah	12	−3	40	Megan	36	−4
16	Alyssa	14	−2	41	Kaylee	50	+9
17	Mia	30	+13	42	Jennifer	38	−4
18	Natalie	19	+1	43	Angelina	60	+17
19	Chloe	23	+4	44	Makayla	47	+3
20	Brianna	17	−3	45	Allison	40	−5
21	Lauren	16	−5	46	Brooke	44	−2
22	Ella	29	+7	47	Maria	45	−2
23	Anna	20	−3	48	Trinity	48	—
24	Taylor	22	−2	49	Lillian	65	+16
25	Kayla	18	−7	50	Mackenzie	43	−7

2005 Rank	Name	2004 Rank	Rank Change	2005 Rank	Name	2004 Rank	Rank Change
51	Faith	53	+2	76	Sara	68	−8
52	Sofia	69	+17	77	Audrey	80	+3
53	Riley	58	+5	78	Brooklyn	101	+23
54	Haley	42	−12	79	Vanessa	75	−4
55	Gabrielle	73	+18	80	Amanda	67	−13
56	Nicole	46	−1	81	Ariana	79	−2
57	Kylie	49	−8	82	Rebecca	72	−10
58	Katelyn	59	+1	83	Caroline	74	−9
59	Zoe	54	−5	84	Amelia	96	+12
60	Paige	51	−9	85	Mariah	113	+28
61	Gabriella	76	+15	86	Jordan	70	−16
62	Jenna	56	−6	87	Jocelyn	84	−3
63	Kimberly	61	−2	88	Arianna	86	−2
64	Stephanie	55	−9	89	Isabel	87	−2
65	Alexa	71	+6	90	Marissa	78	−12
66	Avery	77	+11	91	Autumn	82	−9
67	Andrea	57	−10	92	Melanie	89	−3
68	Leah	64	−4	93	Aaliyah	94	+1
69	Madeline	62	−7	94	Gracie	114	+20
70	Nevaeh	104	+34	95	Claire	98	+3
71	Evelyn	83	+12	96	Isabelle	107	+11
72	Maya	85	+13	97	Molly	97	—
73	Mary	63	−10	98	Mya	116	+18
74	Michelle	66	−8	99	Diana	90	−9
75	Jada	81	+6	100	Katie	103	+3

The 100 Most Popular Boys' Names in 2005

2005 Rank	Name	2004 Rank	Rank Change	2005 Rank	Name	2004 Rank	Rank Change
1	Jacob	1	—	26	Logan	27	+1
2	Michael	2	—	27	Brandon	22	−5
3	Joshua	3	—	28	Gabriel	32	+4
4	Matthew	4	—	29	Zachary	26	−3
5	Ethan	5	—	30	Jose	28	−2
6	Andrew	6	—	31	Elijah	31	—
7	Daniel	7	—	32	Angel	44	+12
8	Anthony	11	+3	33	Kevin	34	+1
9	Christopher	10	+1	34	Jack	41	+7
10	Joseph	9	−1	35	Caleb	33	−2
11	William	8	−3	36	Justin	30	−6
12	Alexander	15	+3	37	Austin	35	−2
13	Ryan	12	−1	38	Evan	39	+1
14	David	14	—	39	Robert	36	−3
15	Nicholas	13	−2	40	Thomas	37	−3
16	Tyler	16	—	41	Luke	42	+1
17	James	17	—	42	Mason	52	+10
18	John	18	—	43	Aidan	40	−3
19	Jonathan	21	+2	44	Jackson	48	+4
20	Nathan	20	—	45	Isaiah	45	—
21	Samuel	23	+2	46	Jordan	43	−3
22	Christian	24	+2	47	Gavin	51	+4
23	Noah	29	+6	48	Connor	38	−10
24	Dylan	19	−5	49	Aiden	60	+11
25	Benjamin	25	—	50	Isaac	46	−4

2005 Rank	Name	2004 Rank	Rank Change	2005 Rank	Name	2004 Rank	Rank Change
51	Jason	47	−4	76	Carter	87	+11
52	Cameron	50	−2	77	Hayden	88	+11
53	Hunter	49	−4	78	Jeremiah	78	—
54	Jayden	62	+8	79	Cole	75	−4
55	Juan	54	−1	80	Brayden	107	+27
56	Charles	56	—	81	Wyatt	90	+9
57	Aaron	53	−4	82	Chase	80	−2
58	Lucas	67	+9	83	Steven	77	−6
59	Luis	57	−2	84	Timothy	79	−5
60	Owen	66	+6	85	Dominic	91	+6
61	Landon	86	+25	86	Sebastian	96	+10
62	Diego	73	+11	87	Xavier	89	+2
63	Brian	59	−4	88	Jaden	83	−5
64	Adam	58	−6	89	Jesse	94	+5
65	Adrian	72	+7	90	Devin	81	−9
66	Kyle	55	−11	91	Seth	82	−9
67	Eric	61	−6	92	Antonio	93	+1
68	Ian	69	+1	93	Richard	92	−1
69	Nathaniel	68	−1	94	Miguel	97	+3
70	Carlos	71	+1	95	Colin	84	−11
71	Alex	63	−8	96	Cody	85	−11
72	Bryan	64	−8	97	Alejandro	99	+2
73	Jesus	70	−3	98	Caden	104	+6
74	Julian	74	—	99	Blake	95	−4
75	Sean	65	−10	100	Carson	101	+1

Changes in Top 100 from 2004 to 2005

Big Gains

Girls		Boys	
Nevaeh	+34	Brayden	+27
Mariah	+28	Landon	+25
Brooklyn	+23	Angel	+12
Gracie	+20	Aiden	+11
Gabrielle	+18	Diego	+11
Mya	+18	Carter	+11
Angelina	+17	Hayden	+11
Sofia	+17	Mason	+10
Ava	+16	Sebastian	+10
Lillian	+16	Lucas	+9

Big Losses

Girls		Boys	
Jordan	−16	Kyle	−11
Amanda	−13	Colin	−11
Haley	−12	Cody	−11
Marissa	−12	Connor	−10
Nicole	−10	Sean	−10
Andrea	−10	Devin	−9
Mary	−10	Seth	−9
Rebecca	−10	Alex	−8
Paige	−9	Bryan	−8
Stephanie	−9	Patrick	−8

New to Top 100

Girls		Boys	
Brooklyn	+23	Brayden	+27
Gracie	+20	Caden	+6
Isabelle	+11	Carson	+1
Katie	+3		
Mariah	+28		
Mya	+18		
Nevaeh	+34		

Out of Top 100

Girls		Boys	
Leslie	−8	Jake	−4
Amber	−14	Ashton	−31
Danielle	−12	Patrick	−8
Melissa	−4		
Sierra	−13		
Bailey	−9		
Erin	−17		

The Most Popular Names for Twins in 2005

Twin Girls	Twin Boys	Twin Girl and Boy
Faith, Hope	Jacob, Joshua	Taylor, Tyler
Hailey, Hannah	Matthew, Michael	Madison, Mason
Madison, Morgan	Daniel, David	Emma, Ethan
Mackenzie, Madison	Ethan, Evan	Emily, Ethan
Ella, Emma	Isaac, Isaiah	Madison, Matthew
Hannah, Sarah	Joseph, Joshua	Ella, Ethan
Faith, Grace	Nathan, Nicholas	Sophia, Samuel
Emily, Sarah	Alexander, Andrew	Ava, Aidan
Olivia, Sophia	Elijah, Isaiah	Alexis, Alexander
Ashley, Emily	Jordan, Justin	Natalie, Nathan
Elizabeth, Emily	Alexander, Nicholas	Brianna, Brian
Elizabeth, Katherine	Caleb, Joshua	Jada, Jaden
Abigail, Allison	Jonathan, Joshua	
Amy, Emily	Alexander, Benjamin	
Gabriella, Isabella	Andrew, Matthew	
Isabella, Sophia	Benjamin, Samuel	
Megan, Morgan	James, John	
Ava, Olivia	Matthew, Nicholas	
Abigail, Emily	Brandon, Brian	
Anna, Emma	Alexander, Zachary	
Haley, Hannah	Dylan, Tyler	
Reagan, Riley	Christian, Christopher	

Names Inspired by People, Places, and Things

Literature

Authors

Female	Male
Anne (Tyler)	Ambrose (Bierce)
Barbara (Kingsolver)	Bram (Stoker)
Carolyn (Keene)	Cormac (McCarthy)
Charlotte (Brontë)	Dan (Brown)
Doris (Lessing)	Ernest (Hemingway)
Elizabeth (Barrett Browning)	George (Orwell)
Emily (Dickinson)	Henry David (Thoreau)
Harper (Lee)	Homer
Harriet (Beecher Stowe)	J. D. (Salinger)
Jane (Austen)	Jules (Verne)
Joanne Kathleen (J. K. Rowling)	Leo (Tolstoy)
Judy (Blume)	Lewis (Carroll)
Katherine (Mansfield)	Mario (Puzo)
Louisa (May Alcott)	Mark (Twain)
Lucy Maud (Montgomery)	Nicholas (Sparks)
Madeleine (L'Engle)	Oscar (Wilde)
Margaret (Atwood)	Ray (Bradbury)
Marge (Piercy)	Scott (Fitzgerald)
Mary (Shelley)	Stephen (King)
Maya (Angelou)	Tennessee (Williams)
Paula (Danziger)	Tom (Clancy)
Rebecca (Wells)	Truman (Capote)
Sylvia (Plath)	Virgil
Virginia (Woolf)	Walt (Whitman)
Willa (Cather)	William (Faulkner)

Fictional Characters

Female	Male
Anna (Karenina)	Atticus (Finch)
Anne (Shirley)	Billy (Coleman)
Antonia (Shimerda)	Boo (Radley)
Bridget (Jones)	Cyrus (Trask)
Cosette (Valjean)	Edmond (Dantés)
Daisy (Buchanan)	Ethan (Frome)
Dorothea (Brooke)	Frodo (Baggins)
Edna (Pontellier)	Guy (Montag)
Elizabeth (Bennet)	Harry (Potter)
Emma (Woodhouse)	Heathcliff
Hermione (Granger)	Henry (Fleming)
Hester (Prynne)	Holden (Caulfield)
Isabel (Archer)	Huck (Finn)
Jane (Eyre)	Jake (Barnes)
Josephine (March)	Jay (Gatsby)
Juliet (Capulet)	Jean (Valjean)
Junie (B. Jones)	John (Proctor)
Mary (Lennox)	Odysseus
Meg (Murry)	Owen (Meany)
Ophelia	Pip (Philip Pirrip)
Phoebe (Caulfield)	Rhett (Butler)
Pippi (Longstocking)	Robinson (Crusoe)
Scarlett (O'Hara)	Romeo (Montague)
Scout (Finch)	Santiago
Serena (Joy)	Victor (Frankenstein)

Movies and TV

Movie Stars

Female	Male
Angelina (Jolie)	Benicio (Del Toro)
Anjelica (Huston)	Bing (Crosby)
Audrey (Hepburn)	Bruce (Willis)
Betty (Grable)	Cary (Grant)
Cameron (Diaz)	Chevy (Chase)
Catherine (Zeta-Jones)	Clark (Gable)
Cher	Clint (Eastwood)
Drew (Barrymore)	Dustin (Hoffman)
Elizabeth (Taylor)	Harrison (Ford)
Emma (Thompson)	Jack (Nicholson)
Gwyneth (Paltrow)	John (Wayne)
Halle (Berry)	Leonardo (DiCaprio)
Jodie (Foster)	Martin (Sheen)
Julia (Roberts)	Mel (Gibson)
Katharine (Hepburn)	Mickey (Rooney)
Liv (Tyler)	Orlando (Bloom)
Meg (Ryan)	Patrick (Swayze)
Meryl (Streep)	Robert (De Niro)
Michelle (Pfeiffer)	Robin (Williams)
Nicole (Kidman)	Rock (Hudson)
Penelope (Cruz)	Russell (Crowe)
Reese (Witherspoon)	Sean (Connery)
Salma (Hayek)	Spencer (Tracy)
Sandra (Bullock)	Sylvester (Stalone)
Shirley (Temple)	Tom (Cruise)

TV Characters

Female	Male
Abby (Lockhart)	Al (Bundy)
Ally (McBeal)	Alex (P. Keaton)
Buffy (Summers)	Archie (Bunker)
Carmela (Soprano)	Arthur ("Fonzie" Fonzarelli)
Carrie (Bradshaw)	Chandler (Bing)
Claire (Kincaid)	Cliff (Huxtable)
Daphne (Moon Crane)	Cosmo (Kramer)
Darlene (Conner-Healy)	Danny ("Danno" Williams)
Donna (Martin Silver)	Dylan (McKay)
Elaine (Benes)	Fox (Mulder)
Erica (Kane)	Frasier (Crane)
Felicity (Porter)	Gil (Grissom)
Fran (Fine)	Jack (McCoy)
Gabrielle (Solis)	Jean-Luc (Picard)
Grace (Adler)	Jed (Bartlet)
Kelly (Bundy)	Joey (Tribbiani)
Kimberly (Shaw Mancini)	John Ross ("J. R." Ewing, Jr.)
Lucy (Ricardo)	Kevin (Arnold)
Marcia (Brady)	Luka (Kovac)
Margaret ("Hot Lips" Houlihan)	Ricky (Ricardo)
Michelle (Tanner)	Sam (Malone)
Rachel (Green)	Tony (Soprano)
Rebecca (Howe)	Vic (Mackey)
Sydney (Bristow)	Will (Truman)
Vanessa (Huxtable)	Zack (Morris)

TV Personalities

Female	Male
Ann (Curry)	Ahmad (Rashad)
Barbara (Walters)	Al (Roker)
Brooke (Burke)	Alex (Trebek)
Connie (Chung)	Bill (O'Reilly)
Diane (Sawyer)	Bob (Barker)
Ellen (DeGeneres)	Carson (Daly)
Jane (Pauley)	Conan (O'Brien)
Jenny (Jones)	Dan (Rather)
Joan (Rivers)	David (Letterman)
Joy (Behar)	Dick (Clark)
Judy ("Judge Judy" Sheindlin)	Geraldo (Rivera)
Kathie (Lee Gifford)	Harry (Caray)
Katie (Couric)	Howard (Stern)
Kelly (Ripa)	Jay (Leno)
Leeza (Gibbons)	Jerry (Springer)
Lisa (Ling)	Jim (Lehrer)
Martha (Stewart)	Johnny (Carson)
Meredith (Vieira)	Larry (King)
Nancy (O'Dell)	Matt (Lauer)
Oprah (Winfrey)	Montel (Williams)
Paige (Davis)	Peter (Jennings)
Ricki (Lake)	Phil (McGraw)
Sally (Jessy Raphaël)	Regis (Philbin)
Star (Jones Reynolds)	Tom (Brokaw)
Vanna (White)	Ty (Pennington)

Music

Pop Artists

Female	Male
Alanis (Morrisette)	Adam (Duritz)
Annie (Lennox)	Billy (Joel)
Avril (Lavigne)	Chris (Martin)
Britney (Spears)	Darius (Rucker)
Celine (Dion)	Dave (Matthews)
Cher	Edwin (McCain)
Christina (Aguilera)	Elton (John)
Dido	Elvis (Presley)
Fiona (Apple)	Enrique (Iglesias)
Gloria (Estefan)	Eric (Clapton)
Gwen (Stefani)	George (Michael)
Janet (Jackson)	Howie (Day)
Jessica (Simpson)	Jack (Johnson)
Jewel	John (Lennon)
Kelly (Clarkson)	Justin (Timberlake)
Madonna	Marc (Anthony)
Mandy (Moore)	Michael (Jackson)
Natalie (Imbruglia)	Nick (Lachey)
Norah (Jones)	Paul (McCartney)
Paula (Abdul)	Prince
Pink	Ricky (Martin)
Sarah (McLachlan)	Ringo (Starr)
Sheryl (Crow)	Rob (Thomas)
Tori (Amos)	Rod (Stewart)
Vanessa (Carlton)	Sting

R&B/Soul Artists

Female	Male
Aaliyah	Aaron (Neville)
Alicia (Keys)	Barry (White)
Aretha (Franklin)	Bill (Withers)
Ashanti	Brian (McKnight)
Beyoncé (Knowles)	Bobby (Brown)
Brandy (Norwood)	Cedric ("K-Ci" Hailey)
Christina (Milian)	Edwin (Starr)
Diana (Ross)	Freddie (Jackson)
Dionne (Warwick)	Ike (Turner)
Faith (Evans)	James (Brown)
Gladys (Knight)	Joel ("Jo-Jo" Hailey)
India (Arie)	Kenneth ("Babyface" Edmonds)
Jennifer (Lopez)	Lionel (Richie)
Kelly (Rowland)	Lou (Rawls)
Lauryn (Hill)	Luther (Vandross)
Macy (Gray)	Marvin (Gaye)
Mariah (Carey)	Michael ("D'Angelo" Archer)
Mary (J. Blige)	Otis (Redding)
Monica (Arnold)	Percy (Sledge)
Mya (Harrison)	Ray (Charles)
Patti (LaBelle)	Robert ("R. Kelly" Kelly)
Tina (Turner)	Ronnie (DeVoe)
Toni (Braxton)	Ruben (Studdard)
Vanessa (Williams)	Stevie (Wonder)
Whitney (Houston)	Usher (Raymond)

Country Artists

Female
Alison (Krauss)
Carolyn Dawn (Johnson)
Chely (Wright)
Crystal (Gayle)
Cyndi (Thomson)
Dolly (Parton)
Faith (Hill)
Gretchen (Wilson)
Jamie (O'Neal)
Jo Dee (Messina)
Julie (Roberts)
LeAnn (Rimes)
Loretta (Lynn)
Martie (Maguire)
Martina (McBride)
Mary (Chapin Carpenter)
Mindy (McCready)
Natalie (Maines)
Patsy (Cline)
Patty (Loveless)
Reba (McEntire)
Sara (Evans)
Shania (Twain)
Tammy (Wynette)
Terri (Clark)

Male
Alan (Jackson)
Billy Ray (Cyrus)
Brad (Paisley)
Charley (Pride)
Chet (Atkins)
Clint (Black)
Darryl (Worley)
Don (Everly)
Garth (Brooks)
Gene (Autry)
George (Strait)
Hank (Williams)
Joe (Nichols)
Johnny (Cash)
Keith (Urban)
Kenny (Chesney)
Kix (Brooks)
Randy (Travis)
Ronnie (Dunn)
Tim (McGraw)
Toby (Keith)
Trace (Adkins)
Vince (Gill)
Waylon (Jennings)
Willie (Nelson)

Latin Artists

Female and Male

Alejandra (Guzmán)
Alejandro (Fernández)
Ana (Gabriel)
Carlos (Santana)
Celia (Cruz)
Cristian (Castro)
Enrique (Iglesias)
Gilberto (Santa Rosa)
Gloria (Estefan)
Graciela (Beltrán)
José (Feliciano)
Juan (Luis Guerra)
Juanes (Juan Esteban Aristizábal Vásquez)
Julio (Iglesias)
Luis (Miguel)
Marco (Antonio Solís)
Olga (Tañón)
Oscar (D'León)
Pancho (Sánchez)
Paulina (Rubio)
Ricardo (Arjona)
Selena (Quintanilla Pérez)
Thalía (Ariadna Thalía Sodi Miranda)
Tito (Puente)
Xavier (Cugat)

Classical Composers and Performers

Female and Male

Andrea (Bocelli)
Antonio (Vivaldi)
Camille (Saint-Saëns)
Claude (Debussy)
Felix (Mendelssohn)
Franz (Schubert)
Frédéric (Chopin)
George (Handel)
Giacomo (Puccini)
Giuseppe (Verdi)
Igor (Stravinsky)
Johann (Sebastian Bach)
José (Carreras)
Joseph (Haydn)
Leonard (Bernstein)
Luciano (Pavarotti)
Ludwig (van Beethoven)
Maria (Callas)
Nikolay (Rimsky-Korsakov)
Plácido (Domingo)
Pyotr (Tchaikovsky)
Renata (Scotto)
Richard (Wagner)
Wolfgang (Mozart)
Yo-Yo (Ma)

History

Presidents	Military Figures
Male	**Female and Male**
Abraham (Lincoln)	Alexander (the Great)
Andrew (Jackson)	Andrew (Johnson)
Bill (Clinton)	Attila (the Hun)
Calvin (Coolidge)	Charles (de Gaulle)
Chester (Arthur)	Che (Guevara)
Dwight (D. Eisenhower)	Deborah
Franklin (D. Roosevelt)	Douglas (MacArthur)
George (Washington)	Dwight (D. Eisenhower)
Gerald (Ford)	Genghis (Khan)
Grover (Cleveland)	George (S. Patton)
Harry (S. Truman)	Ivan (Stepanovich Konev)
Herbert (Hoover)	Jennie (Hodgers)
James (Madison)	Joan (of Arc)
Jimmy (Carter)	Julius (Caesar)
John (F. Kennedy)	Moshe (Dayan)
Lyndon (B. Johnson)	Napoleon (Bonaparte)
Martin (Van Buren)	Norman (Schwarzkopf)
Millard (Fillmore)	Oliver (Cromwell)
Richard (Nixon)	Omar (Bradley)
Ronald (Reagan)	Peter (the Great)
Rutherford (B. Hayes)	Robert (E. Lee)
Thomas (Jefferson)	Tecumseh
Ulysses (S. Grant)	Ulysses (S. Grant)
Warren (G. Harding)	William (Wallace)
Woodrow (Wilson)	Winston (Churchill)

Kings	Queens
Male	**Female**
Albert	Amina
Alexander	Anne
Arthur	Beatrix
Canute	Candace
Charles	Catherine
Cormac	Charlotte
Cyrus	Christina
David	Cleopatra
Edgar	Elizabeth
Edmund	Esther
Edward	Filippa
Ferdinand	Ingrid
Frederick	Isabella
George	Jeanne
Harold	Juliana
Henry	Louise
James	Margaret
John	Marie
Louis	Mary
Magnus	Matilda
Malcolm	Silvia
Niall	Sofia
Phillip	Tamar
Richard	Victoria
William	Zenobia

Religion

Old Testament	New Testament
Male	**Male**
Abel	Agrippa
Abraham	Andrew
Adam	Annas
Cain	Aquila
Caleb	Gabriel
Daniel	Herod
David	James
Eli	Jesus
Esau	John
Ezekiel	Joseph
Ezra	Judas
Isaac	Jude
Isaiah	Luke
Jacob	Mark
Jeremiah	Matthew
Job	Nicolas
Joel	Paul
Joshua	Peter
Moses	Philip
Nemiah	Simon
Noah	Stephen
Samson	Thomas
Samuel	Timothy
Solomon	Titus
	Zechariah

Biblical Women	Saints	
Female	**Female**	**Male**
Abigail	Agatha	Ambrose
Bathsheba	Agnes	Andrew
Deborah	Bernadette	Anslem
Delilah	Bridget	Anthony
Dinah	Candida	Augustine
Eden	Catherine	Bartholomew
Elizabeth	Cecilia	Benedict
Esther	Clare	Christopher
Eve	Florence	Felix
Hagar	Genevieve	Francis
Hannah	Hilary	Gregory
Jezebel	Ingrid	Ignatius
Judith	Joan	Jerome
Julia	Julia	John
Leah	Louise	Jude
Maria	Lucy	Leo
Martha	Lydia	Nicholas
Mary	Margaret	Patrick
Miriam	Maria	Paul
Naomi	Mary	Peter
Phoebe	Monica	Sebastian
Rachel	Regina	Stephen
Rebekah	Rose	Thomas
Ruth	Sylvia	Valentine
Sarah	Teresa	Vincent

Sports

Athletes

Female	Male
Anna (Kournikova)	Andre (Agassi)
Annika (Sorenstam)	Andy (Roddick)
Babe (Didrikson Zaharias)	Babe (Ruth)
Diana (Taurasi)	Bernie (Williams)
Jackie (Joyner-Kersee)	Dale (Earnhardt)
Jennie (Finch)	David (Beckham)
Kerri (Strug)	Elvis (Stojko)
Kristi (Yamaguchi)	Hulk (Hogan)
Florence (Griffith Joyner)	Kasey (Kahne)
Laila (Ali)	Kobe (Bryant)
Lisa (Leslie)	Lance (Armstrong)
Marion (Jones)	Mark (Spitz)
Martina (Hingis)	Michael (Jordan)
Mary Lou (Retton)	Mike (Tyson)
Mia (Hamm)	Muhammad (Ali)
Monica (Seles)	Orenthal James ("O. J." Simpson)
Nadia (Comaneci)	Oscar (De La Hoya)
Oksana (Baiul)	Red (Grange)
Picabo (Street)	Riddick (Bowe)
Rebecca (Lobo)	Rocky (Balboa)
Sarah (Hughes)	Scott (Hamilton)
Serena (Williams)	Tiger (Woods)
Sheryl (Swoopes)	Tony (Hawk)
Steffi (Graf)	Wayne (Gretzky)
Venus (Williams)	Yao (Ming)

Olympians

Female	Male
Amanda (Beard)	Alberto (Tomba)
Bonnie (Blair)	Aleksandr (Popov)
Dominique (Dawes)	Alexei (Yagudin)
Dorothy (Hamill)	Bjørn (Dæhlie)
Dot (Richardson)	Brian (Boitano)
Florence (Griffith Joyner)	Carl (Lewis)
Inge (de Bruijn)	Dan (Jansen)
Irina (Slutskaya)	Dmitri (Bilozerchev)
Jackie (Joyner-Kersee)	Elvis (Stojko)
Janet (Evans)	Eric (Heiden)
Janica (Kostelic)	Gary (Hall, Jr.)
Katarina (Witt)	Greg (Louganis)
Kerri (Strug)	Hermann (Maier)
Kristi (Yamaguchi)	Ian (Thorpe)
Larissa (Latynina)	Ingemar (Stenmark)
Mary Lou (Retton)	Ivar (Ballangrud)
Nadia (Comaneci)	Jonny (Moseley)
Nancy (Kerrigan)	Kurt (Browning)
Oksana (Baiul)	Mark (Spitz)
Olga (Korbut)	Matt (Biondi)
Peggy (Fleming)	Michael (Phelps)
Shannon (Miller)	Paul (Hamm)
Summer (Sanders)	Scott (Hamilton)
Svetlana (Boguinskaya)	Stephan (Eberharter)
Tatyana (Gutsu)	Tamas (Darnyi)

Nature & Places

Flowers	Rocks, Gems, Minerals
Female	**Female and Male**
Angelica	Beryl
Calla	Clay
Dahlia	Coal
Daisy	Coral
Fern	Crystal
Flora	Diamond
Flower	Esmerelda
Holly	Flint
Hyacinth	Garnet
Iris	Gemma
Jasmine	Goldie
Laurel	Jade
Lavender	Jasper
Lilac	Jewel
Lily	Mercury
Marigold	Mica
Pansy	Opal
Poppy	Pearl
Posy	Rock
Rose	Ruby
Sage	Sandy
Tulip	Sapphire
Verbina	Steele
Vine	Stone
Violet	Topaz

Natural Elements		Place Names	
Female	**Male**	**Africa**	**Afton**
Amber	Ash	Asia	Austin
Autumn	Branch	Brooklyn	Boston
Breezy	Bud	Cheyenne	Chad
Blossom	Burr	China	Cleveland
Briar	Canyon	Dakota	Cuba
Brook	Cliff	Florence	Dakota
Delta	Crag	Georgia	Dallas
Gale	Dale	Holland	Denver
Hailey	Eddy	India	Diego
Heather	Field	Italia	Indiana
Ivy	Ford	Jamaica	Israel
Marina	Forest	Kenya	Kent
Rain	Heath	Lourdes	Laramie
Rainbow	Lake	Madison	London
Savannah	Marsh	Montana	Montreal
Sequoia	Moss	Olympia	Nevada
Sierra	Oakes	Paris	Orlando
Skye	Thorne	Regina	Phoenix
Star	Ridge	Savannah	Reno
Summer	River	Siena	Rhodes
Sunny	Rye	Sydney	Rio
Terra	Rock	Tijuana	Sydney
Tempest	Stone	Victoria	Tennessee
Willow	Storm	Vienna	Washington
Windy	Woody		

Pop Culture

Notorious Celebrity Baby Names

Female and Male

Ahmet Emuukha Rodan (son of Frank and Gail Zappa)

Apple Blythe Alison (daughter of Gwyneth Paltrow and Chris Martin)

Audio Science (son of Shannyn Sossamon and Dallas Clayton)

Coco Riley (daughter of Courteney Cox Arquette and David Arquette)

Daisy Boo (daughter of Jamie and Jools Oliver)

Dweezil (son of Frank and Gail Zappa)

Elijah Bob Patricus Guggi Q (son of Bono and Alison Stewart)

Fifi Trixiebelle (daughter of Paula Yates and Bob Geldof)

Hazel Patricia (daughter of Julia Roberts and Danny Moder)

Heavenly Hirani Tiger Lily (daughter of Paula Yates and Michael Hutchence)

Lourdes Maria Ciccone (daughter of Madonna and Carlos Leon)

Moon Unit (daughter of Frank and Gail Zappa)

Moxie CrimeFighter (daughter of Penn and Emily Jillette)

Peaches Honeyblossom (daughter of Paula Yates and Bob Geldof)

Phinnaeus Walter (son of Julia Roberts and Danny Moder)

Pilot Inspektor (son of Jason Lee and Beth Riesgraf)

Pirate Howsmon (son of Jonathan and Deven Davis)

Poppy Honey (daughter of Jamie and Jools Oliver)

Prince Michael (son of Michael Jackson and Debbie Rowe)

Prince Michael II (son of Michael Jackson)

Rocco (son of Madonna and Guy Ritchie)

Rumer Glenn (daughter of Demi Moore and Bruce Willis)

Scout LaRue (daughter of Demi Moore and Bruce Willis)

Seven Sirius (son of Andre 3000 and Erykah Badu)

Tallulah Belle (daughter of Demi Moore and Bruce Willis)

One-Name Wonders	Famous People Known by Initials
Female and Male	**Female and Male**
Ann-Margret	A. A. (Milne)
Beck	A. E. (Housman)
Björk	A. J. (Foyt)
Bono	B. J. (Thomas)
Brandy	C. S. (Lewis)
Cher	D. B. (Cooper)
Dido	D. H. (Lawrence)
Enya	E. E. (Cummings)
Fabio	E. M. (Forster)
Iman	J. D. (Salinger)
Jewel	J. K. (Rowling)
Liberace	J. M. (Barrie)
Madonna	J. P. (Morgan)
Moby	J. R. R. (Tolkien)
Nelly	L. M. (Montgomery)
Pelé	O. J. (Simpson)
Prince	P. J. (Harvey)
Roseanne	P. J. (O'Rourke)
Sade	P. T. (Barnum)
Seal	T. S. (Eliot)
Shakira	V. C. (Andrews)
Sinbad	V. I. (Lennin)
Tiffany	W. C. (Fields)
Twiggy	W. E. B. (DuBois)
Yanni	Y. A. (Tittle)

Other Ideas for Names

Last Names as First Names	Virtue Names
Female and Male	**Female**
Anderson	Amity
Bradshaw	Blythe
Carter	Charity
Chavez	Chastity
Chen	Constance
Foster	Faith
Gallagher	Felicity
Garcia	Fidelity
Harper	Grace
Jackson	Harmony
Johnson	Honora
Keaton	Hope
Kennedy	Innocence
Mackenzie	Joy
Madison	Justice
Meyer	Love
Parker	Mercy
Patterson	Modesty
Ramsey	Passion
Rodriguez	Patience
Sanchez	Prudence
Taylor	Purity
Tennyson	Temperance
Walker	Unity
Wang	Verity

Old-Fashioned Names Now Popular

Female	Male
Abigail	Abraham
Alice	Alexander
Anna	Dominic
Ava	Elijah
Caroline	Ethan
Claire	Gabriel
Claudia	Hector
Elizabeth	Isaac
Emily	Isaiah
Emma	Ivan
Evelyn	Jasper
Grace	Julian
Hannah	Maxwell
Hazel	Nathaniel
Isabella	Noah
Katherine	Omar
Leslie	Oscar
Madeline	Owen
Margaret	Samuel
Maria	Sebastian
Olivia	Vernon
Rebecca	Vincent
Sarah	Wesley
Sofia	Xavier
Victoria	Zachary

Trade Names

Female and Male

Baker
Butcher
Carver
Chandler
Cooper
Cutler
Draper
Fletcher
Fowler
Gardner
Hunter
Marshall
Mason
Miller
Painter
Porter
Ranger
Sawyer
Scribe
Shepherd
Slater
Smith
Stockman
Tailor
Tanner

Names Used for Both Boys and Girls

More for Girls	More for Boys	About Equal
Alexis	Alex	Britt
Ariel	Cameron	Addison
Ashley	Carson	Ashton
Bailey	Chandler	Berwyn
Billie	Chase	Blair
Dominique	Chris	Carey
Guadalupe	Christian	Casey
Holland	Cody	Charley
Jade	Dakota	Derian
Jadyn	Devin	Devyn
Jamie	Drew	Dylan
Kelly	Evan	Gentry
Madison	Hunter	Harley
Morgan	Jaime	Jessie
Payton	Jaylin	Jody
Reagan	Jesse	Kriston
Reese	Jordan	London
Ricki	Logan	Maddox
Robin	Parker	Pat
Shannon	Quinn	Peyton
Shea	Riley	Quincey
Sidney	Ryan	Skylar
Stacy	Skyler	Sunny
Taylor	Terry	Tory
Tegan	Tyler	Tristyn

Girls

A

Aaleyah (Hebrew) a form of Aliya.

Aaliah (Hebrew) a form of Aliya.

Aalisha (Greek) a form of Alisha.

Aaliyah ☙ (Hebrew) a form of Aliya.

Abagail (Hebrew) a form of Abigale.
Abagael, Abagale, Abagil

Abbagail (Hebrew) a form of Abigale.
Abbegail, Abbegale, Abbegayle

Abbey, Abbie, Abby (Hebrew) familiar
forms of Abigail.
Abbe, Abbi, Abbye

Abbygail (Hebrew) a form of Abigale.
Abbygale, Abbygayle

Abegail (Hebrew) a form of Abigail.
Abegale, Abegayle

Abelina (American) a combination of
Abbey + Lina.

Abia (Arabic) great.

Abianne (American) a combination of
Abbey + Ann.

Abida (Arabic) worshiper.

Abigail ☙ (Hebrew) father's joy. Bible:
one of the wives of King David. See also
Gail.
*Abbigail, Abbigale, Abbigayle, Abgail,
Abgale, Abgayle, Abigael, Abigal,
Abigale, Abigayil, Abigayle, Abigel,
Avigail*

Abinaya (American) a form of Abiann.

Abira (Hebrew) my strength.

Abra (Hebrew) mother of many nations.

Abria (Hebrew) a form of Abra.

Abrial (French) open; secure, protected.

Abriana (Italian) a form of Abra.

Abrielle (French) a form of Abrial.

Abril (French) a form of Abrial.

Abygail (Hebrew) a form of Abigail.

Acacia (Greek) thorny. Mythology: the
acacia tree symbolizes immortality and
resurrection. See also Casey.

Ada (German) a short form of Adelaide.
(English) prosperous; happy.
Adabelle, Adan, Adda, Auda

Adah (Hebrew) ornament.

Adair (Greek) a form of Adara.

Adalene (Spanish) a form of Adalia.
Adalina, Adaline

Adalia (German, Spanish) noble.
Adalee

Adama (Phoenician, Hebrew) a form of
Adam (see Boys' Names).

Adamma (Ibo) child of beauty.

Adana (Spanish) a form of Adama.

Adanna (Nigerian) her father's daughter.

Adara (Greek) beauty. (Arabic) virgin.

Adaya (American) a form of Ada.

Addie (Greek, German) a familiar form
of Adelaide, Adrienne.
*Adde, Addey, Addi, Addia, Addy, Adey,
Adi, Adie, Ady, Atti, Attie, Atty*

Addison, Addyson (English) child of
Adam.

Adela (English) a short form of
Adelaide.
Adelia, Adelista, Adella

Adelaide (German) noble and serene.
See also Ada, Adela, Adeline, Adelle,
Ailis, Delia, Della, Ela, Elke, Heidi.
*Adelade, Adelaid, Adelaida, Adelei,
Adelheid, Adeliade, Adelka, Aley,
Laidey, Laidy*

Adele (English) a form of Adelle.
Adel

Adelina (English) a form of Adeline.
Adlena

Adeline (English) a form of Adelaide.
*Adelind, Adelita, Adeliya, Adelyn,
Adelynn, Adlin, Adline*

Adelle (German, English) a short form
of Adelaide, Adeline.
Adell

Adena (Hebrew) noble; adorned.

Adia (Swahili) gift.
Adiah

Adila (Arabic) equal.
Adeela

Adilene (English) a form of Adeline.
Adlene

Adina (Hebrew) a form of Adena. See
also Dina.
Adiana, Adiena, Adinah, Adinna

Adira (Hebrew) strong.

Adison, Adyson (English) forms of
Addison, Addyson.

Aditi (Hindi) unbound. Religion: the
mother of the Hindu sun gods.

Adleigh (Hebrew) my ornament.

Adonia (Spanish) beautiful.

Adora (Latin) beloved. See also Dora.

Adra (Arabic) virgin.

Adreana, Adreanna (Latin) forms of
Adrienne.

Adria (English) a short form of Adriana,
Adriene.
Adrea

Adriana, Adrianna (Italian) forms of
Adrienne.

Adriane, Adrianne (English) forms of
Adrienne.

Adrielle (Hebrew) member of God's
flock.

Adrien, Adriene (English) forms of
Adrienne.

Adrienna (Italian) a form of Adrienne.
See also Edrianna.
Adriena

Adrienne (Greek) rich. (Latin) dark.
See also Hadriane.
Adrie

Adrina (English) a short form of
Adriana.

Adriyanna (American) a form of
Adrienne.

Adya (Hindi) Sunday.

Aerial, Aeriel (Hebrew) forms of Ariel.
Aeriale, Aeriela, Aeryal

Afi (African) born on Friday.

Afra (Hebrew) young doe. (Arabic) earth color. See also Aphra.

Africa (Irish) pleasant. Geography: one of the seven continents.

Afrika (Irish) a form of Africa.

Afrodite, Aphrodite (Greek) Mythology: the goddess of love and beauty.

Afton (English) from Afton, England. *Aftan, Aftine, Aftyn*

Agate (English) a semiprecious stone.

Agatha (Greek) good, kind. Literature: Agatha Christie was a British writer of more than seventy detective novels. See also Gasha.
Agace, Agasha, Agata, Agathi, Agatka, Agota, Agotha, Agueda, Atka

Agathe (Greek) a form of Agatha.

Aggie (Greek) a short form of Agatha, Agnes.

Agnes (Greek) pure. See also Aneesa, Anessa, Anice, Anisha, Ina, Inez, Necha, Nessa, Nessie, Neza, Nyusha, Una, Ynez.
Aganetha, Agna, Agne, Agneis, Agnelia, Agnella, Agnés, Agnesa, Agnesca, Agnese, Agnesina, Agness, Agnesse, Agneta, Agneti, Agnetta, Agnies, Agnieszka, Agniya, Agnola, Aignéis, Aneska

Ahava (Hebrew) beloved.

Ahliya (Hebrew) a form of Aliya.

Aida (Latin) helpful. (English) a form of Ada.

Aidan, Aiden (Latin) forms of Aida.

Aiesha (Swahili, Arabic) a form of Aisha.

Aiko (Japanese) beloved.

Ailani (Hawaiian) chief.

Aileen (Scottish) light bearer. (Irish) a form of Helen. See also Eileen.
Ailean, Ailene, Ailina, Ailinn

Aili (Scottish) a form of Alice. (Finnish) a form of Helen.

Ailis (Irish) a form of Adelaide.
Eilis

Ailsa (Scottish) island dweller. Geography: Ailsa Craig is an island in Scotland.

Ailya (Hebrew) a form of Aliya.

Aimee (Latin) a form of Amy. (French) loved.
Aime, Aimée, Aimey, Aimi, Aimia, Aimie, Aimy

Ainsley (Scottish) my own meadow.
Ainslee, Ainsleigh, Ainslie, Ainsly, Aynslee, Aynsley, Aynslie

Airiana (English) a form of Ariana, Arianna.

Airiél (Hebrew) a form of Ariel.
Aire, Aireal, Airial

Aisha (Swahili) life. (Arabic) woman. See also Asha, Asia, Iesha, Isha, Keisha, Yiesha.
Aesha, Aeshah, Aieshah, Aishah, Aishia, Aishiah, Aysa, Ayse, Aytza

Aislinn, Aislynn (Irish) forms of Ashlyn.

Aiyana (Native American) forever flowering.

Aiyanna (Hindi) a form of Ayanna.

Aja (Hindi) goat.
Ajah, Ajaran, Ajha

Ajanae (American) a combination of the letter A + Janae.

Ajia (Hindi) a form of Aja.

Akayla (American) a combination of the letter A + Kayla.

Akeisha (American) a combination of the letter A + Keisha.

Akela (Hawaiian) noble.

Akeria (American) a form of Akira.

Aki (Japanese) born in autumn.

Akia (American) a combination of the letter A + Kia.

Akiko (Japanese) bright light.

Akilah (Arabic) intelligent.

Akili (Tanzanian) wisdom.

Akina (Japanese) spring flower.

Akira (American) a combination of the letter A + Kira.

Alaina, Alayna (Irish) forms of Alana.
Alaine, Alainna, Alainnah, Alane, Alayne, Aleine, Alleyna, Alleynah, Alleyne

Alair (French) a form of Hilary.

Alamea (Hawaiian) ripe; precious.

Alameda (Spanish) poplar tree.

Alana (Irish) attractive; peaceful. (Hawaiian) offering. See also Lana.
Alanah, Alane, Alania, Alanis, Alawna, Allyn

Alandra, Alandria (Spanish) forms of Alexandra, Alexandria.

Alani (Hawaiian) orange tree. (Irish) a form of Alana.
Alania

Alanna (Irish) a form of Alana.
Alannah

Alanza (Spanish) noble and eager.

Alaysha, Alaysia (American) forms of Alicia.

Alba (Latin) from Alba Longa, an ancient city near Rome, Italy.

Alberta (German, French) noble and bright. See also Auberte, Bertha, Elberta.

Albreanna (American) a combination of Alberta + Breanna (see Breana).

Alcina (Greek) strong-minded.

Alda (German) old; elder.

Alden (English) old; wise protector.

Aldina, Aldine (Hebrew) forms of Alda.

Alea, Aleah (Arabic) high, exalted. (Persian) God's being.
Aleea, Aleeah, Aleia, Allea, Alleea, Alleeah

Aleasha, Aleesha (Greek) forms of Alisha.
Aleashea, Aleeshia

Alecia (Greek) a form of Alicia.
Aleasia, Alecea, Aleecia

Aleela (Swahili) she cries.

Aleena (Dutch) a form of Aleene.
Aleana

Aleene (Dutch) alone.
Aleen, Alene, Alleen

Aleeya (Hebrew) a form of Aliya.
Alee, Aleea

Aleeza (Hebrew) a form of Aliza. See also Leeza.

Alegria (Spanish) cheerful.

Aleisha, Alesha (Greek) forms of Alecia, Alisha.
Aleashea, Aleasia, Aleeshah, Aleeshia, Aleeshya, Aleshia

Alejandra (Spanish) a form of Alexandra.
Alejanda, Alejandr, Alejandrea, Alejandria, Alejandrina

Aleka (Hawaiian) a form of Alice.

Aleksandra (Greek) a form of Alexandra.
Aleksasha

Alena (Russian) a form of Helen.
Alenah, Alene, Aleni, Alenka, Alenna

Alesia, Alessia (Greek) forms of Alice, Alicia, Alisha.
Allesia

Alessa (Greek) a form of Alice.
Allessa

Alessandra (Italian) a form of Alexandra.
Alesandra, Alesandrea, Allesand

Aleta (Greek) a form of Alida. See also Leta.

Alethea (Greek) truth.

Alette (Latin) wing.

Alex (Greek) a short form of Alexander, Alexandra.
Aleix, Aleks, Alexx

Alexa ☽ (Greek) a short form of Alexandra.
Alekia, Aleksa, Aleksha, Aleksi

Alexandra ☽ (Greek) defender of humankind. History: the last czarina of Russia. See also Lexia, Lexie, Olesia, Ritsa, Sandra, Sandrine, Sasha, Shura, Sondra, Xandra, Zandra.
Alexande, Alexina, Alexine, Alexxandra, Aljexi, Alla

Alexandrea (Greek) a form of Alexandria.

Alexandria (Greek) a form of Alexandra. See also Drinka, Xandra, Zandra.
Alexanderia, Alexanderine, Alexandrena, Alexandrie, Alexandrina

Alexandrine (Greek) a form of Alexandra.
Alexandrina

Alexanne (American) a combination of Alex + Anne.

Alexas, Alexes (Greek) short forms of Alexandra.

Alexi, Alexie (Greek) short forms of Alexandra.
Aleksey, Aleksi, Alexey

Alexia (Greek) a short form of Alexandria. See also Lexia.
Aleska, Alexsia, Alka

Alexis ☽ (Greek) a short form of Alexandra.
Alexcis, Alexiou, Alexisia

Alexius, Alexus (Greek) short forms of Alexandra.

Alexsandra (Greek) a form of Alexandra.

Alexsis, Alexxis (Greek) short forms of Alexandra.

Alexys (Greek) a short form of Alexandra.
Alexyss

Alexzandra, Alexzandra (Greek) forms of Alexandra.
Alexzand, Alexzandrea

Aleya, Aleyah (Hebrew) forms of Aliya.

Alfie (English) a familiar form of Alfreda.

Alfreda (English) elf counselor; wise counselor. See also Effie, Elfrida, Freda, Frederica.

Ali, Aly (Greek) familiar forms of Alice, Alicia, Alisha, Alison.
Allea

Alia, Aliah (Hebrew) forms of Aliya. See also Aaliyah, Alea.
Alya

Alice (Greek) truthful. (German) noble. See also Aili, Aleka, Alie, Alisa, Alison, Alli, Alysa, Alyssa, Alysse, Elke.
Adelice, Aleece, Alican, Alicie, Aliece, Alies, Alize, Alla, Alleece, Allice, Allis, Allix

Alicia (English) a form of Alice. See also Elicia, Licia.
Alecea, Aleecia, Alicea, Alicha, Alichia, Alician, Alicja, Alicya, Aliecia, Allicea, Ilysa

Alida (Latin) small and winged. (Spanish) noble. See also Aleta, Lida, Oleda.
Aleda, Alidia, Alleda, Alyda, Alydia

Alie, Allie (Greek) familiar forms of Alice.

Aliesha (Greek) a form of Alisha.
Alieshai

Alika (Hawaiian) truthful. (Swahili) most beautiful.
Alica

Alima (Arabic) sea maiden; musical.

Alina, Alyna (Slavic) bright. (Scottish) fair. (English) short forms of Adeline. See also Alena.
Aliana, Alianna, Allyna

Aline (Scottish) a form of Alina.
Allene, Alline, Allyn, Allyne, Alyne, Alynne

Alisa, Alissa (Greek) a form of Alice. See also Elisa, Ilisa.
Alisza

Alise, Allise (Greek) forms of Alice.
Aliese, Alis, Alisse, Alles, Allesse, Allis, Allisse

Alisha (Greek) truthful. (German) noble. (English) a form of Alicia. See also Elisha, Ilisha, Lisha.
Aliscia, Alishah, Alishay, Alishaye, Alishya, Alitsha

Alishia, Alisia, Alissia (English) forms of Alisha.
Alishea

Alison (English) a form of Alice.

Alita (Spanish) a form of Alida.

Alivia (Latin) a form of Olivia.

Alix (Greek) a short form of Alexandra, Alice.
Allix

Alixandra, Alixandria (Greek) forms of Alexandria.

Aliya (Hebrew) ascender.
Aliyah

Aliye (Arabic) noble.

Aliza (Hebrew) joyful. See also Aleeza, Eliza.
Alieza, Aliezah, Alitza, Alizah, Alize

Alizabeth (Hebrew) a form of Elizabeth.

Allana, Allanah (Irish) forms of Alana.

Allegra (Latin) cheerful.

Allena (Irish) a form of Alana.
Alleen, Alleyna, Alleynah

Alli, Ally (Greek) familiar forms of Alice.

Allia, Alliah (Hebrew) forms of Aliya.

Allison ❦ (English) a form Alice. See also Lissie.
Alicen, Alicyn, Alisann, Alisanne, Alisen, Alisson, Alisun, Alisyn, Alles, Allesse, Allix, Allsun

Allissa (Greek) a form of Alyssa.
Allisa

Alliyah (Hebrew) a form of Aliya.

Allysa, Allyssa (Greek) a form of Alyssa.

Allysha (English) a form of Alisha.

Allyson, Alyson (English) forms of Alison.
Allysen, Allysun

Alma (Arabic) learned. (Latin) soul.
Almah

Almeda (Arabic) ambitious.

Almira (Arabic) aristocratic, princess; exalted. (Spanish) from Almeíra, Spain. See also Elmira, Mira.

Aloha (Hawaiian) loving, kindhearted, charitable.

Aloisa (German) famous warrior.

Aloma (Latin) a short form of Paloma.

Alondra (Spanish) a form of Alexandra.

Alonna (Irish) a form of Alana.

Alonza (English) noble and eager.

Alora (American) a combination of the letter A + Lora.

Alpha (Greek) first-born. Linguistics: the first letter of the Greek alphabet.

Alta (Latin) high; tall.

Althea (Greek) wholesome; healer. History: Althea Gibson was the first African American to win a major tennis title. See also Thea.

Alva (Latin, Spanish) white; light skinned. See also Elva.

Alvina (English) friend to all; noble friend; friend to elves. See also Elva, Vina.

Alyah, Alyiah (Hebrew) forms of Aliya.
Alya

Alycia, Alyssia (English) forms of Alicia.
Allyce, Alycea, Lycia

Alysa, Alyse, Alysse (Greek) forms of Alice.
Allys, Allyse, Allyss, Alys, Alyss

Alysha, Alysia (Greek) forms of Alisha.
*Allysea, Allyscia, Alysea, Alyshia,
Alyssha*

Alyssa ☝ (Greek) rational. Botany:
alyssum is a flowering herb. See also
Alice, Elissa.
Ilyssa, Lyssa, Lyssah

Alysse (Greek) a form of Alice.
Allyce, Allys, Allyse, Allyss, Alys, Alyss

Alyx, Alyxis (Greek) short forms of
Alexandra.

Alyxandra, Alyxandria (Greek) forms
of Alexandria.

Am (Vietnamese) lunar; female.

Ama (African) born on Saturday.

Amabel (Latin) lovable. See also Bel,
Mabel.

Amada (Spanish) beloved.

Amairani (Greek) a form of Amara.

Amal (Hebrew) worker. (Arabic) hopeful.

Amalia (German) a form of Amelia.
Amaliya

Amalie (German) a form of Amelia.

Aman, Amani (Arabic) forms of Imani.

Amanada (Latin) a form of Amanda.

Amanda ☝ (Latin) lovable. See also
Manda.
*Amandah, Amandalee, Amandalyn,
Amandi, Amandie, Amandine,
Amandy*

Amandeep (Punjabi) peaceful light.

Amara (Greek) eternally beautiful. See
also Mara.

Amaranta (Spanish) a flower that never
fades.

Amari (Greek) a form of Amara.

Amaris (Hebrew) promised by God.
Amarissa

Amaryllis (Greek) fresh; flower.

Amaui (Hawaiian) thrush.

Amaya (Japanese) night rain.

Ambar (French) a form of Amber.

Amber (French) amber.
Amberia, Amberise, Ambur

Amberly (American) a familiar form of
Amber.

Amberlyn, Amberlynn (American)
combinations of Amber + Lynn.

Ambria (American) a form of Amber.

Amelia (German) hard working. (Latin)
a form of Emily. History: Amelia
Earhart, an American aviator, was the
first woman to fly solo across the
Atlantic Ocean. See also Ima, Melia,
Millie, Nuela, Yamelia.
*Amaliya, Ameila, Amelina, Ameline,
Amelisa, Amelita, Amella, Amilina,
Amilisa, Amilita, Amilyn, Amylia*

Amelie (German) a familiar form of
Amelia.
Amaley, Amelee, Ameley, Amélie

America (Teutonic) industrious.

Ami, Amie (French) forms of Amy.
Amii, Amiiee, Ammie

Amilia, Amilie (Latin, German) forms
of Amelia.
Amillia

Amina (Arabic) trustworthy, faithful.
History: the mother of the prophet
Muhammad.
*Aminah, Aminda, Amindah, Aminta,
Amintah*

Amira (Hebrew) speech; utterance.
(Arabic) princess. See also Mira.

Amissa (Hebrew) truth.

Amita (Hebrew) truth.

Amity (Latin) friendship.

Amlika (Hindi) mother.

Amma (Hindi) god, godlike. Religion:
another name for the Hindu goddess
Shakti.

Amorie (German) industrious leader.

Amparo (Spanish) protected.

Amrit (Sanskrit) nectar.

Amy (Latin) beloved. See also Aimee,
Emma, Esmé.
*Amata, Ame, Amey, Amia, Amiet,
Amijo, Amiko, Amio, Ammy, Amye,
Amylyn*

An (Chinese) peaceful.

Ana (Hawaiian, Spanish) a form of
Hannah.

Anaba (Native American) she returns
from battle.

Anabel, Anabelle (English) forms of
Annabel.
Anabela

Anahita (Persian) a river and water
goddess.

Anais (Hebrew) gracious.
Anaise, Anaïse

Anala (Hindi) fine.

Analisa, Analise (English) combinations of Ana + Lisa.

Anamaria (English) a combination of
Ana + Maria.

Ananda (Hindi) blissful.

Anastacia (Greek) a form of Anastasia.
Anastace, Anastacie

Anastasia (Greek) resurrection. See also
Nastasia, Stacey, Stacia, Stasya.
*Anastase, Anastasha, Anastashia,
Anastasie, Anastassia, Anastassya,
Anastatia, Anastazia, Anastice,
Annstás*

Anatola (Greek) from the east.

Anci (Hungarian) a form of Hannah.

Andee, Andi, Andie (American) short
forms of Andrea, Fernanda.

Andrea ✹ (Greek) strong; courageous.
See also Ondrea.

Andreana, Andreanna (Greek) forms
of Andrea.

Andreane, Andreanne (Greek) forms
of Andrea.

Andria (Greek) a form of Andrea.

Andriana, Andrianna (Greek) forms of
Andrea.

Aneesa, Aneesha (Greek) forms of
Agnes.

Aneko (Japanese) older sister.

Anela (Hawaiian) angel.
Anelle

Anessa (Greek) a form of Agnes.

Anetra (American) a form of Annette.
Anitra

Anezka (Czech) a form of Hannah.

Angel (Greek) a short form of Angela.
Angele, Angell, Angelle, Angil, Anjel

Angela (Greek) angel; messenger.
Angala, Anganita, Angelanell, Angelanette, Angèle, Angelee, Angeleigh, Angeles, Angeli, Angelita, Angella, Angellita, Anglea, Anjela

Angelia (Greek) a form of Angela.
Angelea, Angeleah

Angelica, Angelika (Greek) forms of Angela.
Angelic, Angelici, Angeliki, Angellica, Angilica

Angelina ☆ (Russian) a form of Angela.
Angalena, Angalina, Angelena, Angeliana, Angeleana, Angellina, Angelyna, Anhelina, Anjelina

Angeline (Russian) a form of Angela.
Angeleen, Angelene, Angelyn, Angelyne, Angelynn, Angelynne

Angelique (French) a form of Angela.
Angeliqua, Angélique, Angilique, Anjelique

Angeni (Native American) spirit.

Angie (Greek) a familiar form of Angela.
Ange, Angee, Angey, Angi, Angy

Ani (Hawaiian) beautiful.

Ania (Polish) a form of Hannah.

Anica, Anika (Czech) familiar forms of Anna.
Anaka, Aneeky, Aneka, Anekah, Anicka, Anik, Anikah, Anikka, Anikke, Aniko, Anikó, Anouska, Anuska

Anice (English) a form of Agnes.
Anis, Anise

Anila (Hindi) Religion: an attendant of the Hindu god Vishnu.

Anisa, Anisah (Arabic) friendly.

Anissa, Anisha (English) forms of Agnes, Ann.
Anis, Anise, Annissa

Anita (Spanish) a form of Ann, Anna. See also Nita.
Aneeta, Aneetah, Aneethah, Anetha, Anitha, Anithah, Anitia, Anitra, Anitte

Anjelica (Greek) a form of Angela.
Anjelika

Anka (Polish) a familiar form of Hannah.
Anke

Ann, Anne (English) gracious.
Annchen, Annze, Anouche

Anna ☆ (German, Italian, Czech, Swedish) gracious. Culture: Anna Pavlova was a famous Russian ballerina. See also Anica, Anissa, Nina.
Anah, Annina, Annora, Anyu, Aska

Annabel (English) a combination of Anna + Bel.

Annabelle (English) a form of Annabel.

Annalie (Finnish) a form of Hannah.

Annalisa, Annalise (English) combinations of Anna + Lisa.

Annamarie, Annemarie, Annmarie, Anne-Marie (English) combinations of Anne + Marie.
Annamaria, Anna-Maria, Anna-Marie, Annmaria

Anneka (Swedish) a form of Hannah.

Annelisa (English) a combination of Ann + Lisa.

Annette (French) a form of Ann. See also Anetra, Nettie.
Anet, Aneta, Anett, Anetta, Anette, Anneth, Annett, Annetta

Annie (English) a familiar form of Ann.
Anni, Anny

Annik, Annika (Russian) forms of Ann.
Aneka, Anekah, Anninka, Anouk

Annjanette (American) a combination of Ann + Janette.

Anona (English) pineapple.

Anouhea (Hawaiian) cool, soft fragrance.

Ansley (Scottish) forms of Ainsley.

Anthea (Greek) flower.
Thia

Antionette (French) a form of Antonia.

Antoinette (French) a form of Antonia. See also Netti, Toinette, Toni.
Anta, Antanette, Antoinella, Antoinet, Antonella, Antonetta, Antonette, Antonieta, Antonietta, Antonique

Antonia (Greek) flourishing. (Latin) praiseworthy. See also Toni, Tonya, Tosha.
Ansonia, Ansonya, Antania, Antona, Antoña, Antonie, Antonina,

Antonine, Antonnea, Antonnia, Antonya

Antonice (Latin) a form of Antonia.

Anya (Russian) a form of Anna.
Anja

Anyssa (English) a form of Anissa.

'Aolani (Hawaiian) heavenly cloud.

Aphra (Hebrew) young doe. See also Afra.

April (Latin) opening. See also Avril.
Aprele, Aprelle, Apriell, Aprielle, Aprila, Aprile, Aprilette, Aprili, Aprill

Apryl (Latin) a form of April.
Apryle

Aquene (Native American) peaceful.

Ara (Arabic) opinionated.

Arabella (Latin) beautiful altar. See also Belle, Orabella.
Arabela, Arabele, Arabelle

Araceli, Aracely (Latin) heavenly altar.

Ardelle (Latin) warm; enthusiastic.

Arden (English) valley of the eagle. Literature: in Shakespeare, a romantic place of refuge.

Ardi (Hebrew) a short form of Arden, Ardice, Ardith.

Ardice (Hebrew) a form of Ardith.

Ardith (Hebrew) flowering field.

Areli, Arely (American) forms of Oralee.

Arella (Hebrew) angel; messenger.

Aretha (Greek) virtuous. See also
Oretha.

Ari, Aria, Arie (Hebrew) short forms of
Ariel.

Ariadne (Greek) holy. Mythology: the
daughter of King Minos of Crete.

Ariana ☝ (Greek) holy.
Aeriana, Arieana

Ariane (French) a form of Ariana,
Arianna.
Arianie, Arien, Arieon, Aryane

Arianna ☝ (Greek) holy.
Aerianna

Arianne (English) form of Ariana,
Arianna.
*Aeriann, Airiann, Ariann, Ariannie,
Arieann, Arienne, Aryanne*

Arica (Scandinavian) a form of Erica.

Ariel (Hebrew) lion of God.
*Aeriale, Aeriela, Aeryal, Aire, Aireal,
Airial, Arial, Ariale, Arieal, Ariela*

Arielle (French) a form of Ariel.
Aeriell, Ariella

Arin (Hebrew) enlightened. (Arabic)
messenger. See also Erin.
Aaren, Arinn

Arista (Greek) best.

Arla (German) a form of Carla.

Arleigh (English) a form of Harley.

Arlene (Irish) pledge. See also Lena,
Lina.

Arlette (English) a form of Arlene.

Arlynn (American) a combination of
Arlene + Lynn.

Armani (Persian) desire, goal.

Armine (Latin) noble. (German) soldier.
(French) a form of Herman (see Boys'
Names).

Arnelle (German) eagle.

Artha (Hindi) wealthy, prosperous.

Artis (Irish) noble; lofty hill. (Scottish)
bear. (English) rock. (Icelandic) follower of Thor.

Aryana, Aryanna (Italian) forms of
Ariana.

Aryn (Hebrew) a form of Arin.

Asa (Japanese) born in the morning.

Asha (Arabic, Swahili) a form of Aisha,
Ashia.

Ashanti (Swahili) from a tribe in West
Africa.

Ashely (English) form of Ashley.
Ashelee, Ashelei, Asheley

Ashia (Arabic) life.
Ashyah

Ashlee, Ashli, Ashlie, Ashly
(English) forms of Ashley.
Ashlea

Ashleigh (English) a form of Ashley.
Asheleigh, Ashlei

Ashley ☝ (English) ash tree meadow.
See also Lee.
*Ashala, Ashalee, Ashalei, Ashaley,
Ashla, Ashlay, Ashleay, Ashlye*

Ashlin (English) a form of Ashlyn.
Ashliann, Ashlianne, Ashline

Ashlyn, Ashlynn (English) ash tree pool. (Irish) vision, dream.
Ashlan, Ashleann, Ashleen, Ashleene, Ashlen, Ashlene, Ashling, Ashlyne, Ashlynne

Ashten, Ashtin (English) forms of Ashton.

Ashton (English) ash-tree settlement.

Ashtyn (English) a form of Ashton.

Asia (Greek) resurrection. (English) eastern sunrise. (Swahili) a form of Aisha.
Aisia, Asiah, Asian, Asya, Aysia, Aysiah, Aysian

Aspen (English) aspen tree.
Aspin, Aspyn

Aster (English) a form of Astra.

Astra (Greek) star.

Astrid (Scandinavian) divine strength.

Atalanta (Greek) mighty huntress. Mythology: an athletic young woman who refused to marry any man who could not outrun her in a footrace. See also Lani.

Atara (Hebrew) crown.

Athena (Greek) wise. Mythology: the goddess of wisdom.
Athenea, Athene, Athina, Atina

Atira (Hebrew) prayer.

Auberte (French) a form of Alberta.

Aubree, Aubrie (French) forms of Aubrey.
Auberi, Aubre, Aubrei, Aubreigh, Aubri

Aubrey (German) noble; bearlike. (French) blond ruler; elf ruler.
Aubary, Aubery, Aubray, Aubrea, Aubreah, Aubrette, Aubria, Aubry, Aubury

Aubriana, Aubrianna (English) combinations of Aubrey + Anna.

Audey (English) a familiar form of Audrey.
Aude, Audi, Audie

Audra (French) a form of Audrey.
Audria

Audreanne (English) a combination of Audrey + Anne.
Audreen, Audrianne

Audree, Audrie (English) forms of Audrey.
Audre, Audri

Audrey ☝ (English) noble strength.
Audray, Audrin, Audriya, Audry, Audrye

Audriana, Audrianna (English) combinations of Audrey + Anna.
Audrina

Audris (German) fortunate, wealthy.

Augusta (Latin) a short form of Augustine. See also Gusta.

Augustine (Latin) majestic. Religion: Saint Augustine was the first archbishop of Canterbury. See also Tina.

'Aulani (Hawaiian) royal messenger.

Aundrea (Greek) a form of Andrea.

Aura (Greek) soft breeze. (Latin) golden. See also Ora.

Aurelia (Latin) golden. See also Oralia.

Aurelie (Latin) a form of Aurelia.

Aurora (Latin) dawn. Mythology: Aurora was the goddess of dawn.
Aurore, Ori, Orie, Rora

Austin (Latin) a short form of Augustine.

Autumn ☝ (Latin) autumn.
Autum

Ava ☝ (Greek) a form of Eva.
Avada, Avae, Ave, Aveen

Avalon (Latin) island.

Avery ☝ (English) a form of Aubrey.

Avis (Latin) bird.

Aviva (Hebrew) springtime. See also Viva.

Avril (French) a form of April.

Axelle (Latin) axe. (German) small oak tree; source of life.

Aya (Hebrew) bird; fly swiftly.

Ayanna (Hindi) innocent.
Ayania

Ayesha (Persian) a form of Aisha.
Ayasha, Ayeshah, Ayisha, Ayishah, Aysha, Ayshah, Ayshe, Ayshea, Aysia

Ayita (Cherokee) first in the dance.

Ayla (Hebrew) oak tree.
Aylana, Aylee, Ayleen, Aylene, Aylie

Aza (Arabic) comfort.
Azia

Aziza (Swahili) precious.

B

Baba (African) born on Thursday.

Babe (Latin) a familiar form of Barbara. (American) a form of Baby.

Babette (French, German) a familiar form of Barbara.

Babs (American) a familiar form of Barbara.

Baby (American) baby.

Bailee, Bailie (English) forms of Bailey.
Baillie

Baileigh, Baleigh (English) forms of Bailey.

Bailey (English) bailiff.
Bailley, Bailly, Baily, Bali

Baka (Hindi) crane.

Bakula (Hindi) flower.

Bambi (Italian) child.

Bandi (Punjabi) prisoner.
Banda, Bandy

Baptista (Latin) baptizer.

Bara, Barra (Hebrew) chosen.

Barb (Latin) a short form of Barbara.

Barbara (Latin) stranger, foreigner. See also Bebe, Varvara, Wava.

Barbie (American) a familiar form of Barbara.
Baubie

Barbra (American) a form of Barbara.

Barrett (German) strong as a bear.

Barrie (Irish) spear; markswoman.

Basia (Hebrew) daughter of God.

Bathsheba (Hebrew) daughter of the oath; seventh daughter. Bible: a wife of King David. See also Sheba.

Batini (Swahili) inner thoughts.

Baylee, Bayleigh, Baylie (English) forms of Bailey.
Bayla

Bayley (English) a form of Bailey.
Bayly

Bayo (Yoruba) joy is found.

Bea, Bee (American) short forms of Beatrice.

Beata (Latin) a short form of Beatrice.

Beatrice (Latin) blessed; happy; bringer of joy. See also Trish, Trixie.
Beatrica, Béatrice, Beatricia, Beatriks, Beatrisa, Beatrise, Beatrissa, Beattie, Beatty

Beatriz (Latin) a form of Beatrice.
Beatris, Beatriss, Beatrix, Beitris

Bebe (Spanish) a form of Barbara, Beatrice.

Becca (Hebrew) a short form of Rebecca.

Becky (American) a familiar form of Rebecca.
Becki, Beckie

Bedelia (Irish) a form of Bridget.

Bel (Hindi) sacred wood of apple trees. A short form of Amabel, Belinda, Isabel.

Bela (Czech) white. (Hungarian) bright.

Belen (Greek) arrow. (Spanish) Bethlehem.

Belicia (Spanish) dedicated to God.

Belinda (Spanish) beautiful. Literature: a name coined by English poet Alexander Pope in *The Rape of the Lock*. See also Blinda, Linda.
Belindra, Belynda

Bella (Latin) beautiful.

Belle (French) beautiful. A short form of Arabella, Belinda, Isabel. See also Billie.

Belva (Latin) beautiful view.

Bena (Native American) pheasant. See also Bina.

Benecia (Latin) a short form of Benedicta.

Benedicta (Latin) blessed.

Benedicte (Latin) a form of Benedicta.

Benita (Spanish) a form of Benedicta.
Benetta, Benitta, Bennita, Neeta

Bennett (Latin) little blessed one.

Benni (Latin) a familiar form of Benedicta.

Bente (Latin) blessed.

Berenice (Greek) a form of Bernice.

Berget (Irish) a form of Bridget.

Berit (German) glorious.
Berta

Berkley (Scottish, English) birch-tree meadow.

Berlynn (English) a combination of Bertha + Lynn.

Bernadette (French) a form of Bernadine. See also Nadette.
Bera, Beradette, Berna, Bernadet, Bernadett, Bernadetta, Bernarda, Bernardette, Bernedet, Bernedette, Bernessa

Bernadine (English, German) brave as a bear.

Berneta (French) a short form of Bernadette.

Berni (English) a familiar form of Bernadine, Bernice.

Bernice (Greek) bringer of victory. See also Bunny, Vernice.
Bernessa

Bertha (German) bright; illustrious; brilliant ruler. A short form of Alberta. See also Birdie, Peke.
Barta, Bartha, Berta, Berthe, Bertita, Bertrona, Bertus

Berti (German, English) a familiar form of Gilberte, Bertina.
Berte

Bertille (French) a form of Bertha.

Bertina (English) bright, shining.

Beryl (Greek) sea green jewel.

Bess, Bessie (Hebrew) familiar forms of Elizabeth.

Beth (Hebrew, Aramaic) house of God. A short form of Bethany, Elizabeth.
Betha, Bethe, Bethia

Bethani, Bethanie (Aramaic) forms of Bethany.
Bethanee, Bethania, Bethannie

Bethann (English) a combination of Beth + Ann.
Bethane

Bethany (Aramaic) house of figs. Bible: the site of Lazarus's resurrection.
Bethaney, Bethanney, Bethanny, Bethena, Betheny, Bethia, Bethina, Bethney

Betsy (American) a familiar form of Elizabeth.
Betsey, Betsi, Betsie

Bette (French) a form of Betty.

Bettina (American) a combination of Beth + Tina.
Betina, Betine, Betti, Bettine

Betty (Hebrew) consecrated to God. (English) a familiar form of Elizabeth.
Betti, Bettye, Bettyjean, Betty-Jean, Bettyjo, Betty-Jo, Bettylou, Betty-Lou, Bety

Betula (Hebrew) girl, maiden.

Beulah (Hebrew) married. Bible: Beulah is a name for Israel.

Bev (English) a short form of Beverly.

Bevanne (Welsh) child of Evan.
Bevan, Bevann, Bevany

Beverly (English) beaver field. See also Buffy.
Bevalee, Beverle, Beverlee, Beverley, Beverlie, Bevlyn, Bevlynn, Bevlynne, Bevvy, Verly

Beverlyann (American) a combination of Beverly + Ann.

Bian (Vietnamese) hidden; secretive.

Bianca (Italian) white. See also Blanca, Vianca.
Biancha, Biancia, Bianey

Bianka (Italian) a form of Bianca.

Bibi (Latin) a short form of Bibiana. (Arabic) lady. (Spanish) a form of Bebe.

Bibiana (Latin) lively.

Biddy (Irish) a familiar form of Bedelia.

Billi, Billy (English) forms of Billie.
Billye

Billie (English) strong willed. (German, French) a familiar form of Belle, Wilhelmina.
Bilee, Bili, Billye

Billie-Jean (American) a combination of Billie + Jean.

Billie-Jo (American) a combination of Billie + Jo.

Bina (Hebrew) wise; understanding. (Swahili) dancer. (Latin) a short form of Sabina. See also Bena.

Binney (English) a familiar form of Benedicta, Bianca, Bina.

Bionca (Italian) a form of Bianca.
Beonca, Beyonca, Bioncha

Birdie (English) bird. (German) a familiar form of Bertha.

Birgitte (Swedish) a form of Bridget.

Blaine (Irish) thin.

Blair (Scottish) plains dweller.

Blaire (Scottish) a form of Blair.
Blayre

Blaise (French) one who stammers.

Blake (English) dark.

Blakely (English) dark meadow.

Blanca (Italian) a form of Bianca.
Bellanca, Blancka, Blanka

Blanche (French) a form of Bianca.

Blinda (American) a short form of Belinda.

Bliss (English) blissful, joyful.

Blodwyn (Welsh) flower. See also Wynne.

Blondelle (French) blond, fair haired.

Blondie (American) a familiar form of Blondell.

Blossom (English) flower.

Blum (Yiddish) flower.

Blythe (English) happy, cheerful.
Blithe, Blyth

Bo (Chinese) precious.

Boacha (Hebrew) blessed.

Bobbette (American) a familiar form of Roberta.

Bobbi, Bobbie (American) familiar forms of Barbara, Roberta.
Baubie, Bobbisue, Bobbijo, Bobbye, Bobi, Bobie

Bobbi-Ann, Bobbie-Ann (American) combinations of Bobbi + Ann.

Bobbi-Jo (American) a combination of Bobbi + Jo.
Bobbiejo, Bobbie-Jo, Bobbijo, Bobby-Jo, Bobijo

Bobbi-Lee (American) a combination of Bobbi + Lee.

Bonita (Spanish) pretty.
Bonnetta

Bonnie, Bonny (English, Scottish) beautiful, pretty. (Spanish) familiar forms of Bonita.
Boni, Bonie, Bonne, Bonnee, Bonnell, Bonney, Bonni, Bonnin

Bonnie-Bell (American) a combination of Bonnie + Belle.

Bradley (English) broad meadow.

Brady (Irish) spirited.

Braeden (English) broad hill.

Braelyn (American) a combination of Braeden + Lynn.

Branda (Hebrew) blessing.

Brandee (Dutch) a form of Brandy.
Brande, Brandea

Branden (English) beacon valley.
Brandyn

Brandi, Brandie (Dutch) forms of Brandy.
Brandei, Brandice, Brandii, Brandily, Brandin, Brandis, Brandise, Brani, Branndie

Brandy (Dutch) an after-dinner drink made from distilled wine.
Brand, Brandace, Brandaise, Brandala, Brandeli, Brandell, Brandye, Brandylee, Brandy-Lee, Brandy-Leigh, Brann, Brantley, Branyell

Brandy-Lynn (American) a combination of Brandy + Lynn.

Braxton (English) Brock's town.

Brea, Bria (Irish) short forms of Breana, Briana.
Breah, Breea, Briah, Brya

Breana, Breanna (Irish) forms of Briana.
Breanda, Bre-Anna, Breawna, Breila

Breann, Breanne (Irish) short forms of Briana.
Bre-Ann, Bre-Anne, Breaunne, Breean, Breeann, Breeanne, Breelyn, Breiann, Breighann, Brieon

Breasha (Russian) a familiar form of Breana.

Breauna, Breunna, Briauna (Irish) forms of Briana.
Breeauna

Breck (Irish) freckled.

Bree (English) broth. (Irish) a short form of Breann. See also Brie.
Breay, Brei, Breigh

Breeana, Breeanna (Irish) forms of Briana.

Breena (Irish) fairy palace. A form of Brina.
Breina

Breiana, Breianna (Irish) forms of Briana.
Breiann

Brenda (Irish) little raven. (English) sword.
Brendell, Brendelle, Brendette, Brendie, Brendyl

Brenda-Lee (American) a combination of Brenda + Lee.

Brenna (Irish) a form of Brenda.
Bren, Brenie, Brenin, Brenn,
Brennah, Brennaugh

Brennan (English) a form of Brendan
(see Boys' Names).

Breona, Breonna (Irish) forms of
Briana.

Brett (Irish) a short form of Brittany. See
also Brita.
Bret, Brette, Brettin, Bretton

Breyana, Breyann, Breyanna (Irish)
forms of Briana.

Breyona, Breyonna (Irish) forms of
Briana.

Briana (Irish) strong; virtuous, honorable.
Brana, Briahna, Briand, Brianda

Brianna ✹ (Irish) strong; virtuous,
honorable.
Briannah, Brianni, Briannon

Brianne (Irish) a form of Briana.
Briane, Briann

Briar (French) heather.
Brear, Brier, Bryar

Bridey (Irish) a familiar form of
Bridget.

Bridget (Irish) strong. See also Bedelia,
Bryga, Gitta.
Brietta

Bridgett, Bridgette (Irish) forms of
Bridget.
Bridgitte, Briggitte, Brigitta

Brie (French) a type of cheese.
Geography: a region in France known
for its cheese. See also Bree.
Briena, Brieon, Brieta, Briette

Brieana, Brieanna (American) combinations of Brie + Anna.

Brieann, Brieanne (American) combinations of Brie + Ann. See also Briana.
Brie-Ann, Brie-Anne

Brielle (French) a form of Brie.

Brienna, Brienne (Irish) forms of
Briana.
Brieon

Brienne (French) a form of Briana.
Brienn

Brigette (French) a form of Bridget.

Brigitte (French) a form of Bridget.
Briggitte, Brigit, Brigita

Brina (Latin) a short form of Sabrina.
(Irish) a familiar form of Briana.
Brinn

Briona (Irish) a form of Briana.

Brisa (Spanish) beloved. Mythology:
Briseis was the Greek name of Achilles's
beloved.

Brita (Irish) a form of Bridget. (English)
a short form of Britany.
Bretta, Brieta, Brietta, Brit

Britaney, Brittaney (English) forms of
Britany, Brittany.
Britanee, Britanny, Britenee, Briteny,
Britianey, British, Britkney, Britley,
Britlyn

Britani, Brittani, Brittanie (English)
forms of Britany.
Brit, Britania, Britanica, Britanie,
Britanii, Britanni, Britannia,
Britatani, Britia, Britini, Brittane,
Brittanee, Brittanni, Brittannia,
Brittannie, Brittenie, Brittiani,
Brittianni

Britany, Brittany (English) from
Britain. See also Brett.
*Britana, Britlyn, Brittainny, Brittainy,
Brittamy, Brittana, Brittania,
Brittanica, Brittany-Ann, Brittanyne,
Brittell, Brittiany, Brittlin, Brittoni,
Brittlynn, Brittony*

Britin, Brittin (English) from Britain.
Britann, Brittan

Britney, Brittney, Brittny (English)
forms of Britany.
*Bittney, Bridnee, Bridney, Britnay,
Britne, Britnee, Britnei, Britny, Britnye,
Brittnay, Brittnaye, Brytnea, Brytni*

Britni, Brittni, Brittnie (English)
forms of Britney, Britany.
Britnie

Briton, Brittin (English) forms of
Britin, Brittin.
Britton

Britt, Britta (Latin) short forms of
Britany, Brittany. (Swedish) strong.
Briet, Brit, Britte

Britteny (English) a form of Britany,
Brittany.
Britten, Brittenee, Britteney, Brittenie

Brittini, Brittiny (English) forms of
Britany, Brittany.

Brittnee (English) a form of Britany,
Brittany.
Brittne, Brittnea, Brittneigh

Briyana, Briyanna (Irish) forms of
Briana.

Brodie (Irish) ditch; canal builder.

Bronnie (Welsh) a familiar form of
Bronwyn.
*Bron, Bronia, Bronney, Bronny,
Bronya*

Bronwyn (Welsh) white breasted.
*Bronwen, Bronwin, Bronwynn,
Bronwynne*

Brook (English) brook, stream.

Brooke ❀ (English) brook, stream.
Brookelle, Brookie, Brooks, Brooky

Brooklyn ❀ (American) a combination of Brook + Lyn.

Brooklynn (American) a combination
of Brook + Lynn.

Bruna (German) a short form of
Brunhilda.

Brunhilda (German) armored warrior.

Bryana, Bryanna, Bryanne (Irish)
short forms of Bryana.
Bryann

Bryce (Welsh) alert; ambitious.

Bryga (Polish) a form of Bridget.

Brylie (American) a combination of the
letter B + Riley.

Bryn, Brynn (Latin) from the boundary
line. (Welsh) mound.
Brinn, Brynee, Brynne

Bryna (Latin, Irish) a form of Brina.
Brynan

Bryona, Bryonna (Irish) forms of
Briana.

Bryttani, Bryttany (English) forms of
Britany.

Buffy (American) buffalo; from the plains.

Bunny (Greek) a familiar form of
Bernice. (English) little rabbit. See also
Bonnie.

Burgundy (French) Geography: a region of France known for its Burgundy wine.

C

Cachet (French) prestigious; desirous.

Cadence (Latin) rhythm.

Cady (English) a form of Kady.

Caeley, Cailey, Cayley (American) forms of Kaylee, Kelly.
Cailee, Cailie, Caily

Caelin, Caelyn (American) forms of Kaelyn.
Caelan, Cailan, Caylan

Cai (Vietnamese) feminine.
Caye

Cailida (Spanish) adoring.

Cailin, Cailyn (American) forms of Caitlin.
Caileen, Cailene, Cailine, Cailynn, Cailynne, Cayleen, Caylene, Caylin, Cayline, Caylyn, Caylyne, Caylynne

Caitlan (Irish) a form of Caitlin.
Caitland, Caitlandt

Caitlin (Irish) pure. See also Kaitlin, Katalina, Katelin, Katelyn, Kaytlyn.
Caitleen, Caitlen, Caitlene, Caitline, Caitlinn, Caitlon, Caitria, Catlee, Catleen, Catleene, Catlin

Caitlyn, Caitlynn (Irish) forms of Caitlin. See also Kaitlyn.
Caitlynne, Catlyn, Catlynn, Catlynne

Cala (Arabic) castle, fortress. See also Callie, Kala.
Calan

Calandra (Greek) lark.
Calan, Calandria, Caleida, Calendra, Calendre, Kalandra, Kalandria

Caleigh, Caley (American) forms of Caeley.

Cali, Calli (Greek) forms of Callie. See also Kali.
Calee

Calida (Spanish) warm; ardent.
Calina

Callie (Greek, Arabic) a familiar form of Cala, Callista. See also Kalli.
Cal, Calie, Callee, Calley, Cally, Caly

Callista (Greek) most beautiful. See also Kallista.

Calvina (Latin) bald.
Calvine, Calvinetta, Calvinette

Calypso (Greek) concealer. Botany: a pink orchid native to northern regions. Mythology: the sea nymph who held Odysseus captive for seven years.
Caly

Cam (Vietnamese) sweet citrus.

Camara (American) a form of Cameron.
Camera, Cameri, Cameria

Camberly (American) a form of Kimberly.

Cambria (Latin) from Wales. See also Kambria.

Camden (Scottish) winding valley.

Camellia (Italian) Botany: a camellia is an evergreen tree or shrub with fragrant roselike flowers.

Cameo (Latin) gem or shell on which a portrait is carved.

Cameron (Scottish) crooked nose. See also Kameron, Kamryn.
Cameran, Cameren

Cami (French) a short form of Camille. See also Kami.
Camey, Camie, Cammi, Cammie, Cammy, Cammye

Camila, Camilla (Italian) forms of Camille. See also Kamila, Mila.
Camia, Camillia, Chamelea, Chamelia, Chamika, Chamila, Chamilia

Camille (French) young ceremonial attendant. See also Millie.
Camill, Cammille, Cammillie, Cammilyn, Cammyl, Cammyll, Chamelle, Chamille, Kamille

Camisha (American) a combination of Cami + Aisha.
Camesha, Cameshia

Camri, Camrie (American) short forms of Camryn. See also Kamri.

Camryn (American) a form of Cameron. See also Kamryn.

Camylle (French) a form of Camille.

Candace (Greek) glittering white; glowing. History: the title of the queens of ancient Ethiopia. See also Dacey, Kandace.
Cace, Canace, Canda, Candas

Candi, Candy (American) familiar forms of Candace, Candice, Candida. See also Kandi.
Candee, Candie

Candice, Candis (Greek) forms of Candace.
Candias, Candies, Candise, Candiss, Candus

Candida (Latin) bright white.

Candra (Latin) glowing. See also Kandra.
Candrea, Candria

Candyce (Greek) a form of Candace.
Candys, Candyse, Cyndyss

Cantara (Arabic) small crossing.

Cantrelle (French) song.

Capri (Italian) a short form of Caprice. Geography: an island off the west coast of Italy. See also Kapri.

Caprice (Italian) fanciful.
Cappi, Caprece, Capricia, Caprina, Caprise, Capritta

Cara (Latin) dear. (Irish) friend. See also Karah.
Caragh, Carah, Caranda

Caralee (Irish) a form of Cara.
Caralea, Caralia, Caralie, Carely

Caralyn (English) a form of Caroline.
Caralin, Caraline, Caralynn, Caralynne

Caressa (French) a form of Carissa.

Carey (Welsh) a familiar form of Cara, Caroline, Karen, Katherine. See also Carrie, Kari.
Caree, Carrey, Cary

Cari, Carie (Welsh) forms of Carey, Kari.

Carina (Italian) dear little one.
(Swedish) a form of Karen. (Greek) a
familiar form of Cora.
Carena

Carine (Italian) a form of Carina.
Carin

Carisa, Carrisa (Greek) forms of
Carissa.
Carisia, Charisa

Carissa (Greek) beloved. See also
Karissa.
Carrissa

Carita (Latin) charitable.

Carla (German) farmer. (English)
strong. (Latin) a form of Carol,
Caroline.
Carila, Carilla, Carleta, Carlia,
Carliqua, Carliyle, Carlonda,
Carlreca, Carlyjo, Carlyle, Carlysle

Carlee, Carleigh, Carley (English)
forms of Carly. See also Karlee.
Carle, Carleah

Carleen, Carlene (English) forms of
Caroline. See also Karlene.
Carlaen, Carlaena, Carleena, Carlen,
Carlena, Carlenna, Carline, Carlyne

Carli, Carlie (English) forms of Carly.
See also Karli.

Carlin (Irish) little champion. (Latin) a
short form of Caroline.
Carlan, Carlina, Carlinda, Carline,
Carling, Carrlin

Carlisa (American) a form of Carlissa.
Carilis, Carilise, Carilyse, Carletha,
Carlethe, Carlicia, Carlyse

Carlissa (American) a combination of
Carla + Lissa.

Carlotta (Italian) a form of Charlotte.
Carliita, Carlota

Carly (English) a familiar form of
Caroline, Charlotte. See also Karli.
Carlye

Carlyn, Carlynn (Irish) forms of Carlin.
Carlynne

Carmela, Carmella (Hebrew) garden;
vineyard. Bible: Mount Carmel in Israel
is often thought of as paradise. See also
Karmel.
Carma, Carmalla, Carmarit,
Carmel, Carmeli, Carmelia,
Carmelina, Carmelle, Carmellia,
Carmellina, Carmesa, Carmesha,
Carmi, Carmie, Carmiel, Carmil,
Carmila, Carmilla, Carmisha, Leeta

Carmelit (Hebrew) a form of Carmela.
Carmaletta, Carmalit, Carmalita,
Carmelita, Carmelitha, Carmelitia,
Carmellit, Carmellita, Carmellitha,
Carmelliitia

Carmen (Latin) song. Religion: Nuestra
Señora del Carmen—Our Lady of
Mount Carmen—is one of the titles of
the Virgin Mary. See also Karmen.
Carma, Carmaine, Carman,
Carmelina, Carmencita, Carmene,
Carmi, Carmia, Carmin, Carmina,
Carmine, Carmita, Carmon,
Carmynn

Carol (German) farmer. (French) song
of joy. (English) strong. See also
Charlene, Kalle, Karoll.
Carel, Cariel, Caro, Carola,
Carolenia, Carolinda, Caroll, Carrol,
Carroll

Carolane, Carolann, Carolanne
(American) combinations of Carol +
Ann. Forms of Caroline.

Carole (English) a form of Carol.
Carolee, Karole, Karrole

Carolina (Italian) a form of Caroline.
See also Karolina.
*Carilena, Carlena, Carlina,
Carrolena*

Caroline ☆ (French) little and strong.
See also Carla, Carleen, Carlin,
Karolina.
*Caralin, Caraline, Carileen, Carilene,
Carilin, Cariline, Carling, Caro,
Caroleen, Carolin, Carrolena,
Carrolene, Carrolin, Carroline, Cary*

Carolyn (English) a form of Caroline.
See also Karolyn.
*Carilyn, Carilynn, Carilynne,
Carlynne, Carolyne, Carolynn,
Carolynne, Carrolyn, Carrolynn,
Carrolynne*

Caron (Welsh) loving, kindhearted,
charitable.
Caronne, Carron

Carra (Irish) a form of Cara.

Carrie (English) a familiar form of
Carol, Caroline. See also Carey, Kari,
Karri.
*Carree, Carrey, Carri, Carria, Carry,
Cary*

Carson (English) child of Carr.

Carter (English) cart driver.

Caryl (Latin) a form of Carol.

Caryn (Danish) a form of Karen.
*Caren, Carren, Carrin, Caryna,
Caryne, Carynn*

Carys (Welsh) love.

Casandra (Greek) a form of Cassandra.
Casandre, Casandrey, Casandri,

*Casandria, Casaundra, Casaundria,
Casondra, Casondre, Casondria*

Casey (Irish) brave. (Greek) a familiar
form of Acacia. See also Kasey.
*Cacy, Cascy, Casse, Cassee, Cassye,
Casy, Cayce, Cayse, Caysee, Caysy*

Casidy (Irish) a form of Cassidy.

Casie (Irish) a form of Casey.
*Caci, Casci, Cascie, Casi, Cayci, Caysi,
Caysie, Cazzi*

Cass (Greek) a short form of Cassandra.

Cassady (Irish) a form of Cassidy.
*Casadee, Casadi, Casadie, Cassadi,
Cassadie, Cassadina*

Cassandra (Greek) helper of men.
Mythology: a prophetess of ancient
Greece whose prophesies were not
believed. See also Kassandra, Sandra,
Sandy, Zandra.
Cassandre, Cassandri, Cassandry

Cassaundra (Greek) a form of
Cassandra.
*Cassaundre, Cassaundri, Cassundra,
Cassundre*

Cassia (Greek) a cinnamon-like spice.
See also Kasia.

Cassidy (Irish) clever. See also Kassidy.
*Casseday, Cassiddy, Cassidee, Cassidi,
Cassidie, Cassity*

Cassie, Cassey, Cassi (Greek) familiar forms of Cassandra, Catherine. See
also Kassie.
Cassee, Cassy, Casy

Cassiopeia (Greek) clever. Mythology:
the wife of the Ethiopian king Cepheus;
the mother of Andromeda.

Cassondra (Greek) a form of
Cassandra.
Cassondre, Cassondri, Cassondria

Catalina (Spanish) a form of Catherine.
See also Katalina.
*Cataleen, Catalena, Catalene,
Catalin, Catalyn, Catalyna, Cateline*

Catarina (German) a form of Catherine.
Catarine, Caterina

Catelyn (Irish) a form of Caitlin.
Cateline

Catharine (Greek) a form of Catherine.
Catharina

Catherine (Greek) pure. (English) a
form of Katherine.
*Cat, Cate, Cathann, Cathanne,
Cathenne, Catheren, Catherene,
Catheria, Catherin, Catherina,
Catheryn, Catlaina, Catreeka,
Catrelle, Catrice, Catricia, Catrika,
Catteeka*

Cathi, Cathy (Greek) familiar forms of
Catherine, Cathleen. See also Kathy.
Catha, Cathe, Cathee, Cathey, Cathie

Cathleen (Irish) a form of Catherine.
See also Caitlin, Kathleen.
*Cathaleen, Cathelin, Cathelina,
Cathelyn, Cathleana, Cathlene,
Cathleyn, Cathlin, Cathlyn, Cathlyne*

Cathrine (Greek) a form of Catherine.

Cathryn (Greek) a form of Catherine.
Catryn

Catrina (Slavic) a form of Catherine,
Katrina.
*Caitriona, Catina, Catreen, Catreena,
Catrene, Catrenia, Catrin, Catrine,
Catrinia, Catriona, Catroina*

Cayla (Hebrew) a form of Kayla.

Caylee, Caylie (American) forms of
Caeley, Cailey, Cayley.
Cayly

Ceara (Irish) a form of Ciara.
Cearaa, Cearra

Cecelia (Latin) a form of Cecilia. See
also Sheila.
*Cacelia, Cece, Ceceilia, Ceceli, Cecely,
Cecelyn, Cecette, Cescelia, Cescelie*

Cecilia (Latin) blind. See also Cicely,
Cissy, Secilia, Selia, Sissy.
*Cacilia, Caecilia, Cecil, Cecila, Cecile,
Cecilea, Cecilija, Cecilla, Cecille,
Cecillia, Ceclia, Cecylia, Cee, Ceila,
Ceilagh, Ceileh, Ceileigh, Ceilena,
Cicelia*

Cecily (Latin) a form of Cecilia.
Cacilie, Ceciley, Cescily, Cilley

Ceil (Latin) a short form of Cecilia.

Ceira, Ceirra (Irish) forms of Ciara.

Celena (Greek) a form of Selena.
Celeena, Celenia

Celene (Greek) a form of Celena.
Celeen

Celeste (Latin) celestial, heavenly.
*Cele, Celense, Celes, Celesia, Celesley,
Celest, Celesta, Celestia, Celestial,
Celestin, Celestina, Celestine,
Celestinia, Celestyn, Celestyna,
Selestina*

Celia (Latin) a short form of Cecilia.
Ceilia, Celie

Celina (Greek) a form of Celena. See
also Selina.
*Caleena, Calena, Calina, Celinda,
Celinka, Celka, Cellina*

Celine (Greek) a form of Celena.
Caline, Celeen, Céline, Cellinn

Cera (French) a short form of Cerise.

Cerella (Latin) springtime.

Cerise (French) cherry; cherry red.

Cesilia (Latin) a form of Cecilia.
Cesia, Cesya

Chablis (French) a dry, white wine.
Geography: a region in France where
wine grapes are grown.

Chadee (French) from Chad, a country
in north-central Africa. See also Sade.

Chai (Hebrew) life.

Chaka (Sanskrit) a form of Chakra. See
also Shaka.

Chakra (Sanskrit) circle of energy.

Chalice (French) goblet.

Chalina (Spanish) a form of Rose.

Chalonna (American) a combination of
the prefix Cha + Lona.

Chambray (French) a lightweight fabric.

Chan (Cambodian) sweet-smelling tree.

Chana (Hebrew) a form of Hannah.

Chancey (English) chancellor; church
official.

Chanda (Sanskrit) short tempered.
Religion: the demon defeated by the
Hindu goddess Chamunda. See also
Shanda.
Chandee, Chandey, Chandi, Chandie

Chandelle (French) candle.
Chandal

Chandler (Hindi) moon. (Old English)
candlemaker.

Chandra (Sanskrit) moon. Religion: the
Hindu god of the moon. See also
Shandra.
*Chandre, Chandrea, Chandrelle,
Chandria*

Chanel (English) channel. See also
Shanel.
Chaneel, Chaneil, Channel

Chanell, Chanelle (English) forms of
Chanel.

Chanise (American) a form of Shanice.

Channa (Hindi) chickpea.

Chantal (French) song.
*Chandal, Chantaal, Chantael,
Chantale, Chantall, Chantalle,
Chantara, Chantarai, Chantasia,
Chanteau, Chantle, Chantoya,
Chantrill*

Chante (French) a short form of
Chantal.
*Chanta, Chantae, Chantai, Chantay,
Chantaye, Chantee, Chantée,
Chaunte, Chauntea, Chauntéa,
Chauntee*

Chantel, Chantell, Chantelle
(French) forms of Chantal. See also
Shantel.
*Chantea, Chanteese, Chantela,
Chantele, Chantella, Chanter,
Chantey, Chantez, Chantrel,
Chantrell, Chantrelle*

Chantilly (French) fine lace. See also
Shantille.
*Chantiel, Chantielle, Chantil,
Chantila, Chantill, Chantille*

Chantrea (Cambodian) moon; moonbeam.
Chantra, Chantri

Chantrice (French) singer. See also
Shantrice.
Chantress

Chardae, Charde (Punjabi) charitable.
(French) short forms of Chardonnay.
See also Shardae.
*Charda, Chardai, Charday, Chardea,
Chardee, Chardée, Chardese*

Chardonnay (French) a dry white wine.
Char

Charis (Greek) grace; kindness.
*Charese, Chari, Charice, Charie,
Charish*

Charissa, Charisse (Greek) forms of
Charity.
*Charesa, Charese, Charisa, Charise,
Charisha, Charissee, Charista*

Charity (Latin) charity, kindness.
*Chariety, Charista, Charita, Chariti,
Sharity*

Charla (French, English) a short form of
Charlene, Charlotte.
Char, Charlea

Charlaine (English) a form of Charlene.
Charlaina

Charlee, Charley (German, English)
forms of Charlie.
Charle, Charleigh

Charlene (English) a form of Caroline.
See also Carol, Karla, Sharlene.
*Charleen, Charleesa, Charlena,
Charlesena, Charline, Charlyn,
Charlyne, Charlynn, Charlynne,
Charlzina, Charoline*

Charlie (German, English) strong.
Charli, Charyl, Chatty, Sharli, Sharlie

Charlotte (French) a form of Caroline.
Literature: Charlotte Brontë was a
British novelist and poet best known for
her novel *Jane Eyre*. See also Karlotte,
Lotte, Sharlotte, Tottie.
*Chara, Charil, Charl, Charlet,
Charlett, Charletta, Charlette,
Charlisa, Charlita, Charlott, Charlotta,
Charlotty, Charolet, Charolette,
Charolot, Charolotte*

Charmaine (French) a form of Carmen.
See also Sharmaine.
*Charamy, Charma, Charmain,
Charmalique, Charman, Charmane,
Charmar, Charmara, Charmayane,
Charmeen, Charmene, Charmese,
Charmian, Charmin, Charmine,
Charmion, Charmisa, Charmon,
Charmyn*

Charnette (American) a combination of
Charo + Annette.

Charnika (American) a combination of
Charo + Nika.

Charo (Spanish) a familiar form of
Rosa.

Charyanna (American) a combination
of Charo + Anna.
Cheryn

Chasidy, Chassidy (Latin) forms of
Chastity.
*Chasa Dee, Chasadie, Chasady,
Chassedi*

Chasity (Latin) a form of Chastity.
Chasiti, Chassey, Chassie, Chassity,
Chassy

Chastity (Latin) pure.
Chasta, Chastady, Chastidy, Chastin,
Chastitie, Chastney, Chasty

Chauntel (French) a form of Chantal.
Chaunta, Chauntay, Chaunte,
Chauntell, Chauntelle, Chawntel,
Chawntell, Chawntelle, Chontelle

Chava (Hebrew) life. (Yiddish) bird.
Religion: the original name of Eve.

Chavella (Spanish) a form of Isabel.

Chavi (Gypsy) girl.

Chavon (Hebrew) a form of Jane.

Chavonne (Hebrew) a form of Chavon.
(American) a combination of the prefix
Cha + Yvonne.

Chaya (Hebrew) life; living.

Chelci, Chelcie (English) forms of
Chelsea.
Chelcy

Chelsea (English) seaport. See also
Kelsi, Shelsea.
Chelese, Chelesia, Chelsa, Chelsae,
Chelse, Chelsia, Chesea, Cheslee

Chelsee (English) a form of Chelsea.
Chelsei

Chelsey, Chelsy (English) forms of
Chelsea. See also Kelsey.
Chelcy, Chelsay, Chesley

Chelsie (English) a form of Chelsea.
Chelli, Chellie, Chellise, Chellsie, Chelsi,
Cheslie, Chessie

Chenelle (English) a form of Chanel.

Chenoa (Native American) white dove.

Cher (French) beloved, dearest.
(English) a short form of Cherilyn.

Cherelle, Cherrelle (French) forms of
Cheryl. See also Sherelle.
Charell, Charelle

Cherese (Greek) a form of Cherish.
Chereese, Cheresa, Cheresse, Cherice

Cheri, Cherie (French) familiar forms
of Cher.
Chérie

Cherilyn (English) a combination of
Cheryl + Lynn.
Cherylene, Cheryline, Sherilyn

Cherise (French) a form of Cherish. See
also Sharice, Sherice.
Charisa, Charise, Cherece, Chereese,
Cheresa, Cherice

Cherish (English) dearly held, precious.
Charish, Charisha, Cheerish, Cherishe,
Cherrish, Sherish

Cherokee (Native American) a tribal
name.

Cherry (Latin) a familiar form of
Charity. (French) cherry; cherry red.

Cheryl (French) beloved. See also Sheryl.
Charel, Charil, Charyl, Cheryl-
Ann, Cheryl-Anne, Cheryle, Cherylee,
Cheryll, Cherylle, Cheryl-Lee

Chesarey (American) a form of Desiree.

Chesna (Slavic) peaceful.

Chessa (American) a short form of
Chesarey.
Chessie

Cheyanne (Cheyenne) a form of Cheyenne.
Cheyan, Cheyana, Cheyann

Cheyenne (Cheyenne) a tribal name. See also Shaianne, Sheyenne, Shianne, Shyann.
Cheyene, Cheyenna, Chi, Chi-Anna, Chie

Cheyla (American) a form of Sheila.

Cheyna (American) a short form of Cheyenne.
Chey

Chiara (Italian) a form of Clara.

Chika (Japanese) near and dear.

Chiku (Swahili) chatterer.

China (Chinese) fine porcelain. Geography: a country in eastern Asia. See also Ciana, Shina.

Chinira (Swahili) God receives.

Chinue (Ibo) God's own blessing.

Chiquita (Spanish) little one. See also Shiquita.
Chaqueta, Chaquita, Chica, Chickie, Chicky, Chikata, Chikita, Chiqueta, Chiquila, Chiquite, Chiquitha, Chiquithe, Chiquitia, Chiquitta

Chiyo (Japanese) eternal.

Chloe ♛ (Greek) blooming, verdant. Mythology: another name for Demeter, the goddess of agriculture.
Chloé, Chlöe, Chloee

Chloris (Greek) pale. Mythology: the only daughter of Niobe to escape the vengeful arrows of Apollo and Artemis. See also Loris.

Cho (Korean) beautiful.

Cholena (Native American) bird.

Chriki (Swahili) blessing.

Chris (Greek) a short form of Christina. See also Kris.

Chrissa (Greek) a short form of Christina. See also Khrissa.

Chrissy (English) a familiar form of Christina.
Chrisie, Chrissee, Chrissie, Crissie, Khrissy

Christa (German) a short form of Christina. History: Christa McAuliffe, an American school teacher, was the first civilian on a U. S. space flight. See also Krista.
Chrysta

Christabel (Latin, French) beautiful Christian.
Kristabel

Christain (Greek) a form of Christina.

Christal (Latin) a form of Crystal. (Scottish) a form of Christina.
Christalene, Christalin, Christaline, Christall, Christalle, Christalyn

Christelle (French) a form of Christal.
Christel, Chrystel

Christen, Christin (Greek) forms of Christina. See also Kristen.
Christan, Chrystan, Chrysten, Chrystyn, Crestienne

Christena, Christen (Greek) forms of Christina.

Christi, Christie (Greek) short forms of Christina, Christine. See also Kristi.
Chrysti, Chrystie, Chrysty

Christian, Christiana, Christianna
(Greek) forms of Christina. See also
Kristian, Krystian.
*Christiane, Christiann, Christi-Ann,
Christianne, Christi-Anne, Christianni,
Christienne, Christy-Ann, Christy-
Anne, Chrystyann, Chrystyanne,
Crystiann, Crystianne*

Christin (Greek) a short form of
Christina.
Chrystin

Christina (Greek) Christian; anointed.
See also Khristina, Kristina, Stina, Tina.
*Christeena, Christella, Christinea,
Christinna, Christna, Christyna,
Chrystina, Chrystyna, Cristeena,
Cristena, Chrystena*

Christine (French, English) a form of
Christina. See also Kirsten, Kristen,
Kristine.
*Chrisa, Christeen, Christene, Chrystine,
Cristeen, Cristene, Crystine*

Christophe (Greek) Christ-bearer.

Christy (English) a short form of
Christina, Christine.

Christyn (Greek) a form of Christina.

Chrys (English) a form of Chris.

Chrystal (Latin) a form of Christal.

Chu Hua (Chinese) chrysanthemum.

Chumani (Lakota) dewdrops.

Chun (Burmese) nature's renewal.

Chyanne, Chyenne (Cheyenne) forms
of Cheyenne.
Chyann, Chyanna

Chyna, Chynna (Chinese) forms of
China.

Ciana (Chinese) a form of China.
(Italian) a form of Jane.

Ciara, Ciarra (Irish) black. See also
Sierra.
*Cearia, Ciaara, Ciarrah, Cieara,
Ciearra, Ciearria*

Cicely (English) a form of Cecilia. See
also Sissy.
Cicelia, Cilla

Cidney (French) a form of Sydney.

Ciera, Cierra (Irish) forms of Ciara.
Cierrah

Cinderella (French, English) little
cinder girl. Literature: a fairy tale heroine.

Cindy (Greek) moon. (Latin) a familiar
form of Cynthia. See also Sindy.
Cindee, Cindi, Cindl

Cinthia, Cinthya (Greek) forms of
Cynthia.

Cira (Spanish) a form of Cyrilla.

Cissy (American) a familiar form of
Cecelia, Cicely.

Claire ★ (French) a form of Clara.
Clair, Klaire, Klarye

Clairissa (Greek) a form of Clarissa.

Clara (Latin) clear; bright. Music: Clara
Shumann was a famous nineteenth-
century German composer. See also
Chiara, Klara.
Claresta, Clarina, Clarinda, Clarine

Clarabelle (Latin) bright and beautiful.
Claribel

Clare (English) a form of Clara.

Clarie (Latin) a familiar form of Clara.
Clarey, Clari, Clary

Clarice (Italian) a form of Clara.

Clarisa (Greek) a form of Clarissa.
Claresa

Clarissa (Greek) brilliant. (Italian) a
form of Clara. See also Klarissa.
*Clarecia, Claressa, Claresta, Clarissia,
Claritza, Clarizza, Clarrisa, Clarrissa,
Clerissa*

Clarita (Spanish) a form of Clara.
Clairette, Clarette, Claritza

Claudette (French) a form of Claudia.

Claudia (Latin) lame. See also Gladys,
Klaudia.
*Claudeen, Claudelle, Claudex,
Claudiane, Claudie-Anne, Claudina,
Claudine*

Claudie (Latin) a form of Claudia.
Claudee

Clea (Greek) a form of Cleo, Clio.

Clementine (Latin) merciful.

Cleo (Greek) a short form of Cleopatra.

Cleone (Greek) famous.

Cleopatra (Greek) her father's fame.
History: a great Egyptian queen.

Cleta (Greek) illustrious.

Clio (Greek) proclaimer; glorifier.
Mythology: the Muse of history.

Cloe (Greek) a form of Chloe.
Clo, Cloey

Clotilda (German) heroine.

Coco (Spanish) coconut. See also Koko.

Codi, Cody (English) cushion. See also
Kodi.
Coady, Codee, Codey, Codie

Colby (English) coal town. Geography: a
region in England known for cheese-
making. See also Kolby.
Cobi, Cobie, Colbi, Colbie

Colette (Greek, French) a familiar form
of Nicole.
*Coe, Coetta, Coletta, Collet, Collete,
Collett, Colletta, Collette, Kolette,
Kollette*

Colleen (Irish) girl. See also Kolina.
*Coe, Coel, Cole, Coleen, Colene, Coley,
Coline, Colleene, Collen, Collene,
Collie, Colline, Colly*

Collina (Irish) a form of Colleen.
Colena, Colina, Colinda

Concetta (Italian) pure.

Conchita (Spanish) conception.

Concordia (Latin) harmonious.
Mythology: the goddess governing the
peace after war.
Con

Connie (Latin) a familiar form of
Constance.
*Con, Connee, Conni, Conny, Konnie,
Konny*

Connor (Scottish) wise. (Irish) praised;
exhalted.

Constance (Latin) constant; firm.
History: Constance Motley was the first
African-American woman to be
appointed as a U.S. federal judge. See
also Konstance, Kosta.
*Constancia, Constancy, Constanta,
Constantia, Constantina, Constantine*

Constanza (Spanish) a form of
Constance.

Consuelo (Spanish) consolation.
Religion: Nuestra Señora del
Consuelo—Our Lady of Consolation—
is a name for the Virgin Mary.

Cora (Greek) maiden. Mythology: Kore is
another name for Persephone, the
goddess of the underworld. See also
Kora.
Corra

Corabelle (American) a combination of
Cora + Belle.
Corabel, Corabella

Coral (Latin) coral. See also Koral.
Corral

Coralee (American) a combination of
Cora + Lee.
Coraline, Coralyn

Coralie (American) a form of Coralee.

Corazon (Spanish) heart.

Corbin (Latin) raven.

Cordasha (American) a combination of
Cora + Dasha.

Cordelia (Latin) warm-hearted. (Welsh)
sea jewel. See also Delia, Della.

Cordi (Welsh) a short form of Cordelia.

Coretta (Greek) a familiar form of Cora.

Corey, Cory (Irish) from the hollow.
(Greek) familiar forms of Cora. See also
Kori.
Coree, Correy, Correye, Corry

Cori, Corie, Corrie (Irish) forms of
Corey.

Coriann, Corianne (American) combi-
nations of Cori + Ann, Cori + Anne.
*Corian, Cori-Ann, Corri, Corrie-Ann,
Corrianne, Corrie-Anne*

Corina, Corinna (Greek) familiar forms
of Corinne. See also Korina.
Coreena, Corinda, Correna, Corrinna

Corinne (Greek) maiden.
*Coreen, Coren, Corin, Corine,
Corinee, Corinn, Coryn, Corynn,
Corynna*

Corissa (Greek) a familiar form of Cora.
Coresa, Coressa, Corisa, Korissa

Corliss (English) cheerful; goodhearted.

Cornelia (Latin) horn colored. See also
Kornelia, Nelia, Nellie.

Corrina, Corrine (Greek) forms of
Corinne.
*Correen, Corren, Corrin, Corrinn,
Corrinna, Corrinne, Corrinne,
Corryn*

Cortney (English) a form of Courtney.
*Cortnea, Cortnee, Cortneia, Cortni,
Cortnie, Cortny, Corttney*

Cosette (French) a familiar form of
Nicole.

Courtenay (English) a form of
Courtney.
Courteney

Courtnee, Courtnie (English) forms of
Courtney.
Courtnée, Courtnei, Courtni

Courtney (English) from the court. See
also Kortney, Kourtney.
*Courtena, Courtene, Courtnae,
Courtnay, Courtny, Courtonie*

Crisbell (American) a combination of Crista + Belle.

Crista, Crysta (Italian) forms of Christa.

Cristal (Latin) a form of Crystal.
Cristalie, Cristalina, Cristalle, Cristel, Cristela, Cristelia, Cristella, Cristelle, Cristhie, Cristle

Cristen, Cristin (Irish) forms of Christen, Christin. See also Kristin.
Cristan, Cristyn, Crystan, Crysten, Crystin, Crystyn

Cristina, Cristine (Greek) forms of Christina. See also Kristina.
Cristiona

Cristy (English) a familiar form of Cristina. A form of Christy. See also Kristy.
Cristey, Cristi, Cristie, Crysti, Crystie, Crysty

Crystal (Latin) clear, brilliant glass. See also Kristal, Krystal.
Chrystal-Lynn, Chrystel, Crystala, Crystale, Crystalee, Crystall, Crystaly, Crystel, Crystelia, Crysthelle, Crystl, Crystle, Crystol, Crystole, Crystyl

Crystalin (Latin) crystal pool.
Crystal-Ann, Crystal-Anne, Cristalina

Crystina (Greek) a form of Christina.
Crystin, Crystine, Crystyn, Crystyna

Curran (Irish) heroine.

Cybele (Greek) a form of Sybil.

Cydney (French) a form of Sydney.

Cyerra (Irish) a form of Ciara.

Cyndi (Greek) a form of Cindy.
Cynda, Cyndal, Cyndale, Cyndall,
Cyndee, Cyndel, Cyndia, Cyndie,
Cyndle, Cyndy

Cynthia (Greek) moon. Mythology: another name for Artemis, the moon goddess. See also Hyacinth, Kynthia.
Cyneria, Cynethia, Cynithia, Cynthea, Cynthiana, Cynthiann, Cynthie, Cynthria, Cynthy, Cynthya, Cyntreia, Cythia

Cyrilla (Greek) noble.

D

Dacey (Irish) southerner. (Greek) a familiar form of Candace.

Dacia (Irish) a form of Dacey.

Dae (English) day. See also Dai.

Daeja (French) a form of Déja.

Daelynn (American) a combination of Dae + Lynn.

Daeshandra (American) a combination of Dae + Shandra.

Daeshawna (American) a combination of Dae + Shawna.

Daeshonda (American) a combination of Dae + Shonda.

Dafny (American) a form of Daphne.

Dagmar (German) glorious.

Dagny (Scandinavian) day.

Dahlia (Scandinavian) valley. Botany: a perennial flower. See also Daliah.

Dai (Japanese) great. See also Dae.

Daija, Daijah (French) forms of Déja.

Daisha (American) a form of Dasha.
Daisia

Daisy (English) day's eye. Botany: a
white and yellow flower.
*Daisee, Daisey, Daisi, Daisia, Daisie,
Dasey, Dasi, Dasie, Dasy*

Daja, Dajah (French) forms of Déja.

Dakayla (American) a combination of
the prefix Da + Kayla.

Dakira (American) a combination of the
prefix Da + Kira.

Dakota (Native American) a tribal
name.
*Dakotah, Dakotha, Dekoda, Dekota,
Dekotah, Dekotha*

Dale (English) valley.
*Dael, Dahl, Daile, Daleleana,
Dalena, Dalina*

Dalia, Daliah (Hebrew) branch. See
also Dahlia.
Dalialah

Dalila (Swahili) gentle.

Dalisha (American) a form of Dallas.
Dalishya, Dalisia, Dalissia

Dallas (Irish) wise.
Dallys, Dalyce, Dalys

Damaris (Greek) gentle girl. See also
Maris.
*Damar, Damara, Damarius,
Damary, Damarys, Dameress,
Dameris, Damiris, Dammaris,
Dammeris, Damris, Demaras,
Demaris*

Damiana (Greek) tamer, soother.

Damica (French) friendly.

Damita (Spanish) small noblewoman.

Damonica (American) a combination
of the prefix Da + Monica.
Diamonique

Dana (English) from Denmark; bright as
day.
*Daina, Dainna, Danah, Danaia,
Danan, Danarra, Dane, Danean*

Danae (Greek) Mythology: the mother of
Perseus.
*Danaë, Danay, Danayla, Danai,
Danea, Danee, Dannae, Denee*

Danalyn (American) a combination of
Dana + Lynn.
Danalee

Daneil (Hebrew) a form of Danielle.

Danella (American) a form of Danielle.
Danayla, Donnella

Danelle (Hebrew) a form of Danielle.
*Danael, Danalle, Danel, Danele,
Danell, Donelle, Donnelle*

Danesha, Danisha (American) forms
of Danessa.

Danessa (American) a combination of
Danielle + Vanessa. See also Doneshia.

Danessia (American) a form of
Danessa.

Danette (American) a form of Danielle.
Danetra, Danett, Danetta, Donnita

Dani (Hebrew) a familiar form of
Danielle.
*Danee, Danie, Danne, Dannee,
Danni, Dannie, Danny, Dannye,
Dany*

Dania, Danya (Hebrew) short forms of
Danielle.
Daniah, Danja, Dannia, Danyae

Danica, Danika (Slavic) morning star.
(Hebrew) forms of Danielle.
*Daneeka, Danikla, Danneeka,
Dannica, Dannika, Donnaica,
Donnica, Donnika*

Danice (American) a combination of
Danielle + Janice.

Daniela (Italian) a form of Danielle.
Dannilla, Danijela

Danielan (Spanish) a form of Danielle.

Daniella (English) a form of Dana.
Danka, Danniella, Danyella

Danielle (Hebrew, French) God is my
judge.
*Daneen, Daneille, Danial, Danialle,
Daniele, Danielka, Daniell, Danilka*

Danille (American) a form of Danielle.

Danit (Hebrew) a form of Danielle.
Danett

Danna (Hebrew) a short form of
Danella.
Dannah, Dannon

Dannielle (Hebrew, French) a form of
Danielle.
Danniele, Danniell

Danyel, Danyell, Danyelle
(American) forms of Danielle.
*Daniyel, Danyae, Danyail, Danyaile,
Danyal, Danyale, Danyea, Danyele,
Danyle, Donnyale, Donnyell,
Donyale, Donyell*

Daphne (Greek) laurel tree.
Daphane, Daphany, Dapheney,

*Daphna, Daphnique, Daphnit,
Daphny*

Daphnee (Greek) a form of Daphne.
*Daphaney, Daphanie, Daphney,
Daphnie*

Dara (Hebrew) compassionate.
*Dahra, Darah, Daraka, Daralea,
Daralee, Darda, Darice, Darisa,
Darissa, Darja, Darra, Darrah*

Darby (Irish) free. (Scandinavian) deer
estate.
Darb, Darbi, Darbie, Darbra

Darcelle (French) a form of Darci.

Darci, Darcy (Irish) dark. (French)
fortress.
*Darcee, Darcey, Darcie, Darsey,
Darsi, Darsie*

Daria (Greek) wealthy.
Dari, Darria, Darya

Darian, Darrian (Greek) forms of
Daron.
Darianne

Darielle (French) a form of Daryl.

Darien, Darrien (Greek) forms of
Daron.

Darilynn (American) a form of Darlene.
Darilyn, Darlin

Darion, Darrion (Irish) forms of Daron.

Darla (English) a short form of Darlene.
*Darli, Darlice, Darlie, Darlis, Darly,
Darlys*

Darlene (French) little darling. See also
Daryl.
*Darlean, Darleen, Darlena,
Darlenia, Darletha, Darlin, Darline,
Darling*

Darnee (Irish) a familiar form of Darnelle.

Darnelle (English) hidden place.

Darnesha, Darnisha (American) forms of Darnelle.

Daron (Irish) great.

Darselle (French) a form of Darcelle.

Daru (Hindi) pine tree.

Daryl (English) beloved. (French) a short form of Darlene.
Darelle, Daril, Darrel, Darrell, Darrelle, Darreshia, Darryl, Darryll

Daryn (Greek) gifts. (Irish) great.

Dasha, Dasia (Russian) forms of Dorothy.

Dashawna (American) a combination of the prefix Da + Shawna.

Dashiki (Swahili) loose-fitting shirt worn in Africa.

Dashonda (American) a combination of the prefix Da + Shonda.

Davalinda (American) a combination of Davida + Linda.

Davalynda (American) a form of Davalinda.

Davalynn (American) a combination of Davida + Lynn.

Davida (Hebrew) beloved. Bible: David was the second king of Israel. See also Vida.

Davina (Scottish) a form of Davida. See also Vina.
Dava, Davannah, Davean, Davee, Daveen, Daveena, Davene, Daveon,
Davey, Davi, Daviana, Davie, Davin, Davine, Davineen, Davinia, Davinna, Davria, Devean, Deveen, Devene, Devina

Davisha (American) a combination of the prefix Da + Aisha.

Davonna (Scottish, English) a form of Davina, Devonna.

Dawn (English) sunrise, dawn.
Dawana, Dawandrea, Dawanna, Dawin, Dawne, Dawnee, Dawnetta, Dawnlynn, Dawnn, Dawnrae

Dawna (English) a form of Dawn.
Dawnna, Dawnya

Dawnyelle (American) a combination of Dawn + Danielle.
Dawnele, Dawnell, Dawnelle, Dawnyel, Dawnyella

Dawnisha (American) a form of Dawn.

Dayana (Latin) a form of Diana.
Dayanna

Dayle (English) a form of Dale.

Dayna (Scandinavian) a form of Dana.
Dayne, Daynna

Daysha (American) a form of Dasha.

Daysi, Deysi (English) forms of Daisy.
Daysee, Daysie, Daysy

Dayton, Daytona (English) day town; bright, sunny town.

Deana (Latin) divine. (English) valley.
Deane, Deanielle, Deanisha, Deeann, Deeanna

Deandra (American) a combination of
Dee + Andrea.
*Deandre, Deandré, Deandrea,
Deandree, Deandria, Deanndra,
Deondra, Diandra, Diandre,
Diandrea*

Deangela (Italian) a combination of
the prefix De + Angela.

Deanna (Latin) a form of Deana, Diana.
*Deaana, Deahana, Deandre,
Déanna, Deannia, Deeanna*

Deanne (Latin) a form of Diane.
*Deahanne, Deane, Deann, Déanne,
Deeann, Deeanne*

Debbie (Hebrew) a short form of
Deborah.
*Debbee, Debbey, Debbi, Debby,
Debee, Debi, Debie*

Deborah (Hebrew) bee. Bible: a great
Hebrew prophetess.
*Deb, Debbora, Debborah, Deberah,
Debor, Debora, Deboran, Deborha,
Deborrah, Debrena, Debrina,
Debroah, Dobra*

Debra (American) a form of Deborah.
*Debbra, Debbrah, Debrah, Debrea,
Debria*

Dedra (American) a form of Deirdre.
Deeddra, Deedra, Deedrea, Deedrie

Dedriana (American) a combination of
Dedra + Adriana.

Dee (Welsh) black, dark.
De, Dea, Didi

Deena (American) a form of Deana,
Dena, Dinah.

Deidra, Deidre (Irish) forms of Deirdre.
Deidrea, Deidrie, Diedre, Dierdra

Deirdre (Irish) sorrowful; wanderer.
*Deerdra, Deerdre, Deirdree, Didi,
Dierdre, Diérdre, Dierdrie*

Deisy (English) a form of Daisy.

Deitra (Greek) a short form of Demetria.

Déja (French) before.

Dejanae (French) a form of Déja.

Dejon (French) a form of Déja.

Deka (Somali) pleasing.

Delacy (American) a combination of
the prefix De + Lacy.

Delainey (Irish) a form of Delaney.

Delana (German) noble protector.
Dalena, Dalina

Delaney (Irish) descendant of the challenger. (English) a form of Adeline.
Del

Delanie (Irish) a form of Delaney.

Delfina (Greek) a form of Delphine.
(Spanish) dolphin.

Delia (Greek) visible; from Delos, Greece.
(German, Welsh) a short form of
Adelaide, Cordelia. Mythology: a festival
of Apollo held in ancient Greece.
*Dehlia, Delea, Deli, Delinda, Dellia,
Dellya, Delya*

Delicia (English) delightful.
Delya

Delilah (Hebrew) brooder. Bible: the
companion of Samson. See also Lila.
Dalialah, Daliliah, Delila, Delilia

Della (English) a short form of Adelaide, Cordelia, Delaney.
Del, Dela, Dell, Delle, Delli, Dellie, Dells

Delores (Spanish) a form of Dolores.
Delora, Delore, Deloria, Delories, Deloris, Delorise

Delphine (Greek) from Delphi, Greece. See also Delfina.

Delsie (English) a familiar form of Delores.

Delta (Greek) door. Linguistics: the fourth letter in the Greek alphabet. Geography: a triangular land mass at the mouth of a river.

Demetria (Greek) cover of the earth. Mythology: Demeter was the Greek goddess of the harvest.
Demeta, Demeteria, Demetra, Demetrice, Demetris, Demita, Demitra, Dymitra

Demi (French) half. (Greek) a short form of Demetria.
Demiah

Dena (English, Native American) valley. (Hebrew) a form of Dinah. See also Deana.
Deane, Deeyn, Dene, Denea, Deney, Denna

Denae (Hebrew) a form of Dena.
Denaé, Denay, Denee, Deneé

Deni (French) a short form of Denise.
Deney, Denie, Denni, Dennie, Denny, Dinnie, Dinny

Denica, Denika (Slavic) forms of Danica.

Denise (French) Mythology: follower of Dionysus, the god of wine.
Danise, Denese, Denice, Deniece, Denize, Dennise, Dennys, Denyce, Denys, Denyse

Denisha (American) a form of Denise.
Deneesha, Deneichia, Denesha, Deneshia, Deniesha, Denishia

Denisse (French) a form of Denise.

Deonna (English) a form of Dena.
Deona, Deondra, Deonne

Derika (German) ruler of the people.

Derry (Irish) redhead.

Deryn (Welsh) bird.

Desarae (French) a form of Desiree.
Desara, Desarai, Desaraie, Desaray, Desare, Desaré, Desarea, Desaree, Desarie

Deserae, Desirae (French) forms of Desiree.
Desera, Deserai, Deseray, Desere, Deseree, Deseret, Deseri, Deserie, Deserrae, Deserray, Deserré, Dessirae, Dezeray, Dezere, Dezerea, Dezrae, Dezyrae

Deshawna (American) a combination of the prefix De + Shawna.

Deshawnda (American) a combination of the prefix De + Shawnda.

Desi (French) a short form of Desiree.

Desiree (French) desired, longed for. See also Dessa.
Desirah, Desirai, Desiray, Desire, Desirea, Desirée, Désirée, Desirey, Desiri, Desray, Desree, Dessie, Dessire

Dessa (Greek) wanderer. (French) a
form of Desiree.

Desta (Ethiopian) happy. (French) a
short form of Destiny.
Desty

Destany (French) a form of Destiny.
Destanee, Destanie, Destannie

Destinee, Destini, Destinie (French)
forms of Destiny.
Desteni, Destinée, Destnie

Destiney (French) a form of Destiny.

Destiny ☝ (French) fate.
Desnine, Destin

Destynee, Destyni (French) forms of
Destiny.
Desty, Destyn, Destyne

Deva (Hindi) divine.

Devan (Irish) a form of Devin.
Devane, Devanie, Devany

Devi (Hindi) goddess. Religion: the
Hindu goddess of power and destruction.

Devin (Irish) poet.
*Deven, Devena, Devenje, Deveny,
Devine, Devinne*

Devon (English) a short form of Devonna.
(Irish) a form of Devin.
Devonne

Devonna (English) from Devonshire.

Devora (Hebrew) a form of Deborah.

Devyn (Irish) a form of Devin.
Deveyn

Dextra (Latin) adroit, skillful.

Dezarae, Dezirae, Deziree (French)
forms of Desiree.
Dezerie, Dezirée, Dezorae, Dezra

Di (Latin) a short form of Diana, Diane.

Dia (Latin) a short form of Diana, Diane.

Diamond (Latin) precious gem.
*Diamonda, Diamonia, Diamonique,
Diamonte, Diamontina*

Diana (Latin) divine. Mythology: the
goddess of the hunt, the moon, and
fertility. See also Deanna, Deanne, Dyan.
*Daiana, Daianna, Dayanna, Dianah,
Dianalyn, Dianarose, Dianatris,
Dianca, Diandra, Dianelis, Diania,
Dianielle, Dianita, Dianys, Didi*

Diane, Dianne (Latin) short forms of
Diana.
*Deane, Deeane, Deeanne, Diahann,
Dian, Diani, Dianie, Diann*

Dianna (Latin) a form of Diana.
Diahanna

Diantha (Greek) divine flower.
Diandre

Diedra (Irish) a form of Deirdre.
Diedre

Dillan (Irish) loyal, faithful.

Dilys (Welsh) perfect; true.

Dina (Hebrew) a form of Dinah.

Dinah (Hebrew) vindicated. Bible: a
daughter of Jacob and Leah.

Dinka (Swahili) people.

Dionna (Greek) a form of Dionne.
*Deona, Deondra, Deonia, Deonyia,
Diona, Diondra, Diondrea*

Dionne (Greek) divine queen.
Mythology: Dione was the mother of
Aphrodite, the goddess of love.
*Deonjala, Deonne, Dion, Dione,
Dionee, Dionis, Dionte*

Dior (French) golden.

Dita (Spanish) a form of Edith.

Divinia (Latin) divine.
Devina

Dixie (French) tenth. (English) wall;
dike. Geography: a nickname for the
American South.
Dix, Dixee, Dixi, Dixy

Diza (Hebrew) joyful.

Dodie (Hebrew) beloved. (Greek) a
familiar form of Dorothy.

Dolly (American) a short form of
Dolores, Dorothy.

Dolores (Spanish) sorrowful. Religion:
Nuestra Señora de los Dolores—Our
Lady of Sorrows—is a name for the
Virgin Mary. See also Lola.
Deloria, Dolorcitas, Dolorita, Doloritas

Dominica, Dominika (Latin) belonging to the Lord. See also Mika.

Dominique, Domonique (French)
forms of Dominica, Dominika.
*Domanique, Domeneque,
Domenique, Domineque, Dominiqua,
Dominoque, Dominuque, Domique,
Domminique, Domoniqua*

Domino (English) a short form of
Dominica, Dominique.

Dona (English) world leader; proud ruler.
(Italian) a form of Donna.

Doña (Italian) a form of Donna.

Donata (Latin) gift.
Donnita

Dondi (American) a familiar form of
Donna.

Doneshia, Donisha (American) forms
of Danessa.
Donnisha

Donna (Italian) lady.
*Donnalee, Donnalen, Donnay,
Donnell, Donni, Donnie, Donnise,
Donny, Dontia, Donya*

Donniella (American) a form of
Danielle.
Donnella

Dora (Greek) gift. A short form of Adora,
Eudora, Pandora, Theodora.
*Doralia, Doralie, Doralisa, Doraly,
Doran, Dorchen, Dore, Dorece, Doree,
Doreece, Dorelia, Dorella, Dorelle,
Doresha, Doressa, Dorika, Doriley,
Dorilis, Dorion, Dorita, Doro*

Doralynn (English) a combination of
Dora + Lynn.

Doreen (Irish) moody, sullen. (French)
golden. (Greek) a form of Dora.
*Doreena, Dorena, Dorene, Dorina,
Dorine*

Doretta (American) a form of Dora,
Dorothy.

Dori, Dory (American) familiar forms of
Dora, Doria, Doris, Dorothy.
Dore

Doria (Greek) a form of Dorian.

Dorian (Greek) from Doris, Greece.
Dorina

Dorinda (Spanish) a form of Dora.

Doris (Greek) sea. Mythology: wife of
Nereus and mother of the Nereids or sea
nymphs.
Dorice, Dorisa, Dorise, Dorris,
Dorrise, Dorrys, Dorys

Dorothea (Greek) a form of Dorothy.
See also Thea.

Dorothy (Greek) gift of God. See also
Dasha, Dodie, Lolotea, Theodora.
Dasya, Do, Doa, Doe, Dorathy, Dordi,
Dorika, Doritha, Dorlisa, Doro,
Dorosia, Dorota, Dorothee, Dorottya,
Dorte, Dortha, Dorthy, Dosi, Dossie,
Dosya

Dorrit (Greek) dwelling. (Hebrew) generation.
Dorita

Dottie, Dotty (Greek) familiar forms of
Dorothy.

Drew (Greek) courageous; strong.
(Latin) a short form of Drusilla.
Dru, Drue

Drinka (Spanish) a form of Alexandria.

Drusi (Latin) a short form of Drusilla.

Drusilla (Latin) descendant of Drusus,
the strong one. See also Drew.

Dulce (Latin) sweet.

Dulcinea (Spanish) sweet. Literature: Don
Quixote's love interest.

Duscha (Russian) soul; sweetheart; term
of endearment.

Dusti, Dusty (English) familiar forms
of Dustine.
Dustee, Dustie

Dustine (German) valiant fighter.
(English) brown rock quarry.
Dustina, Dustyn

Dyamond, Dymond (Latin) forms of
Diamond.

Dyana (Latin) a form of Diana. (Native
American) deer.

Dylan (Welsh) sea.

Dyllis (Welsh) sincere.

Dynasty (Latin) powerful ruler.

Dyshawna (American) a combination
of the prefix Dy + Shawna.

E

Earlene (Irish) pledge. (English) noblewoman.

Eartha (English) earthy.

Easter (English) Easter time. History: a
name for a child born on Easter.

Ebone, Ebonee (Greek) forms of
Ebony.
Ebanee, Ebonnee

Eboni, Ebonie (Greek) forms of Ebony.
Ebanie, Ebonni, Ebonnie

Ebony (Greek) a hard, dark wood.
Eban, Ebanie, Ebany, Ebbony,
Eboney, Ebonique, Ebonisha,
Ebonye, Ebonyi

Echo (Greek) repeated sound.
Mythology: the nymph who pined for
the love of Narcissus until only her
voice remained.
Echoe, Ekko, Ekkoe

Eda (Irish, English) a short form of Edana, Edith.

Edana (Irish) ardent; flame.

Edda (German) a form of Hedda.

Eddy (American) a familiar form of Edwina.

Edeline (English) noble; kind.

Eden (Babylonian) a plain. (Hebrew) delightful. Bible: the earthly paradise.
Ede, Edena, Edene, Edenia, Edin, Edyn

Edie (English) a familiar form of Edith.

Edith (English) rich gift. See also Dita.
Eadith, Ede, Edetta, Edette, Edit, Edita, Edite, Editha, Edithe, Editta, Ediva, Edyta, Edyth, Edytha, Edythe

Edna (Hebrew) rejuvenation. Religion: the wife of Enoch, according to the Book of Enoch.
Ednah, Edneisha, Ednita

Edrianna (Greek) a form of Adrienne.

Edwina (English) prosperous friend. See also Winnie.

Effia (Ghanaian) born on Friday.

Effie (Greek) spoken well of. (English) a short form of Alfreda, Euphemia.

Eileen (Irish) a form of Helen. See also Aileen, Ilene.
Eilean, Eilena, Eilene, Eiley, Eilidh, Eilleen, Eillen, Eilyn, Eleen, Elene

Ekaterina (Russian) a form of Katherine.

Ela (Polish) a form of Adelaide.

Elaina (French) a form of Helen.
Elainia, Elainna

Elaine (French) a form of Helen. See also Lainey, Laine.
Elain, Elan, Elane, Elania, Elanie, Elanit, Elauna, Ellaine

Elana (Greek) a short form of Eleanor. See also Ilana, Lana.
Elan, Elani, Elania, Elanie, Elanna

Elayna (French) a form of Elaina.
Elayn, Elayne

Elberta (English) a form of Alberta.

Eldora (Spanish) golden, gilded.

Eleanor (Greek) light. History: Anna Eleanor Roosevelt was a U. S. delegate to the United Nations, a writer, and the thirty-second First Lady of the United States. See also Elana, Ella, Ellen, Leanore, Lena, Lenore, Leonore, Leora, Nellie, Nora, Noreen.
Elanor, Elanore, Eleanore, Elenor, Elenorah, Elenore, Eleonor, Eleonore, Elianore, Elinor, Elinore, Elladine, Ellenor, Elliner, Ellinor, Ellinore, Elna, Elnore, Elynor, Elynore

Eleanora (Greek) a form of Eleanor. See also Lena.

Electra (Greek) shining; brilliant. Mythology: the daughter of Agamemnon, leader of the Greeks in the Trojan War.

Elena (Greek) a form of Eleanor. (Italian) a form of Helen.
Eleana, Eleen, Eleena, Elen, Elene, Elenitsa, Elenka, Elenoa, Elenola, Elina, Ellena

Eleni (Greek) a familiar form of Eleanor.
Eleny

Eleora (Hebrew) the Lord is my light.

Elexis (Greek) a form of Alexis.

Elexus (Greek) a form of Alexius, Alexus.

Elfrida (German) peaceful. See also Freda.

Elga (Norwegian) pious. (German) a form of Helga.

Elia (Hebrew) a short form of Eliana.

Eliana (Hebrew) my God has answered me. See also Iliana.

Eliane (Hebrew) a form of Eliana.

Elicia (Hebrew) a form of Elisha. See also Alicia.
Elisia, Ellicia

Elida, Elide (Latin) forms of Alida.

Elisa (Spanish, Italian, English) a short form of Elizabeth. See also Alisa, Ilisa.
Elecea, Eleesa, Elesa, Elesia, Elisia, Elisya, Ellisa, Ellisia, Ellissa, Ellissia, Ellissya, Ellisya, Elysa, Elyssia, Elyssya, Elysya

Elisabeth (Hebrew) a form of Elizabeth.
Elisabet, Elisabeta, Elisabethe, Elisabetta, Elisabette, Elisebet, Elisheba, Elisheva

Elise (French, English) a short form of Elizabeth, Elysia. See also Ilise, Liese, Lisette, Lissie.
Eilis, Eilise, Elese, Élise, Elisee, Elisie, Elisse, Elizé, Ellise, Ellyce, Ellyse, Ellyze, Elsey, Elsy, Elyce, Elyci, Elyze, Lisel, Lisl, Lison

Elisha (Hebrew) consecrated to God. (Greek) a form of Alisha. See also

Ilisha, Lisha.
Elisheva, Elysha

Elissa, Elyssa (Greek, English) forms of Elizabeth. Short forms of Melissa. See also Alissa, Alyssa, Lissa.
Ellissa, Ellyssa, Ilissa, Ilyssa

Elita (Latin, French) chosen. See also Lida, Lita.

Eliza (Hebrew) a short form of Elizabeth. See also Aliza.
Eliz, Elizaida, Elizalina, Elize, Elizea

Elizabet (Hebrew) a form of Elizabeth.
Elizabete

Elizabeth ❦ (Hebrew) consecrated to God. Bible: the mother of John the Baptist. See also Bess, Beth, Betsy, Betty, Elsa, Ilse, Libby, Liese, Liesel, Lisa, Lisbeth, Lisette, Lissa, Lissie, Liz, Liza, Lizabeta, Lizabeth, Lizbeth, Lizina, Lizzy, Veta, Yelisabeta, Zizi.
Eliabeth, Elizabee, Elizebeth, Elsabeth, Elysabeth, Elzbieta, Erzsébet, Ilizzabet

Elizaveta (Polish, English) a form of Elizabeth.

Elka (Polish) a form of Elizabeth.

Elke (German) a form of Adelaide, Alice.

Ella ❦ (English) elfin; beautiful fairy-woman. (Greek) a short form of Eleanor.
Ellamae, Ellia

Elle (Greek) a short form of Eleanor. (French) she.

Ellen (English) a form of Eleanor, Helen.
Elen, Elenee, Eleny, Elin, Elina, Elinda, Ellan, Ellena, Ellene, Ellin, Ellon, Ellyn, Ellynn, Elyn

Ellice (English) a form of Elise.
Ellyce, Elyce

Ellie, Elly (English) short forms of
Eleanor, Ella, Ellen.

Elma (Turkish) sweet fruit.

Elmira (Arabic, Spanish) a form of
Almira.

Elnora (American) a combination of
Ella + Nora.

Elodie (American) a form of Melody.
(English) a form of Alodie.

Eloise (French) a form of Louise.
Eloisa

Elora (American) a short form of Elnora.

Elsa (German) noble. (Hebrew) a short
form of Elizabeth. See also Ilse.
Ellsa, Ellse, Else, Elsje

Elsbeth (German) a form of Elizabeth.
Elsbet, Elzbieta

Elsie (German) a familiar form of Elsa,
Helsa.
Ellsie, Ellsy, Elsi, Elsy

Elspeth (Scottish) a form of Elizabeth.
Elspet, Elspie

Elva (English) elfin. See also Alva,
Alvina.

Elvina (English) a form of Alvina.

Elvira (Latin) white; blond. (German)
closed up. (Spanish) elfin. Geography:
the town in Spain that hosted a
Catholic synod in 300 A.D.
Vira

Elyse (Latin) a form of Elysia.
Ellyse, Elyce

Elysia (Greek) sweet; blissful. Mythology:
Elysium was the dwelling place of
happy souls.
Ellicia, Ilysha, Ilysia

Elyssa (Latin) a form of Elysia.
Ellyssa

Emalee (Latin) a form of Emily.
Emaili, Emalia, Emalie

Emani (Arabic) a form of Iman.

Emanuelle (Hebrew) a form of
Emmanuelle.

Ember (French) a form of Amber.

Emelia, Emelie (Latin) forms of Emily.

Emely (Latin) a form of Emily.

Emerald (French) bright green gemstone.
Emelda

Emery (German) industrious leader.

Emilee, Emilie (English) forms of
Emily.
Émilie, Emillie, Emméie, Emmélie

Emilia (Italian) a form of Amelia, Emily.
Emalia, Emila

Emily ❀ (Latin) flatterer. (German)
industrious. See also Amelia, Emma,
Millie.
*Eimile, Em, Emaily, Emeli, Emelita,
Emiley, Emili, Émilie, Emilis, Emilka,
Emillie, Emilly, Emmaly, Emmélie,
Emmey, Emmi, Emmie, Emmilly,
Emmye, Emyle*

Emilyann (American) a combination of
Emily + Ann.

Emma ⚝ (German) a short form of
Emily. See also Amy.
Em, Ema

Emmalee (American) a combination of
Emma + Lee. A form of Emily.

Emmaline (French) a form of Emily.
Emeline, Emilienne

Emmalynn (American) a combination
of Emma + Lynn.

Emmanuelle (Hebrew) God is with us.

Emmy (German) a familiar form of
Emma.
Emi, Emiy, Emmi, Emmie, Emmye

Emmylou (American) a combination of
Emmy + Lou.
Emmalou

Ena (Irish) a form of Helen.

Enid (Welsh) life; spirit.

Enrica (Spanish) a form of Henrietta.
See also Rica.

Eppie (English) a familiar form of
Euphemia.

Erica (Scandinavian) ruler of all.
(English) brave ruler. See also Arica,
Rica, Ricki.
Ericca, Ericha, Errica, Eryka

Ericka, Erika (Scandanavian) forms of
Erica.
Erikka, Errika, Erykka

Erin (Irish) peace. History: another name
for Ireland. See also Arin.
*Eran, Eren, Erena, Erene, Ereni, Eri,
Erian, Erina, Erine, Erinetta*

Erinn (Irish) a form of Erin.
Erinna, Erinne

Erma (Latin) a short form of Ermine,
Hermina. See also Irma.

Ermine (Latin) a form of Hermina.

Erna (English) a short form of Ernestine.

Ernestine (English) earnest, sincere.

Eryn (Irish) a form of Erin.
Erynn, Erynne

Eshe (Swahili) life.

Esmé (French) a familiar form of
Esmeralda. A form of Amy.

Esmeralda (Greek, Spanish) a form of
Emerald.
Emelda

Esperanza (Spanish) hope. See also
Speranza.

Essence (Latin) life; existence.

Essie (English) a short form of Estelle,
Esther.

Estee (English) a short form of Estelle,
Esther.

Estefani, Estefania, Estefany
(Spanish) forms of Stephanie.

Estelle (French) a form of Esther. See
also Stella, Trella.
*Estel, Estela, Estele, Estelina, Estelita,
Estell, Estella, Estellina, Estellita,
Esthella*

Estephanie (Spanish) a form of
Stephanie.

Esther (Persian) star. Bible: the Jewish
captive whom Ahasuerus made his
queen. See also Hester.
Ester, Esthur, Eszter, Eszti

Estrella (French) star.
Estrela

Ethana (Hebrew) strong; firm.

Ethel (English) noble.

Étoile (French) star.

Etta (German) little. (English) a short form of Henrietta.

Eudora (Greek) honored gift. See also Dora.

Eugenia (Greek) born to nobility. See also Gina.
Eugenina, Eugina, Evgenia

Eugenie (Greek) a form of Eugenia.
Eugénie

Eulalia (Greek) well spoken. See also Ula.

Eun (Korean) silver.

Eunice (Greek) happy; victorious. Bible: the mother of Saint Timothy. See also Unice.
Euna, Eunique, Eunise, Euniss

Euphemia (Greek) spoken well of, in good repute. History: a fourth-century Christian martyr.

Eurydice (Greek) wide, broad. Mythology: the wife of Orpheus.

Eustacia (Greek) productive. (Latin) stable; calm. See also Stacey.

Eva (Greek) a short form of Evangelina. (Hebrew) a form of Eve. See also Ava, Chava.
Éva, Evah, Evalea, Evalee, Evike

Evaline (French) a form of Evelyn.
Evalyn, Evalynn, Eveleen, Eveline

Evangelina (Greek) bearer of good news.
Evangelia, Evangelica, Evangeline, Evangelique

Evania (Irish) young warrior.

Eve (Hebrew) life. Bible: the first woman created by God. (French) a short form of Evonne. See also Chava, Hava, Naeva, Vica, Yeva.
Evyn, Ewa

Evelin (English) a form of Evelyn.
Eveline

Evelyn ❊ (English) hazelnut.
Aveline, Evaleen, Evalene, Evalyn, Evalynn, Evalynne, Eveleen, Evelyne, Evelynn, Evelynne, Ewalina

Everett (German) courageous as a boar.

Evette (French) a form of Yvette. A familiar form of Evonne. See also Ivette.
Evett

Evie (Hungarian) a form of Eve.
Evey, Evi, Evicka, Evike, Evvie, Evvy, Evy, Ewa

Evita (Spanish) a form of Eve.

Evline (English) a form of Evelyn.

Evonne (French) a form of Yvonne. See also Ivonne.
Evyn

Ezri (Hebrew) helper; strong.

F

Fabia (Latin) bean grower.

Fabiana (Latin) a form of Fabia.

Fabienne (Latin) a form of Fabia.

Fabiola, Faviola (Latin) forms of Fabia.

Faith ✷ (English) faithful; fidelity. See also Faye, Fidelity.
Fayth, Faythe

Faizah (Arabic) victorious.

Falda (Icelandic) folded wings.

Faline (Latin) catlike.
Falin, Fallyn

Fallon (Irish) grandchild of the ruler.
Falan, Falen, Fallan, Fallonne, Falon, Falyn, Falynn, Falynne

Fancy (French) betrothed. (English) whimsical; decorative.

Fannie, Fanny (American) familiar forms of Frances.
Fan, Fanette, Fani, Fania, Fannee, Fanney, Fanni, Fannia, Fanya

Fantasia (Greek) imagination.

Farah, Farrah (English) beautiful; pleasant.
Fara, Farra, Fayre

Faren, Farren (English) wanderer.
Faran, Fare, Farin, Faron, Farrahn, Farran, Farrand, Farrin, Farron, Farryn, Farye, Faryn, Feran, Ferin, Feron, Ferran, Ferren, Ferrin, Ferryn

Fatima (Arabic) daughter of the Prophet. History: the daughter of Muhammad. Religion: Fátima is a village in Portugal were the Virgin Mary was reported to appear.
Fatema, Fathma, Fatimah, Fatime, Fatma, Fattim

Fawn (French) young deer.
Faun, Fawne

Fawna (French) a form of Fawn.
Fauna, Fawnia, Fawnna

Faye (French) fairy; elf. (English) a form of Faith.
Fae, Fay, Fayann, Fayanna, Fayette, Fayina, Fey

Fayola (Nigerian) lucky.
Fayla, Estela

Felecia (Latin) a form of Felicia.
Flecia

Felica (Spanish) a short form of Felicia.
Falisa, Felisa, Felisca, Felissa, Feliza

Felice (Latin) a short form of Felicia.
Felicie

Felicia (Latin) fortunate; happy. See also Lecia, Phylicia.
Falecia, Faleshia, Falicia, Fela, Felicidad, Feliciona, Felicya, Felisiana, Felita, Felixia, Felizia, Felka, Fellcia, Felysia, Fleasia, Fleichia, Fleishia, Flichia

Felicity (English) a form of Felicia.

Felisha (Latin) a form of Felicia.
Faleisha, Falesha, Falisha, Falleshia, Feleasha, Feleisha, Felesha, Felishia, Fellishia, Flisha

Femi (French) woman. (Nigerian) love me.

Feodora (Greek) gift of God.

Fern (English) fern. (German) a short form of Fernanda.

Fernanda (German) daring, adventurous. See also Andee, Nan.

Fiala (Czech) violet.

Fidelia (Latin) a form of Fidelity.

Fidelity (Latin) faithful, true. See also Faith.

Fifi (French) a familiar form of Josephine.

Filippa (Italian) a form of Philippa.

Filomena (Italian) a form of Philomena.

Fiona (Irish) fair, white.
Fionna

Fionnula (Irish) white shouldered. See also Nola, Nuala.

Flair (English) style; verve.

Flannery (Irish) redhead. Literature: Flannery O'Connor was a renowned American writer.

Flavia (Latin) blond, golden haired.

Flavie (Latin) a form of Flavia.

Fleur (French) flower.

Flo (American) a short form of Florence.

Flora (Latin) flower. A short form of Florence. See also Lore.
Fiora, Fiore, Fiorenza, Flor, Florann, Florella, Florelle, Floren, Floriana, Florianna, Florica, Florimel

Florence (Latin) blooming; flowery; prosperous. History: Florence Nightingale, a British nurse, is considered the founder of modern nursing. See also Florida.
Fiorenza, Florance, Florencia, Florency, Florendra, Florentia, Florentina, Florentyna, Florenza, Floretta, Florette, Florina, Florine

Floria (Basque) a form of Flora.

Florida (Spanish) a form of Florence.

Florie (English) a familiar form of Florence.

Floris (English) a form of Florence.

Flossie (English) a familiar form of Florence.

Fola (Yoruba) honorable.

Fonda (Latin) foundation. (Spanish) inn.

Fontanna (French) fountain.

Fortuna (Latin) fortune; fortunate.

Fran (Latin) a short form of Frances.

Frances (Latin) free; from France. See also Paquita.
Franca, France, Francee, Francena, Francess, Francesta, Franceta, Francetta, Francette, Frankie

Francesca (Italian) a form of Frances.
Franceska, Francessca, Francesta, Franzetta

Franchesca (Italian) a form of Francesca.
Cheka, Chekka, Chesca, Cheska, Francheca, Francheka, Franchelle, Franchesa, Francheska, Franchessca, Franchesska

Franci (Hungarian) a familiar form of Francine.

Francine (French) a form of Frances.
Franceen, Franceine, Franceline, Francene, Francenia, Francin, Francina, Francyne

Francis (Latin) a form of Frances.
Francise

Francisca (Italian) a form of Frances.
Franciska, Franciszka, Frantiska, Franziska

Françoise (French) a form of Frances.

Frankie (American) a familiar form of Frances.
Francka, Francki, Franka, Frankeisha, Frankey, Franki, Frankia, Franky

Frannie, Franny (English) familiar forms of Frances.

Freda, Freida, Frida (German) short forms of Alfreda, Elfrida, Frederica, Sigfreda.

Freddi, Freddie (English) familiar forms of Frederica, Winifred.

Frederica (German) peaceful ruler. See also Alfreda, Rica, Ricki.

Frederika (German) a form of Frederica.

Frederike (German) a form of Frederica.

Frederique (French) a form of Frederica.

Freja (Scandinavian) a form of Freya.

Freya (Scandinavian) noblewoman. Mythology: the Norse goddess of love.

Fritzi (German) a familiar form of Frederica.

G

Gabriel, Gabriele (French) forms of Gabrielle.
Gabreil, Gabrial

Gabriela ❦ (Italian) a form of Gabrielle.
Gabriala, Gabrielia, Gabrila

Gabriella (Italian) a form of Gabrielle.
Gabrialla, Gabriellia, Gabrilla

Gabrielle ❦ (French) devoted to God.
Gabielle, Gabriana, Gabriell, Gabrille, Gabrina

Gaby (French) a familiar form of Gabrielle.

Gada (Hebrew) lucky.

Gaea (Greek) planet Earth. Mythology: the Greek goddess of Earth.

Gaetana (Italian) from Gaeta. Geography: a city in southern Italy.

Gagandeep (Sikh) sky's light.

Gail (Hebrew) a short form of Abigail. (English) merry, lively.
Gael, Gaela, Gaelle, Gaila, Gaile, Gale, Gayla

Gala (Norwegian) singer.

Galen (Greek) healer; calm. (Irish) little and lively.
Gaelen, Gaellen, Galyn

Galena (Greek) healer; calm.

Gali (Hebrew) hill; fountain; spring.

Galina (Russian) a form of Helen.

Ganesa (Hindi) fortunate. Religion: Ganesha was the Hindu god of wisdom.

Ganya (Hebrew) garden of the Lord. (Zulu) clever.

Gardenia (English) Botany: a sweet-smelling flower.

Garland (French) wreath of flowers.

Garnet (English) dark red gem.

Garyn (English) spear carrier.

Gasha (Russian) a familiar form of Agatha.

Gavriella (Hebrew) a form of Gabrielle.

Gay (French) merry.

Gayle (English) a form of Gail.
Gayla

Gayna (English) a familiar form of Guinevere.

Geela (Hebrew) joyful.
Gila

Geena (American) a form of Gena.

Gelya (Russian) angelic.

Gema, Gemma (Latin, Italian) jewel, precious stone. See also Jemma.
Gem, Gemmey, Gemmie, Gemmy

Gemini (Greek) twin.

Gen (Japanese) spring. A short form of names beginning with "Gen."

Gena (French) a form of Gina. A short form of Geneva, Genevieve, Iphigenia.
Geanna, Geenah, Genah, Genea, Geni, Genia, Genie

Geneen (Scottish) a form of Jeanine.

Genell (American) a form of Jenelle.

Genesis (Latin) origin; birth.

Geneva (French) juniper tree. A short form of Genevieve. Geography: a city in Switzerland.
Geneive, Geneve, Ginneva, Janeva, Jeaneva, Jeneva

Genevieve (German, French) a form of Guinevere. See also Gwendolyn.
Genaveve, Genavieve, Genavive, Geneveve, Genevie, Geneviéve, Genevievre, Genevive, Gineveve, Ginevieve, Ginevive, Guinevieve, Guinivive, Gwenevieve, Gwenivive

Genevra (French, Welsh) a form of Guinevere.
Genever, Genevera, Ginevra

Genice (American) a form of Janice.

Genita (American) a form of Janita.

Genna (English) a form of Jenna.
Gennae, Gennay, Genni, Gennie, Genny

Gennifer (American) a form of Jennifer.

Genovieve (French) a form of Genevieve.

Georgeanna (English) a combination of Georgia + Anna.

Georgeanne (English) a combination of Georgia + Anne.

Georgene (English) a familiar form of Georgia.
Georgena, Georgine

Georgette (French) a form of Georgia.
Georgeta, Georgett, Georgetta, Georjetta

Georgia (Greek) farmer. Art: Georgia O'Keeffe was an American painter known especially for her paintings of flowers. Geography: a southern American state; a country in Eastern Europe. See also Jirina, Jorja.
Giorgia

Georgianna (English) a form of Georgeanna.

Georgie (English) a familiar form of Georgeanne, Georgia, Georgianna.
Georgi, Giorgi

Georgina (English) a form of Georgia.
Georgena, Georgine, Giorgina

Geraldine (German) mighty with a spear. See also Dena, Jeraldine.
Geralda, Geraldina, Geraldyna, Geraldyne, Gerhardine, Gerianna, Gerianne, Gerrilee, Giralda

Geralyn (American) a combination of Geraldine + Lynn.

Gerardo (English) brave spearwoman.

Gerda (Norwegian) protector. (German) a familiar form of Gertrude.

Geri (American) a familiar form of Geraldine. See also Jeri.
Gerri, Gerrie, Gerry

Germaine (French) from Germany. See also Jermaine.

Gertie (German) a familiar form of Gertrude.

Gertrude (German) beloved warrior. See also Trudy.

Gervaise (French) skilled with a spear.

Gessica (Italian) a form of Jessica.

Geva (Hebrew) hill.

Ghada (Arabic) young; tender.

Ghita (Italian) pearly.

Gianna (Italian) a short form of Giovanna. See also Jianna, Johana.
Geona, Geonna, Gia, Giana, Gianella, Gianetta, Gianina, Giannella, Giannetta, Gianni, Giannina, Gianny, Gianoula

Gigi (French) a familiar form of Gilberte.

Gilana (Hebrew) joyful.
Gila

Gilberte (German) brilliant; pledge; trustworthy. See also Berti.

Gilda (English) covered with gold.

Gill (Latin, German) a short form of Gilberte, Gillian.
Gili, Gillie, Gilly

Gillian (Latin) a form of Jillian.
Gila, Gilenia, Gili, Gilian, Gilliana, Gilliane, Gilliann, Gillianna, Gillianne, Gillie, Gilly, Gillyan, Gillyane, Gillyann, Gillyanne, Gyllian

Gin (Japanese) silver. A short form of names beginning with "Gin."

Gina (Italian) a short form of Angelina, Eugenia, Regina, Virginia. See also Jina.
Ginah, Ginea

Ginette (English) a form of Genevieve.
Ginata

Ginger (Latin) flower; spice. A familiar
form of Virginia.
Ginja, Ginjer

Ginia (Latin) a familiar form of Virginia.

Ginnifer (English) white; smooth; soft.
(Welsh) a form of Jennifer.

Ginny (English) a familiar form of
Ginger, Virginia. See also Jin, Jinny.
Gini, Ginney, Ginni, Ginnie, Giny

Giordana (Italian) a form of Jordana.

Giorgianna (English) a form of
Georgeanna.
Giorgina

Giovanna (Italian) a form of Jane.
Giavanna, Giavonna, Giovana

Gisa (Hebrew) carved stone.

Gisela (German) a form of Giselle.
Gisella, Gissella

Giselle (German) pledge; hostage. See
also Jizelle.
Gisel, Gisele, Giséle, Gisell, Gissell

Gissel, Gisselle (German) forms of
Giselle.
Gissell

Gita (Yiddish) good. (Polish) a short
form of Margaret.

Gitana (Spanish) gypsy; wanderer.

Gitta (Irish) a short form of Bridget.

Giulia (Italian) a form of Julia.

Gizela (Czech) a form of Giselle.

Gladis (Irish) a form of Gladys.
Gladi, Gladiz

Gladys (Latin) small sword. (Irish)
princess. (Welsh) a form of Claudia.
Glad, Gladness, Gladwys, Gwladys

Glenda (Welsh) a form of Glenna.
Glanda, Glennda, Glynda

Glenna (Irish) valley, glen. See also
Glynnis.
*Glenetta, Glenina, Glenine, Glenn,
Glennie, Glenora, Gleny, Glyn*

Glennesha (American) a form of
Glenna.

Gloria (Latin) glory. History: Gloria
Steinem, a leading American feminist,
founded *Ms.* magazine.
*Gloresha, Gloriah, Gloribel, Gloriela,
Gloriella, Glorielle, Gloris, Glorisha,
Glorvina*

Glorianne (American) a combination of
Gloria + Anne.

Glory (Latin) a form of Gloria.

Glynnis (Welsh) a form of Glenna.

Golda (English) gold. History: Golda
Meir was a Russian-born politician who
served as prime minister of Israel.

Goldie (English) a familiar form of
Golda.

Goma (Swahili) joyful dance.

Grace ❀ (Latin) graceful.
*Engracia, Graca, Graciela, Graciella,
Gracinha, Grata, Gratia, Gray,
Grayce*

Graceanne (English) a combination of
Grace + Anne.

Gracia (Spanish) a form of Grace.
Gracea

Gracie 𝕎 (English) a familiar form of Grace.
Gracey, Graci, Gracy

Grant (English) great; giving.

Grayson (English) bailiff's child.

Grazia (Latin) a form of Grace.

Grecia (Latin) a form of Grace.

Greer (Scottish) vigilant.

Greta (German) a short form of Gretchen, Margaret.
Greatal, Greatel, Greeta, Gretal, Grete, Gretel, Gretha, Grethal, Grethe, Grethel, Gretta, Grette, Grieta, Gryta, Grytta

Gretchen (German) a form of Margaret.
Gretchin

Gricelda (German) a form of Griselda.

Grisel (German) a short form of Griselda.

Griselda (German) gray woman warrior. See also Selda, Zelda.

Guadalupe (Arabic) river of black stones. See also Lupe.
Guadulupe

Gudrun (Scandinavian) battler. See also Runa.

Guillerma (Spanish) a short form of Guillermina.

Guinevere (French, Welsh) white wave; white phantom. Literature: the wife of King Arthur. See also Gayna, Genevieve, Genevra, Jennifer, Winifred, Wynne.

Gunda (Norwegian) female warrior.

Gurit (Hebrew) innocent baby.

Gurleen (Sikh) follower of the guru.

Gurpreet (Punjabi) religion.

Gusta (Latin) a short form of Augusta.

Gwen (Welsh) a short form of Guinevere, Gwendolyn.
Gwenesha, Gweness, Gweneta, Gwenetta, Gwenette, Gweni, Gwenisha, Gwenita, Gwenn, Gwenna, Gwennie, Gwenny

Gwenda (Welsh) a familiar form of Gwendolyn.

Gwendolyn (Welsh) white wave; white browed; new moon. Literature: Gwendoloena was the wife of Merlin, the magician. See also Genevieve, Gwyneth, Wendy.
Guendolen, Gwendalin, Gwendalee, Gwendaline, Gwendalyn, Gwendela, Gwendolen, Gwendolene, Gwendolin, Gwendoline, Gwendolyne, Gwendolynn, Gwendolynne, Gwendylan

Gwyn (Welsh) a short form of Gwyneth.

Gwyneth (Welsh) a form of Gwendolyn. See also Winnie, Wynne.
Gwenith

Gypsy (English) wanderer.

H

Habiba (Arabic) beloved.

Hachi (Japanese) eight; good luck.

Hadara (Hebrew) adorned with beauty.

Hadassah (Hebrew) myrtle tree.

Hadiya (Swahili) gift.

Hadley (English) field of heather.

Hadriane (Greek, Latin) a form of Adrienne.

Haeley (English) a form of Hailey.

Hagar (Hebrew) forsaken; stranger. Bible: Sarah's handmaiden, the mother of Ishmael.

Haidee (Greek) modest.

Haiden (English) heather-covered hill.

Hailee (English) a form of Hayley.

Hailey ※ (English) a form of Hayley.
Hailea, Hailley, Hailly

Haili, Hailie (English) forms of Hayley.

Haldana (Norwegian) half-Danish.

Halee (English) a form of Haley.

Haleigh (English) a form of Haley.

Haley ※ (Scandinavian) heroine. See also Hailey, Hayley.

Hali, Halie (English) forms of Haley.

Halia (Hawaiian) in loving memory.

Halimah (Arabic) gentle; patient.

Halina (Hawaiian) likeness. (Russian) a form of Helen.
Halena

Halla (African) unexpected gift.

Halley (English) a form of Haley.
Hally, Hallye

Hallie (Scandinavian) a form of Haley.
Hallee, Hallei, Halli

Halona (Native American) fortunate.

Halsey (English) Hall's island.

Hama (Japanese) shore.

Hana, Hanah (Japanese) flower. (Arabic) happiness. (Slavic) forms of Hannah.
Hanan, Haneen, Hanin, Hanita

Hanako (Japanese) flower child.

Hania (Hebrew) resting place.
Hanja

Hanna (Hebrew) a form of Hannah.

Hannah ※ (Hebrew) gracious. Bible: the mother of Samuel. See also Anci, Anezka, Ania, Anka, Ann, Anna, Annalie, Anneka, Chana, Nina, Nusi.
Hannalore, Hanneke, Hannele, Hannon, Honna

Hanni (Hebrew) a familiar form of Hannah.

Happy (English) happy.

Hara (Hindi) tawny. Religion: another name for the Hindu god Shiva, the destroyer.

Harlee, Harleigh, Harlie (English) forms of Harley.

Harley (English) meadow of the hare. See also Arleigh.

Harleyann (English) a combination of Harley + Ann.

Harmony (Latin) harmonious.
Harmon, Harmoni, Harmonia, Harmonie

Harpreet (Punjabi) devoted to God.

Harriet (French) ruler of the household. (English) a form of Henrietta. Literature: Harriet Beecher Stowe was an American writer noted for her novel *Uncle Tom's Cabin*.
Harri, Harrie, Harriett, Harrietta, Harriette, Harriot, Harriott

Haru (Japanese) spring.

Hasana (Swahili) she arrived first. Culture: a name used for the first-born female twin. See also Huseina.

Hasina (Swahili) good.

Hateya (Moquelumnan) footprints.

Hattie (English) familiar forms of Harriet, Henrietta.

Hausu (Moquelumnan) like a bear yawning upon awakening.

Hava (Hebrew) a form of Chava. See also Eve.

Haven (English) a form of Heaven.

Haviva (Hebrew) beloved.

Hayden (English) a form of Haiden.

Hayfa (Arabic) shapely.

Haylee, Hayleigh, Haylie (English) forms of Hayley.
Hayli

Hayley (English) hay meadow. See also Hailey, Haley.
Hayly

Hazel (English) hazelnut tree; commanding authority.
Hazal, Hazaline, Haze, Hazeline, Hazell, Hazelle, Hazen, Hazyl

Heather (English) flowering heather.
Heath, Heatherlee, Heatherly

Heaven (English) place of beauty and happiness. Bible: where God and angels are said to dwell.
Heavenly, Heavin, Heavyn, Heven

Hedda (German) battler. See also Edda, Hedy.
Heida

Hedy (Greek) delightful; sweet. (German) a familiar form of Hedda.

Heidi, Heidy (German) short forms of Adelaide.
Heida, Heide, Heidie, Hidee, Hidi, Hiede, Hiedi

Helen (Greek) light. See also Aileen, Aili, Alena, Eileen, Elaina, Elaine, Eleanor, Ellen, Galina, Ila, Ilene, Ilona, Jelena, Leanore, Leena, Lelya, Lenci, Lene, Liolya, Nellie, Nitsa, Olena, Onella, Yalena, Yelena.
Hela, Hele, Helle, Hellen, Helli, Hellin, Hellon, Helon

Helena (Greek) a form of Helen. See also Ilena.
Halena, Helaina, Helana, Helayna, Heleana, Heleena, Helenna, Helina, Hellanna, Hellenna, Helona, Helonna

Helene (French) a form of Helen.
Helaine, Helayne, Heleen, Héléne, Helenor, Heline, Hellenor

Helga (German) pious. (Scandinavian) a form of Olga. See also Elga.

Helki (Native American) touched.
Helkey, Helkie, Helky

Helma (German) a short form of Wilhelmina.

Heloise (French) a form of Louise.

Helsa (Danish) a form of Elizabeth.

Heltu (Moquelumnan) like a bear reaching out.

Henna (English) a familiar form of Henrietta.

Henrietta (English) ruler of the household. See also Enrica, Etta, Yetta.

Hera (Greek) queen; jealous. Mythology: the queen of heaven and the wife of Zeus.

Hermia (Greek) messenger.

Hermina (Latin) noble. (German) soldier. See also Erma, Ermine, Irma.

Hermione (Greek) earthy.

Hermosa (Spanish) beautiful.

Hertha (English) child of the earth.

Hester (Dutch) a form of Esther.

Hestia (Persian) star. Mythology: the Greek goddess of the hearth and home.

Heta (Native American) racer.

Hetta (German) a form of Hedda. (English) a familiar form of Henrietta.

Hettie (German) a familiar form of Henrietta, Hester.

Hilary, Hillary (Greek) cheerful, merry. See also Alair.
Hilaree, Hilari, Hilaria, Hilarie, Hilery, Hiliary, Hillaree, Hillari, Hillarie, Hilleary, Hilleree, Hilleri, Hillerie, Hillery, Hillianne, Hilliary, Hillory

Hilda (German) a short form of Brunhilda, Hildegarde.
Helle

Hildegarde (German) fortress.

Hinda (Hebrew) hind; doe.

Hisa (Japanese) long lasting.

Hiti (Eskimo) hyena.

Hoa (Vietnamese) flower; peace.

Hola (Hopi) seed-filled club.

Holley (English) a form of Holly.
Hollee

Holli, Hollie (English) forms of Holly.

Hollis (English) near the holly bushes.

Holly (English) holly tree.
Hollina

Hollyann (English) a combination of Holly + Ann.

Hollyn (English) a short form of Hollyann.

Honey (English) sweet. (Latin) a familiar form of Honora.

Hong (Vietnamese) pink.

Honora (Latin) honorable. See also Nora, Onora.

Hope (English) hope.
Hopey, Hopi, Hopie

Hortense (Latin) gardener. See also Ortensia.

Hoshi (Japanese) star.

Hua (Chinese) flower.

Huata (Moquelumnan) basket carrier.

Hunter (English) hunter.

Huong (Vietnamese) flower.

Huseina (Swahili) a form of Hasana.

Hyacinth (Greek) Botany: a plant with colorful, fragrant flowers. See also Cynthia, Jacinda.

Hydi, Hydeia (German) forms of Heidi.

Hye (Korean) graceful.

Ian (Hebrew) God is gracious.

Ianthe (Greek) violet flower.

Icess (Egyptian) a form of Isis.

Ida (German) hard working. (English) prosperous.
Idaia, Idalia, Idamae, Idania, Idarina, Idarine, Idaya, Ide, Idette, Idys

Idalina (English) a combination of Ida + Lina.
Idaleena, Idaleene, Idalena, Idalene, Idaline

Idalis (English) a form of Ida.

Ideashia (American) a combination of Ida + Iesha.

Idelle (Welsh) a form of Ida.

Iesha (American) a form of Aisha.
Ieachia, Ieaisha, Ieasha, Ieesha, Ieeshia, Ieisha, Ieishia, Ieshia

Ignacia (Latin) fiery, ardent.

Ikia (Hebrew) God is my salvation. (Hawaiian) a form of Isaiah (see Boys' Names).
Ikaisha, Ikea, Ikeisha, Ikeishi, Ikeishia, Ikesha, Ikeshia

Ila (Hungarian) a form of Helen.

Ilana (Hebrew) tree.
Ilane, Ilani, Ilania, Ilainie, Illana, Illane, Illani, Illanie, Ilanit

Ileana (Hebrew) a form of Iliana.

Ilena (Greek) a form of Helena.

Ilene (Irish) a form of Helen. See also Aileen, Eileen.

Iliana (Greek) from Troy.

Ilima (Hawaiian) flower of Oahu.

Ilisa (Scottish, English) a form of Alisa, Elisa.
Ilissa, Ilysa, Ilysia, Ilyssa

Ilise (German) a form of Elise.

Ilisha (Hebrew) a form of Alisha, Elisha. See also Lisha.
Ilysha

Ilka (Hungarian) a familiar form of Ilona.

Ilona (Hungarian) a form of Helen.

Ilse (German) a form of Elizabeth. See also Elsa.

Ima (Japanese) presently. (German) a familiar form of Amelia.

Imala (Native American) strong-minded.

Iman (Arabic) believer.

Imani (Arabic) a form of Iman.

Imelda (German) warrior.

Imena (African) dream.

Imogene (Latin) image, likeness.

Ina (Irish) a form of Agnes.

India (Hindi) from India.
Indi, Indie, Indy, Indya

Indigo (Latin) dark blue color.

Indira (Hindi) splendid. History: Indira
Nehru Gandhi was an Indian politician
and prime minister.

Ines, Inez (Spanish) forms of Agnes. See
also Ynez.

Inga (Scandinavian) a short form of
Ingrid.
Inge

Ingrid (Scandinavian) hero's daughter;
beautiful daughter.
Inger

Inoa (Hawaiian) name.

Ioana (Romanian) a form of Joan.

Iola (Greek) dawn; violet colored.
(Welsh) worthy of the Lord.

Iolana (Hawaiian) soaring like a hawk.

Iolanthe (English) a form of Yolanda.
See also Jolanda.

Iona (Greek) violet flower.

Iphigenia (Greek) sacrifice. Mythology:
the daughter of the Greek leader
Agamemnon. See also Gena.

Irene (Greek) peaceful. Mythology: the
goddess of peace. See also Orina, Rena,
Rene, Yarina.
Irén, Irien

Irina (Russian) a form of Irene.
*Eirena, Erena, Ira, Irana, Iranda,
Iranna, Irena, Irenea, Irenka, Iriana*

Iris (Greek) rainbow. Mythology: the
goddess of the rainbow and messenger
of the gods.
Irisa, Irisha, Irissa, Irita

Irma (Latin) a form of Erma.

Isabeau (French) a form of Isabel.

Isabel ☀ (Spanish) consecrated to
God. See also Bel, Belle, Chavella,
Ysabel.
*Isabal, Isabeli, Isabelita, Ishbel,
Izabel, Izabele*

Isabella ☀ (Italian) a form of Isabel.
Isabela

Isabelle ☀ (French) a form of Isabel.

Isadora (Latin) gift of Isis.

Isela (Scottish) a form of Isla.

Isha (American) a form of Aisha.

Ishi (Japanese) rock.

Isis (Egyptian) supreme goddess.
Mythology: the goddess of nature and
fertility.

Isla (Scottish) Geography: the River Isla
is in Scotland.

Isobel (Spanish) a form of Isabel.

Isoka (Benin) gift from god.

Isolde (Welsh) fair lady. Literature: a
princess in the Arthurian legends, also
known as Iseult.

Issie (Spanish) a familiar form of Isabel.
Isa, Issi, Issy, Iza

Ita (Irish) thirsty.

Italia (Italian) from Italy.

Itamar (Hebrew) palm island.

Itzel (Spanish) protected.

Iva (Slavic) a short form of Ivana.

Ivana (Slavic) God is gracious. See also
Yvanna.

Iverem (Tiv) good fortune; blessing.

Iverna (Latin) from Ireland.

Ivette (French) a form of Yvette. See also
Evette.
Ivete, Iveth, Ivetha, Ivetta

Ivonne (French) a form of Yvonne. See
also Evonne.

Ivory (Latin) made of ivory.
Ivori, Ivorine, Ivree

Ivria (Hebrew) from the land of
Abraham.

Ivy (English) ivy tree.
Ivey, Ivie

Iyabo (Yoruba) mother has returned.

Iyana, Iyanna (Hebrew) forms of Ian.

Izabella (Spanish) a form of Isabel.
Izabelle

Izusa (Native American) white stone.

J

Jabrea, Jabria (American) combinations of the prefix Ja + Brea.

Jacalyn (American) a form of
Jacqueline.
Jacolyn, Jacolyne, Jacolynn

Jacelyn (American) a form of Jocelyn.
*Jacelyne, Jacelynn, Jacilyn, Jacilyne,
Jacilynn, Jacylyn, Jacylyne, Jacylynn*

Jacey, Jacy (Greek) familiar forms of
Jacinda. (American) combinations of
the initials J. + C.
Jace, Jac-E, Jacèe, Jacylin

Jaci, Jacie (Greek) forms of Jacey.
Jacia, Jaciel

Jacinda, Jacinta (Greek) beautiful,
attractive. (Spanish) forms of Hyacinth.
Jacenda, Jacenta, Jakinda, Jaxine

Jacinthe (Spanish) a form of Jacinda.
Jacinth, Jacintha

Jackalyn (American) a form of
Jacqueline.

Jackeline, Jackelyn (American)
forms of Jacqueline.
Jockeline

Jacki, Jackie (American) familiar
forms of Jacqueline.
Jackee, Jackia, Jackielee, Jacky

Jacklyn (American) a form of
Jacqueline.
*Jacklin, Jackline, Jacklyne, Jacklynn,
Jacklynne*

Jackquel (French) a short form of
Jacqueline.
Jackquelin, Jackqueline, Jackquiline

Jaclyn (American) a short form of
Jacqueline.
*Jacleen, Jaclin, Jacline, Jaclyne,
Jaclynn*

Jacobi (Hebrew) supplanter, substitute.
Bible: Jacob was the son of Isaac,
brother of Esau.

Jacqualine (French) a form of
Jacqueline.
*Jacqualin, Jacqualyn, Jacqualyne,
Jacqualynn*

Jacquelin (French) a form of
Jacqueline.

Jacqueline (French) supplanter, substi-
tute; little Jacqui.
*Jacqueleen, Jacquelene, Jacquine,
Jocqueline*

Jacquelyn, Jacquelynn (French)
forms of Jacqueline.
Jacquelyne

Jacqui (French) a short form of
Jacqueline.

Jacqulin, Jacqulyn (American) forms
of Jacqueline.
Jackquilin

Jacquiline (French) a form of
Jacqueline.
*Jacquil, Jacquilin, Jacquilyn,
Jacquilyne, Jacquilynn*

Jacynthe (Spanish) a form of Jacinda.
Jacynth

Jada ☀ (Spanish) a form of Jade.
*Jadah, Jadda, Jadzia, Jadziah, Jaeda,
Jaedra*

Jade ☀ (Spanish) jade.
*Jadea, Jadeann, Jadee, Jadera, Jadi,
Jadie, Jadienne, Jady, Jaedra*

Jadelyn (American) a combination of
Jade + Lynn.
Jadielyn

Jaden (Spanish) a form of Jade.

Jadyn (Spanish) a form of Jade.

Jae (Latin) jaybird. (French) a familiar
form of Jacqueline.

Jael (Hebrew) mountain goat; climber.
See also Yael.

Jaelyn, Jaelynn (American) combinations of Jae + Lynn.
Jayleen

Jaffa (Hebrew) a form of Yaffa.

Jaha (Swahili) dignified.

Jai (Tai) heart. (Latin) a form of Jaye.

Jaida, Jaide (Spanish) forms of Jade.

Jaiden, Jaidyn (Spanish) forms of
Jade.

Jailyn (American) a form of Jaelyn.

Jaime (French) I love.
Jaima, Jaimey, Jaimini, Jaimy

Jaimee (French) a form of Jaime.

Jaimie (French) a form of Jaime.
Jaimi, Jaimmie

Jaira (Spanish) Jehovah teaches.

Jakeisha (American) a combination of
Jakki + Aisha.

Jakelin (American) a form of
Jacqueline.

Jakki (American) a form of Jacki.

Jaleesa (American) a form of Jalisa.

Jalena (American) a combination of Jane + Lena.

Jalesa, Jalessa (American) forms of Jalisa.

Jalia, Jalea (American) combinations of Jae + Leah.

Jalila (Arabic) great.

Jalisa, Jalissa (American) combinations of Jae + Lisa.

Jalyn, Jalynn (American) combinations of Jae + Lynn. See also Jaylyn.

Jalysa (American) a form of Jalisa.

Jamaica (Spanish) Geography: an island in the Caribbean.
Jamika

Jamani (American) a form of Jami.

Jamaria (American) combinations of Jae + Maria.

Jamecia (Spanish) a form of Jamaica.

Jamee (French) a form of Jaime.

Jameika, Jameka (Spanish) forms of Jamaica.

Jamesha (American) a form of Jami.
Jamiesha, Jammesha, Jammisha

Jamey (English) a form of Jami, Jamie.

Jami, Jamie (Hebrew, English) supplanter, substitute.
Jama, Jamay, Jamii, Jamis, Jamise, Jamy, Jamye

Jamia (English) a form of Jami, Jamie.
Jamea, Jamya

Jamica (Spanish) a form of Jamaica.
Jamika

Jamila (Arabic) beautiful. See also Yamila.
Jahmela, Jahmelia, Jahmil, Jahmilla, Jameela, Jameelah, Jameeliah, Jameila, Jamela, Jamelia, Jameliah, Jamell, Jamella, Jamelle, Jamely, Jamelya, Jamiela, Jamielee, Jamilah, Jamilee, Jamilia, Jamiliah, Jamilla, Jamillah, Jamille, Jamillia, Jamilya, Jamyla, Jemeela, Jemelia, Jemila, Jemilla

Jamilynn (English) a combination of Jami + Lynn.
Jamielin, Jamieline, Jamielyn, Jamielyne, Jamielynn, Jamielynne, Jamilin, Jamiline, Jamilyn, Jamilyne, Jamilynne

Jammie (American) a form of Jami.
Jammi, Jammice

Jamonica (American) a combination of Jami + Monica.

Jamylin (American) a form of Jamilynn.

Jan (English) a short form of Jane, Janet, Janice.
Jania, Jandy

Jana (Hebrew) gracious, merciful. (Slavic) a form of Jane. See also Yana.
Janalee, Janalisa, Janne

Janae, Janay (American) forms of Jane.
Janaé, Janaea, Janaeh, Janah, Janaya, Janaye, Janea, Janee, Janée, Jannae, Jannay, Jenay, Jenaya, Jennae, Jennay, Jennaya, Jennaye

Janai (American) a form of Janae.

Janalynn (American) a combination of Jana + Lynn.

Janan (Arabic) heart; soul.

Jane (Hebrew) God is gracious. See also Chavon, Jean, Joan, Juanita, Seana, Shana, Shawna, Sheena, Shona, Shunta, Sinead, Zaneta, Zanna, Zhana.
Jaine, Janen, Jania, Janka

Janel, Janell (French) forms of Janelle.
Janiel, Jannel, Jannell, Janyll, Jaynel, Jaynell

Janelle (French) a form of Jane.
Janela, Janele, Janelis, Janella, Janelli, Janellie, Janelly, Janely, Janelys, Janielle, Janille, Jannelle, Jannellies, Jaynelle

Janesha (American) a form of Janessa.
Janiesha, Janisha, Jannesha, Jannisha, Jenisha, Jennisha

Janessa (American) a form of Jane.
Janeesa, Janesa, Janesia, Janeska, Janiesa, Janissa, Jannesa, Jannessa, Jannisa, Jannissa, Jenesa, Jenissa, Jennisa, Jennissa

Janet (English) a form of Jane. See also Jessie, Yanet.
Janeta, Janete, Janett, Jannet, Janot, Jante, Janyte

Janeth (English) a form of Janet.
Janith, Janneth

Janette, Jannette (French) forms of Janet.
Janett, Janetta, Jannetta

Janice (Hebrew) God is gracious. (English) a familiar form of Jane. See also Genice.
Janece, Janecia, Janeice, Janizzette,

Jannice, Janniece, Janyce, Jenice, Jynice

Janie (English) a familiar form of Jane.
Janey, Jani, Jany

Janika (Slavic) a form of Jane.
Janaca, Janique, Janka, Jannika, Jenika, Jennica, Jennika

Janine (French) a form of Jane.
Janean, Janeann, Janeen, Janenan, Janene, Janina, Jannina, Jannine, Jannyne, Janyne, Jeannine

Janis (English) a form of Jane.
Janees, Janese, Janesey, Janesse, Janise, Jannis, Jenesse, Jenis, Jennise, Jennisse

Janita (American) a form of Juanita. See also Genita.
Janitza, Janneta, Jaynita, Jennita

Janna (Arabic) harvest of fruit. (Hebrew) a short form of Johana.
Janaya, Janaye, Jannae

Jannie (English) a familiar form of Jan, Jane.

Jaquana (American) a combination of Jacqueline + Anna.

Jaquelen (American) a form of Jacqueline.

Jaquelin, Jaqueline (French) forms of Jacqueline.

Jaquelyn (French) a form of Jacqueline.
Jaquelyne, Jaquelynn

Jardena (Hebrew) a form of Jordan. (French, Spanish) garden.

Jarian (American) a combination of Jane + Marian.

Jarita (Arabic) earthen water jug.

Jas (American) a short form of Jasmine.

Jasia (Polish) a form of Jane.

Jasleen, Jaslyn (Latin) forms of Jocelyn.

Jasmain (Persian) a short form of Jasmine.
Jasmaine, Jassmain, Jassmaine

Jasmarie (American) a combination of Jasmine + Marie.

Jasmin (Persian) a form of Jasmine.
Jasman, Jasmeen, Jasmon, Jassmin

Jasmine ✚ (Persian) jasmine flower.
See also Jessamine, Yasmin.
Jasma, Jasme, Jasmeet, Jasmene, Jasmina, Jasmira, Jasmit, Jassma, Jassmin, Jassmine, Jassmit, Jassmon, Jassmyn

Jasmyn, Jasmyne (Persian) forms of Jasmine.
Jassmyn

Jaspreet (Punjabi) virtuous.
Jaspar, Jasparit, Jasparita, Jasper, Jasprit, Jasprita, Jasprite

Jatara (American) a combination of Jane + Tara.

Javana (Malayan) from Java.

Javiera (Spanish) owner of a new house. See also Xaviera.
Viera

Javona, Javonna (Malayan) forms of Javana.

Jaya (Hindi) victory.

Jaycee (American) a combination of the initials J. + C.
Jacee

Jayda (Spanish) a form of Jada.

Jayde (Spanish) a form of Jade.

Jaydee (American) a combination of the initials J. + D.
Jadee, Jadi, Jadie, Jady

Jayden (Spanish) a form of Jade.

Jaye (Latin) jaybird.
Jay

Jayla (American) a short form of Jaylene.
Jaylah

Jaylene (American) forms of Jaylyn.
Jayelene, Jaylan, Jayleana, Jaylee, Jayleen

Jaylin (American) a form of Jaylyn.

Jaylyn, Jaylynn (American) combinations of Jaye + Lynn. See also Jalyn.

Jayme, Jaymie (English) forms of Jami.
Jaymia, Jaymine, Jaymini

Jaymee, Jaymi (English) forms of Jami.

Jayna (Hebrew) a form of Jane.
Jaynae

Jayne (Hindi) victorious. (English) a form of Jane.
Jayn, Jaynne

Jaynie (English) a familiar form of Jayne.
Jaynee, Jayni

Jazlyn (American) a combination of Jazmin + Lynn.

Jazmin, Jazmine (Persian) forms of
Jasmine.
Jazman, Jazmen, Jazminn, Jazmon,
Jazzmit

Jazmyn, Jazmyne (Persian) forms of
Jasmine.
Jazzmyn

Jazzmin, Jazzmine (Persian) forms of
Jasmine.
Jazzman, Jazzmen, Jazzmon

Jean, Jeanne (Scottish) God is gra-
cious. See also Kini.
Jeanann, Jeancie, Jeane, Jeaneia,
Jeaneva, Jeanice, Jeanmarie, Jeanné,
Jeannita, Jeannot, Jeantelle

Jeana, Jeanna (Scottish) forms of
Jean.

Jeanette, Jeannett (French) forms of
Jean.
Jeanete, Jeanett, Jeanetta, Jeanita,
Jeannete, Jeannetta, Jeannette,
Jeannita, Jenet, Jenett, Jenette, Jennet,
Jennett, Jennetta, Jennette, Jennita,
Jinetta, Jinette

Jeanie, Jeannie (Scottish) familiar
forms of Jean.
Jeannee, Jeanney, Jeani, Jeanny,
Jeany

Jeanine, Jenine (Scottish) forms of
Jean. See also Geneen.
Jeaneane, Jeaneen, Jeanene, Jeanina,
Jeannina, Jeannine, Jennine

Jelena (Russian) a form of Helen. See
also Yelena.

Jelisa (American) a combination of
Jean + Lisa.
Jillisa, Jillissa

Jem (Hebrew) a short form of Jemima.
Gem

Jemima (Hebrew) dove.

Jemma (Hebrew) a short form of
Jemima. (English) a form of Gemma.

Jena, Jenae (Arabic) forms of Jenna.
Jenah, Jenai, Jenal, Jenay, Jenaya

Jendaya (Zimbabwean) thankful.

Jenelle (American) a combination of
Jenny + Nelle.
Jeanell, Jeanelle, Jenall, Jenalle, Jenel,
Jenell, Jenille, Jennel, Jennell,
Jennelle, Jennielle, Jennille

Jenessa (American) a form of Jenisa.
Jenesa

Jenica (Romanian) a form of Jane.
Jenika, Jennica, Jennika

Jenifer, Jeniffer (Welsh) forms of
Jennifer.
Jenefer

Jenilee (American) a combination of
Jennifer + Lee.
Jenalea, Jenalee, Jenaleigh, Jenaly,
Jenelea, Jenelee, Jeneleigh, Jenely,
Jenelly, Jenileigh, Jenily, Jennely,
Jennielee, Jennilea, Jennilie

Jenisa (American) a combination of
Jennifer + Nisa.
Jenisha, Jenissa, Jennisa, Jennise,
Jennisha, Jennissa, Jennisse

Jenka (Czech) a form of Jane.

Jenna ✶ (Arabic) small bird. (Welsh)
a short form of Jennifer. See also Gen.
Jennae, Jennah, Jennat, Jennay,
Jennaya, Jennaye, Jhenna

Jenni, Jennie (Welsh) familiar forms of Jennifer.
Jeni, Jenne, Jenné, Jennee, Jenney, Jennia, Jennier, Jennita, Jennora, Jensine

Jennifer ✧ (Welsh) white wave; white phantom. A form of Guinevere. See also Gennifer, Ginnifer, Yenifer.
Jen, Jenipher, Jennafer, Jenniferanne, Jenniferlee, Jenniffe, Jenniffer, Jenniffier, Jennifier, Jenniphe, Jennipher

Jennilee (American) a combination of Jenny + Lee.
Jennielee, Jennilea, Jennilie

Jennilyn, Jennilynn (American) combinations of Jenni + Lynn.

Jenny (Welsh) a familiar form of Jennifer.
Jenney, Jeny

Jennyfer (Welsh) a form of Jennifer.

Jeraldine (English) a form of Geraldine.
Jeraldeen, Jeraldene, Jeraldina, Jeraldyne, Jeralee

Jereni (Russian) a form of Irene.
Jerina

Jeri, Jerri, Jerrie (American) short forms of Jeraldine. See also Geri.
Jera, Jerae, Jeree, Jeriel, Jerilee, Jerinda, Jerra, Jerrece, Jerriann, Jerrilee, Jerrine, Jerry, Jerrylee, Jerryne, Jerzy

Jerica (American) a combination of Jeri + Erica.
Jerice, Jericka, Jerika, Jerrice

Jerilyn (American) a combination of Jeri + Lynn.
Jeralin, Jeraline, Jeralyn, Jeralyne,

Jeralynn, Jeralynne, Jerelin, Jereline, Jerelyn, Jerelyne, Jerelynn, Jerelynne, Jerilin, Jeriline, Jerilyne, Jerilynn, Jerilynne, Jerrilin, Jerriline, Jerrilyn, Jerrilyne, Jerrilynn, Jerrilynne

Jermaine (French) a form of Germaine.

Jerrica (American) a form of Jerica.
Jerreka, Jerricca, Jerricka, Jerrika

Jerusha (Hebrew) inheritance.

Jesenia, Jessenia (Arabic) flower.
Jescenia

Jesica, Jesika (Hebrew) forms of Jessica.

Jessa (American) a short form of Jessalyn, Jessamine, Jessica.
Jessah

Jessalyn (American) a combination of Jessica + Lynn.
Jesalin, Jesaline, Jesalyn, Jesalyne, Jesalynn, Jesalynne, Jesilin, Jesiline, Jesilyn, Jesilyne, Jesilynn, Jesilynne, Jessalin, Jessaline, Jessalyne, Jessalynn, Jessalynne, Jesseline, Jesselyn, Jesselyne, Jesselynn, Jesselynne

Jessamine (French) a form of Jasmine.

Jesse, Jessi (Hebrew) forms of Jessie.
Jesi

Jesseca (Hebrew) a form of Jessica.

Jessica ✧ (Hebrew) wealthy. Literature: a name perhaps invented by Shakespeare for a character in his play *The Merchant of Venice*. See also Gessica, Yessica.
Jessaca, Jessca, Jesscia, Jessia, Jessicca, Jessicia, Jessicka, Jessiqua, Jezeca, Jezica, Jezika, Jezyca

Jessie, Jessy (Hebrew) short forms of
Jessica. (Scottish) forms of Janet.
*Jescie, Jesey, Jess, Jessé, Jessee, Jessey,
Jessia, Jessiya, Jessye*

Jessika (Hebrew) a form of Jessica.
Jessieka

Jesslyn (American) a short form of
Jessalyn.

Jessyca, Jessyka (Hebrew) forms of
Jessica.

Jésusa (Hebrew, Spanish) God is my
salvation.

Jetta (English) jet black mineral.
(American) a familiar form of Jevette.

Jevette (American) a combination of
Jean + Yvette.

Jewel (French) precious gem.
Juel, Jule

Jezebel (Hebrew) unexalted; impure.
Bible: the wife of King Ahab.

Jianna (Italian) a form of Gianna.
Jianni, Jiannini

Jibon (Hindi) life.

Jill (English) a short form of Jillian.
Jil, Jilli, Jillie, Jilly

Jillaine (Latin) a form of Jillian.

Jilleen (Irish) a form of Jillian.
Jiline, Jilline, Jillyn

Jillian (Latin) youthful. See also Gillian.
*Jilian, Jiliana, Jiliann, Jilianna,
Jilianne, Jilienna, Jilienne, Jilliana,
Jilliane, Jilliann, Jillianne, Jillien,
Jillienne, Jillion, Jilliyn*

Jimi (Hebrew) supplanter, substitute.

Jimisha (American) a combination of
Jimi + Aisha.

Jin (Japanese) tender. (American) a short
form of Ginny, Jinny.

Jina (Swahili) baby with a name.
(Italian) a form of Gina.

Jinny (Scottish) a familiar form of
Jenny. (American) a familiar form of
Virginia. See also Ginny.

Jirina (Czech) a form of Georgia.

Jizelle (American) a form of Giselle.

Jo (American) a short form of Joanna,
Jolene, Josephine.
Joangie, Joetta, Joette, Joey

Joan (Hebrew) God is gracious. History:
Joan of Arc was a fifteenth-century hero-
ine and resistance fighter. See also Ioana,
Jean, Juanita, Siobhan.
*Joane, Joaneil, Joanel, Joanelle,
Joanmarie, Joann, Joannanette,
Joannel*

Joana, Joanna (English) a form of
Joan. See also Yoanna.
*Janka, Jo-Ana, Joandra, Joananna,
Jo-Anie, Joanka, Jo-Anna, Joannah,
Jo-Annie, Joeana, Joeanna*

Joanie, Joannie (Hebrew) familiar
forms of Joan.
Joani, Joanni, Joenie

Joanne (English) a form of Joan.
*Joanann, Joananne, Joann, Jo-Ann,
Jo-Anne, Joayn, Joeann, Joeanne*

Joanny (Hebrew) a familiar form of
Joan.
Joany

Joaquina (Hebrew) God will establish.

Jobeth (English) a combination of Jo + Beth.

Joby (Hebrew) afflicted. (English) a familiar form of Jobeth.

Jocacia (American) a combination of Joy + Acacia.

Jocelin, Joceline (Latin) forms of Jocelyn.

Jocelyn ✡ (Latin) joyous. See also Yocelin, Yoselin.
Jocelle, Jocelynn, Joci, Jocia, Jocinta

Jocelyne (Latin) a form of Jocelyn.
Jocelynne

Jodi, Jodie, Jody (American) familiar forms of Judith.
Jodee, Jodele, Jodell, Jodelle, Jodevea, Jodilee, Jodi-Lee, Jodilynn, Jodi-Lynn

Jodiann (American) a combination of Jodi + Ann.
Jodene, Jodine, Jodyne

Joelle (Hebrew) God is willing.
Joel, Joela, Joelee, Joeli, Joell, Joella, Joëlle, Joelly, Joyelle

Joelynn (American) a combination of Joelle + Lynn.
Joeleen, Joelene, Joeline, Joellen, Joellyn, Joelyn, Joelyne

Johana, Johanna, Johannah (German) forms of Joana.
Johanah, Johanka, Johanne, Johonna, Joyhanna, Joyhannah

Johanie, Johannie (Hebrew) forms of Joanie.
Johani, Johanni

Johnna, Jonna (American) forms of Johana, Joanna.
Jahna, Jahnaya, Jhona, Jhonna, Johna, Johnda, Johnnielynn, Johnnie-Lynn, Johnnquia, Johnnquita, Joncie, Jonda, Jondell, Jondrea, Jonnica, Jonnika, Jutta

Johnnie (Hebrew) a form of Joanie.
Johni, Johnie, Johnni, Johnny

Johnnessa (American) a combination of Johnna + Nessa.
Johneatha

Joi (Latin) a form of Joy.
Joie

Jokla (Swahili) beautiful robe.

Jolanda (Greek) a form of Yolanda. See also Iolanthe.

Joleen, Joline (English) forms of Jolene.
Jolleen, Jollene

Jolene (Hebrew) God will add, God will increase. (English) a form of Josephine.
Jolaine, Jolana, Jolane, Jolanna, Jolanne, Jolanta, Jolayne, Jole, Jolean, Joleane, Jolena, Joléne, Jolenna, Jolin, Jolina, Jolinda, Jolinna, Jolleane, Jolleen, Jolline

Jolie (French) pretty.
Jole, Jolee, Joley, Jolye

Jolisa (American) a combination of Jo + Lisa.

Jolynn (American) a combination of Jo + Lynn.

Jonatha (Hebrew) gift of God.

Jonelle (American) a combination of Joan + Elle.
Jahnel, Jahnell, Jahnelle, Johnel, Johnell, Johnella, Johnelle, Jonel, Jonell, Jonella, Jonyelle, Jynell, Jynelle

Jonesha, Jonisha (American) forms of Jonatha.
Joneisha, Jonessa, Jonisa

Joni (American) a familiar form of Joan.
Jona, Jonae, Jonai, Jonann, Jonati, Joncey, Jonci, Joncie, Joneen, Jonice, Jonie, Jonilee, Joni-lee, Jonis, Jony

Jonika (American) a form of Janika.
Johnica, Johnique, Joneeka, Joneika, Jonica, Joniqua, Jonique

Jonina (Hebrew) dove. See also Yonina.
Jona

Jonita (Hebrew) a form of Jonina. See also Yonita.
Johnetta, Johnette, Johnita, Johnittia, Jonati, Jonetia, Jonetta, Jonette, Jonit, Jonnita

Jonni, Jonnie (American) familiar forms of Joan.
Jonny

Jonquil (Latin, English) Botany: an ornamental plant with fragrant yellow flowers.

Jontel (American) a form of Johnna.

Jora (Hebrew) autumn rain.

Jordan ☀ (Hebrew) descending. See also Jardena.
Jordain, Jordane, Jordann, Jordanne, Jordi

Jordana, Jordanna (Hebrew) forms of Jordan. See also Giordana, Yordana.
Jordonna, Jourdana, Jourdanna

Jorden, Jordin, Jordon (Hebrew) forms of Jordan.
Jordenne, Jordine

Jordyn (Hebrew) a form of Jordan.
Jordyne

Jori, Jorie (Hebrew) familiar forms of Jordan.

Joriann (American) a combination of Jori + Ann.

Jorja (American) a form of Georgia.

Josalyn (Latin) a form of Jocelyn.
Josalene

Joscelin, Joscelyn (Latin) forms of Jocelyn.

Josee, Josée (American) familiar forms of Josephine.
Joesee, Josi, Josiann, Josina, Josy, Jozee

Josefina (Spanish) a form of Josephine.
Josefa, Josefena, Josefine

Joselin, Joseline (Latin) forms of Jocelyn.
Josielina

Joselle (American) a form of Jizelle.
Joesell, Jozelle

Joselyn, Joslyn (Latin) forms of Jocelyn.
Joselene, Josiline, Josilyn

Josephine (French) God will add, God will increase. See also Fifi, Pepita, Yosepha.
Fina, Joey, Josepha, Josephe, Josephene, Josephin, Josephina, Josephyna, Josephyne

Josette (French) a familiar form of Josephine.
Joesette, Jozette

Josey, Josie (Hebrew) familiar forms of Josephine.
Josi, Josy, Josye

Joshann (American) a combination of Joshlyn + Ann.

Joshlyn (Latin) a form of Jocelyn.
(Hebrew) God is my salvation.

Josiane, Josianne (American) combinations of Josie + Anne.

Josilin, Joslin (Latin) forms of Jocelyn.
*Josielina, Josiline, Josilyn, Josilyne,
Josilynn, Josilynne, Josline, Joslyne,
Joslynn, Joslynne*

Jossalin (Latin) a form of Jocelyn.

Josselyn (Latin) a form of Jocelyn.

Jourdan (Hebrew) a form of Jordan.
Jourdann, Jourdanne

Jovana (Latin) a form of Jovanna.

Jovanna (Latin) majestic. (Italian) a
form of Giovanna. Mythology: Jove, also
known as Jupiter, was the supreme
Roman god.

Jovannie (Italian) a familiar form of
Jovanna.

Jovita (Latin) jovial.

Joy (Latin) joyous.
*Joya, Joye, Joyeeta, Joyia, Joyous,
Joyvina*

Joyanne (American) a combination of
Joy + Anne.
Joyan, Joyann, Joyanna

Joyce (Latin) joyous. A short form of
Joycelyn.
Joice, Joycey, Joycie, Joyous, Joysel

Joycelyn (American) a form of Jocelyn.

Joylyn (American) a combination of Joy
+ Lynn.
*Joylin, Joyline, Joylyne, Joylynn,
Joylynne*

Jozie (Hebrew) a familiar form of
Josephine.
Jozee

Juana (Spanish) a short form of Juanita.
Juanna

Juandalyn (Spanish) a form of Juanita.

Juanita (Spanish) a form of Jane, Joan.
See also Kwanita, Nita, Waneta, Wanika.
*Juaneice, Juanequa, Juanesha,
Juanice, Juanicia, Juaniqua,
Juanisha, Juanishia*

Juci (Hungarian) a form of Judy.
Jucika

Judith (Hebrew) praised. Mythol-ogy: the
slayer of Holofernes, according to ancient
Jewish legend. See also Yehudit, Yudita.
*Giuditta, Ioudith, Jude, Judine, Judit,
Judita, Judite, Juditha, Judithe,
Judyta, Jutka*

Judy (Hebrew) a familiar form of Judith.
Judi, Judie, Judye

Judyann (American) a combination of
Judy + Ann.
Judana

Jula (Polish) a form of Julia.

Julene (Basque) a form of Julia. See
also Yulene.
Julina, Juline

Julia ☀ (Latin) youthful. See also
Giulia, Jill, Jillian, Sulia, Yulia.
*Iulia, Julica, Julija, Julina, Juline,
Julyssa*

Juliana, Julianna (Czech, Spanish,
Hungarian) forms of Julia.
Julliana, Jullianna

Juliann, Julianne (English) forms of Julia.
Juliane, Julieann, Julie-Ann, Julieanne, Julie-Anne, Julien, Juliene, Julienne

Julie (English) a form of Julia.
Juel, Jule, Julee, Juli, Julie-Lynn, Julie-Mae, Jullie, July

Juliet, Juliette (French) forms of Julia.
Julet, Julieta, Julietta, Jullet, Julliet, Jullietta

Julisa, Julissa (Latin) forms of Julia.
Julyssa

Julita (Spanish) a form of Julia.

Jumaris (American) a combination of Julie + Maris.

Jun (Chinese) truthful.

June (Latin) born in the sixth month.
Juna, Junell, Junelle, Junette, Junia, Junie, Juniet, Junieta, Junietta, Juniette, Junina, Junita

Juno (Latin) queen. Mythology: the supreme Roman goddess.

Justice (Latin) just, righteous.

Justina (Italian) a form of Justine.
Jestena, Jestina, Justinna, Justyna

Justine (Latin) just, righteous.
Giustina, Jestine, Juste, Justi, Justie, Justinn, Justy, Justyne

K

Kacey, Kacy (Irish) brave. (American) forms of Casey. Combinations of the initials K. + C.
K. C., Kace, Kacee, Kaicee, Kaicey, Kayci, Kaycie

Kachina (Native American) sacred dancer.

Kaci, Kacie (American) forms of Kacey, Kacy.
Kasci, Kaycie, Kaysie

Kacia (Greek) a short form of Acacia.

Kadedra (American) a combination of Kady + Dedra.

Kadejah (Arabic) a form of Kadijah.

Kadelyn (American) a combination of Kady + Lynn.

Kadesha (American) a combination of Kady + Aisha.

Kadie (English) a form of Kady.

Kadijah (Arabic) trustworthy.

Kadisha (American) a form of Kadesha.

Kady (English) a form of Katy. A combination of the initials K. + D. See also Cady.

Kaedé (Japanese) maple leaf.

Kaela (Hebrew, Arabic) beloved, sweetheart. A short form of Kalila, Kelila.
Kaelea, Kaeleah

Kaelee, Kaeli (American) forms of
Kaela.
Kaeleigh, Kaelie

Kaelin (American) a form of Kaelyn.
Kaeleen, Kaelene, Kaelinn, Kalan

Kaelyn (American) a combination of
Kae (see Kay) + Lynn. See also Caelin,
Kaylyn.
Kaelan, Kaelen, Kaelynn, Kaelynne

Kaetlyn (Irish) a form of Kaitlin.
Kaetlin, Kaetlynn

Kagami (Japanese) mirror.

Kahsha (Native American) fur robe.

Kai (Hawaiian) sea. (Hopi, Navaho)
willow tree.
Kae

Kaia (Greek) earth. Mythology: Gaea was
the earth goddess.

Kaila (Hebrew) laurel; crown.
Kailah, Kailea, Kaileah

Kailee, Kailey (American) familiar
forms of Kaila. Forms of Kaylee.
Kaile, Kaileigh, Kaili

Kailyn, Kailynn (American) forms of
Kaitlin.
Kaileen, Kailen, Kailene, Kailynne

Kairos (Greek) last, final, complete.
Mythology: the last goddess born to
Jupiter.
Kaira

Kaishawn (American) a combination of
Kai + Shawna.

Kaitlin (Irish) pure. See also Katelin.
*Kaitlan, Kaitland, Kaitleen, Kaitlen,
Kaitlind, Kaitlinn, Kaitlon*

Kaitlyn ★ (Irish) a form of Caitlyn.

Kaitlynn (Irish) a form of Caitlyn.
Kaitlynne

Kaiya (Japanese) forgiveness.

Kala (Arabic) a short form of Kalila. A
form of Cala.

Kalama (Hawaiian) torch.

Kalani (Hawaiian) chieftain; sky.

Kalare (Latin, Basque) bright; clear.

Kalea (Hawaiian) bright; clear.
Kailea, Kaileah, Kaylea, Kayleah

Kalee, Kaleigh, Kaley, Kalie
(American) forms of Caley, Kaylee.
Kalleigh, Kalley, Kally, Kaly

Kalei (Hawaiian) flower wreath.
Kaylei

Kalena (Hawaiian) pure. See also
Kalina.
Kaleena

Kalere (Swahili) short woman.

Kali (Hindi) the black one. (Hawaiian)
hesitating. Religion: a form of the
Hindu goddess Devi. See also Cali.
Kallee, Kalley, Kally, Kallye, Kaly

Kalia (Hawaiian) a form of Kalea.

Kalifa (Somali) chaste; holy.

Kalila (Arabic) beloved, sweetheart. See
also Kaela.

Kalina (Slavic) flower. (Hawaiian) a form
of Karen. See also Kalena.

Kalinda (Hindi) sun.

Kalisa (American) a combination of Kate + Lisa.

Kalisha (American) a combination of Kate + Aisha.

Kaliska (Moquelumnan) coyote chasing deer.

Kallan (Slavic) stream, river.
Kalan

Kalle (Finnish) a form of Carol.

Kalli, Kallie (Greek) forms of Callie. Familiar forms of Kalliope, Kallista, Kalliyan.
Kallee, Kalley, Kallita, Kally

Kalliope (Greek) a form of Calliope.

Kallista (Greek) a form of Callista.

Kalliyan (Cambodian) best.

Kaltha (English) marigold, yellow flower.

Kaluwa (Swahili) forgotten one.

Kalyca (Greek) rosebud.
Kaly

Kalyn, Kalynn (American) forms of Kaylyn.

Kama (Sanskrit) loved one. Religion: the Hindu god of love.

Kamala (Hindi) lotus.

Kamali (Mahona) spirit guide; protector.

Kamaria (Swahili) moonlight.

Kamata (Moquelumnan) gambler.

Kambria (Latin) a form of Cambria.

Kamea (Hawaiian) one and only; precious.

Kameke (Swahili) blind.

Kameko (Japanese) turtle child. Mythology: the turtle symbolizes longevity.

Kameron (American) a form of Cameron.

Kami (Japanese) divine aura. (Italian, North African) a short form of Kamila, Kamilah. See also Cami.
Kammi, Kammie, Kammy, Kamy

Kamila (Slavic) a form of Camila. See also Millie.
Kamille

Kamilah (North African) perfect.

Kamiya (Hawaiian) a form of Kamea.

Kamri (American) a short form of Kameron. See also Camri.

Kamryn (American) a short form of Kameron. See also Camryn.

Kanani (Hawaiian) beautiful.

Kanda (Native American) magical power.

Kandace, Kandice (Greek) glittering white; glowing. (American) forms of Candace, Candice.
Kandas, Kandess, Kandis, Kandise, Kandiss, Kandus, Kandyce, Kandys, Kandyse

Kandi (American) a familiar form of Kandace, Kandice. See also Candi.

Kandra (American) a form of Kendra. See also Candra.

Kane (Japanese) two right hands.

Kaneisha, Kanisha (American) forms of Keneisha.

Kanene (Swahili) a little important thing.

Kani (Hawaiian) sound.

Kanika (Mwera) black cloth.

Kannitha (Cambodian) angel.

Kanoa (Hawaiian) free.

Kanya (Hindi) virgin. (Tai) young lady. Religion: a form of the Hindu goddess Devi.

Kapri (American) a form of Capri.

Kapua (Hawaiian) blossom.

Kapuki (Swahili) first-born daughter.

Kara (Greek, Danish) pure.
Kaira, Kairah, Karalea, Karaleah, Karalee, Karalie

Karah (Greek, Danish) a form of Kara. (Irish, Italian) a form of Cara.
Karrah

Karalynn (English) a combination of Kara + Lynn.
Karalyn, Karalynne

Karelle (American) a form of Carol.

Karen (Greek) pure. See also Carey, Carina, Caryn.
Kaaren, Karaina, Karan, Karna, Karon, Karren, Karron, Kerron, Koren

Karena (Scandinavian) a form of Karen.

Karessa (French) a form of Caressa.

Kari (Greek) pure. (Danish) a form of Caroline, Katherine. See also Carey, Cari, Carrie.
Karee, Karey, Karie, Karrey, Karry, Kary

Kariane, Karianne (American) combinations of Kari + Ann.
Kariann, Karianna

Karida (Arabic) untouched, pure.

Karilynn (American) a combination of Kari + Lynn.
Karilyn, Karilynne

Karimah (Arabic) generous.

Karin (Scandinavian) a form of Karen.
Kaarin, Karinne, Karrin, Kerrin

Karina (Russian) a form of Karen.
Kaarina, Karinna, Karrina, Karryna, Karyna

Karine (Russian) a form of Karen.
Karrine, Karryne, Karyne

Karis (Greek) graceful.

Karissa (Greek) a form of Carissa.
Karese, Karesse, Karisa, Karisha, Karishma, Karisma, Karissimia, Kariza, Karrisa, Karrissa, Karyssa

Karla (German) a form of Carla. (Slavic) a short form of Karoline.
Karila, Karilla, Karle, Karlenn, Karlicka, Karlinka, Karlisha, Karlisia, Karlitha, Karlla, Karlon

Karlee, Karleigh (American) forms of Karley, Karly. See also Carlee.

Karlene, Karlyn (American) forms of Karla. See also Carleen.
Karleen, Karlen, Karlena, Karlign, Karlin, Karlina, Karlyan, Karlynn, Karlynne

Karley, Karly (Latin) little and strong. (American) forms of Carly.
Karlyan, Karlye

Karli, Karlie (American) forms of Karley, Karly. See also Carli.

Karlotte (American) a form of Charlotte. *Karlita, Karletta*

Karma (Hindi) fate, destiny; action.

Karmel (Hebrew) a form of Carmela.

Karmen (Latin) song. *Karman, Karmencita, Karmin, Karmina, Karmine, Karmita, Karmon, Karmyn, Karmyne*

Karolane (American) a combination of Karoll + Anne.

Karolina, Karoline (Slavic) forms of Caroline. See also Carolina. *Karleen, Karlen, Karlena, Karling*

Karoll (Slavic) a form of Carol. *Karilla, Karole*

Karolyn (American) a form of Carolyn. *Karalyn, Karalyna, Karalynne, Karilyn, Karilyna, Karilynne, Karlynn, Karlynne, Karolyna, Karolynn, Karolynne, Karrolyn, Karrolyna, Karrolynn, Karrolynne*

Karri, Karrie (American) forms of Carrie. *Karie, Karry, Kary*

Karsen, Karsyn (English) child of Kar. Forms of Carson.

Karuna (Hindi) merciful.

Karyn (American) a form of Karen. *Karyne, Karynn, Kerrynn, Kerrynne*

Kasa (Hopi) fur robe.

Kasandra (Greek) a form of Kassandra. *Kasander, Kasandria, Kasaundra, Kasondra, Kasoundra*

Kasey, Kasie (Irish) brave. (American) forms of Casey, Kacey. *Kaisee, Kaisie, Kasci, Kascy, Kasee, Kassey, Kasy, Kasya, Kaysci, Kaysea, Kaysee, Kaysey, Kaysi, Kaysie, Kaysy*

Kashawna (American) a combination of Kate + Shawna.

Kashmir (Sanskrit) Geography: a region located between India and Pakistan.

Kasi (Hindi) from the holy city.

Kasia (Polish) a form of Katherine. See also Cassia. *Kasienka, Kassia, Kasya*

Kasinda (Umbundu) our last baby.

Kassandra (Greek) a form of Cassandra. *Kassandr, Kassandre, Kassandré, Kassaundra, Kazandra, Khrisandra, Krisandra, Krissandra*

Kassi, Kassie (American) familiar forms of Kassandra, Kassidy. See also Cassie. *Kassey, Kassia, Kassy*

Kassidy (Irish) clever. (American) a form of Cassidy. *Kassadee, Kassadi, Kassadie, Kassadina, Kassady, Kasseday, Kassedee, Kassiddy, Kassidee, Kassidi, Kassidie, Kassity*

Katalina (Irish) a form of Caitlin. See also Catalina. *Kataleena, Katalin, Katalyn*

Katarina (Czech) a form of Katherine. *Kata, Katarin, Kataryna, Katrika*

Kate (Greek) pure. (English) a short form of Katherine. *Kait, Kata, Katica*

Katee, Katey (English) familiar forms of Kate, Katherine.

Katelin (Irish) a form of Caitlin. See also Kaitlin.
Kaetlin, Katalin, Katelan, Kateland, Kateleen, Katelen, Katelene, Katelind, Katelinn, Katelun

Katelyn ☀ (Irish) a form of Caitlin.

Katelynn (Irish) a form of Caitlin.
Kaetlynn, Kaetlynne, Kaytlynn, Kaytlynne

Katerina (Slavic) a form of Katherine.
Katerine, Katerini

Katharine (Greek) a form of Katherine.
Katharaine, Katharin, Katharina, Katharyn

Katherine ☀ (Greek) pure. See also Carey, Catherine, Ekaterina, Kara, Karen, Kari, Kasia, Katerina, Yekaterina.
Ekatrinna, Kasienka, Kasin, Kat, Katchen, Kathann, Kathanne, Kathereen, Katheren, Katherene, Katherenne, Katherin, Katherina, Katheryn, Katheryne, Kathyrine, Katina, Katlaina, Katoka, Katreeka

Kathi, Kathy (English) familiar forms of Katherine, Kathleen. See also Cathi.
Kaethe, Katha, Kathe, Kathee, Kathey, Kathie, Katla, Kató

Kathleen (Irish) a form of Katherine. See also Cathleen.
Katheleen, Kathelene, Kathileen, Kathlyn, Kathlyne, Kathlynn, Katleen

Kathrine (Greek) a form of Katherine.

Kathryn (English) a form of Katherine.
Kathren, Kathryne

Kati (Estonian) a familiar form of Kate.
Katja

Katia, Katya (Russian) forms of Katherine.
Cattiah, Kattiah

Katie ☀ (English) a familiar form of Kate.
Kayte

Katilyn (Irish) a form of Katlyn.

Katlin (Irish) a form of Katlyn.

Katlyn (Greek) pure. (Irish) a form of Katelin.
Kaatlain, Katland, Katlynd, Katlynn, Katlynne

Katriel (Hebrew) God is my crown.
Katrelle, Katri

Katrina (German) a form of Katherine. See also Catrina, Trina.
Katreen, Katreena, Katrene, Katri, Katrice, Katricia, Katrien, Katrin, Katrine, Katrinia, Katriona, Katryn, Katryna, Kattrina, Kattryna

Katy (English) a familiar form of Kate. See also Cady.
Kayte

Kaulana (Hawaiian) famous.

Kaveri (Hindi) Geography: a sacred river in India.

Kavindra (Hindi) poet.

Kawena (Hawaiian) glow.

Kay (Greek) rejoicer. (Teutonic) a fortified place. (Latin) merry. A short form of Katherine.
Caye, Kae, Kaye

Kaya (Hopi) wise child. (Japanese) resting place.

Kaycee (American) a combination of the initials K. + C.
Kaysee, Kaysey, Kaysi, Kaysie

Kaydee (American) a combination of the initials K. + D.

Kayla ⚜ (Arabic, Hebrew) laurel; crown. A form of Kaela, Kaila. See also Cayla.
Kaylea, Kaylia

Kaylah (Arabic, Hebrew) a form of Kayla.
Kayleah, Kaylia

Kaylan, Kaylen (Hebrew) forms of Kayleen.

Kaylee ⚜ (American) a form of Kayla. See also Caeley, Kalee.
Kayle

Kayleen, Kaylene (Hebrew) beloved, sweetheart. Forms of Kayla.

Kayleigh (American) a form of Kaylee.
Kaylei

Kayley, Kayli, Kaylie (American) forms of Kaylee.

Kaylin (American) a form of Kaylyn.
Kaylon

Kaylyn, Kaylynn (American) combinations of Kay + Lynn. See also Kaelyn.
Kaylynne

Kaytlin, Kaytlyn (Irish) forms of Kaitlin.
Kaytlynn, Kaytlynne

Keaira (Irish) a form of Keara.

Keala (Hawaiian) path.

Keana, Keanna (German) bold; sharp. (Irish) beautiful.

Keandra, Keondra (American) forms of Kenda.

Keara (Irish) dark; black. Religion: an Irish saint.
Kearia, Kearra, Keera, Keerra, Kera

Kearsten, Keirsten (Greek) forms of Kirstin.
Keirstan

Keeley, Keely (Irish) forms of Kelly.
Kealee, Kealey, Keali, Kealie, Keallie, Kealy, Keela, Keelan, Keelee, Keeleigh, Keeli, Keelie, Keellie, Keighla, Keilee, Keileigh, Keiley, Keilly, Kiela, Kieley, Kielly, Kiely

Keelyn (Irish) a form of Kellyn.
Kealyn, Keelin, Keilan, Kielyn

Keena (Irish) brave.
Keenya

Keesha (American) a form of Keisha.

Kei (Japanese) reverent.

Keiana, Keianna (Irish) forms of Keana. (American) forms of Kiana.

Keiki (Hawaiian) child.

Keiko (Japanese) happy child.

Keila (Arabic, Hebrew) a form of Kayla.

Keilani (Hawaiian) glorious chief.
Keilan

Keira (Irish) a form of Keara.
Keirra, Kera

Keisha (American) a short form of Keneisha.
Keishaun, Keishauna, Keishawn, Kiesha, Kisha, Kishanda

Keita (Scottish) woods; enclosed place.

Kekona (Hawaiian) second-born child.

Kelcey, Kelci, Kelcie (Scottish) forms
of Kelsey.
Kelcy

Kelila (Hebrew) crown, laurel. See also
Kaela, Kayla, Kalila.

Kelley (Irish) a form of Kelly.

Kelli, Kellie (Irish) familiar forms of
Kelly.
Keli, Kelia, Kellia, Kellisa

Kelly (Irish) brave warrior. See also
Caeley.
Kellye

Kellyanne (Irish) a combination of
Kelly + Anne.
Kelliann, Kellianne, Kellyann

Kellyn (Irish) a combination of Kelly +
Lyn.
*Kelleen, Kellen, Kellene, Kellina,
Kelline, Kellynn, Kellynne*

Kelsea (Scottish) a form of Kelsey.
Kelsa

Kelsey (Scandinavian, Scottish) ship
island. (English) a form of Chelsea.
*Kelda, Kellsee, Kellsei, Kellsey, Kellsie,
Kellsy, Kelsei, Keslie*

Kelsi, Kelsie, Kelsy (Scottish) forms
of Chelsea.

Kenda (English) water baby. (Dakota)
magical power.

Kendal (English) a form of Kendall.
Kendahl, Kendel, Kendele, Kindal

Kendall (English) ruler of the valley.
*Kendalla, Kendalle, Kendell,
Kendelle, Kendera, Kendia, Kinda,
Kindall, Kindi, Kindle, Kynda*

Kendra (English) a form of Kenda.
*Kendre, Kenndra, Kentra, Kentrae,
Kindra, Kyndra*

Kendyl (English) a form of Kendall.
Kendyle, Kendyll

Keneisha (American) a combination of
the prefix Ken + Aisha.

Kenenza (English) a form of Kennice.

Kenia (Hebrew) a form of Kenya.
Kennia

Kenisha (American) a form of Keneisha.

Kenna (Irish) a short form of Kennice.

Kennedy (Irish) helmeted chief. History:
John F. Kennedy was the thirty-fifth U.
S. president.

Kennice (English) beautiful.

Kenya (Hebrew) animal horn.
Geography: a country in Africa.
Keenya, Kenja

Kenyatta (American) a form of Kenya.

Kenzie (Scottish) light skinned. (Irish) a
short form of Mackenzie.
Kenzy, Kinzie

Keona, Keonna (Irish) forms of Keana.

Keosha (American) a short form of
Keneisha.

Kerani (Hindi) sacred bells. See also
Rani.
Kera

Keren (Hebrew) animal's horn.
Kerrin, Keryn

Kerensa (Cornish) a form of Karenza.

Keri, Kerri, Kerrie (Irish) forms of Kerry.
Keriann, Kerianne, Kerriann, Kerrianne

Kerry (Irish) dark haired. Geography: a county in Ireland.
Keree, Kerey, Kerryann, Kerryanne

Kerstin (Scandinavian) a form of Kirsten.

Kesare (Latin) long haired. (Russian) a form of Caesar (see Boys' Names).

Kesha (American) a form of Keisha.

Keshia (American) a form of Keisha. A short form of Keneisha.
Kecia, Keishia, Keschia, Kesia, Kesiah, Kessiah

Kesi (Swahili) born during difficult times.

Kessie (Ashanti) chubby baby.

Kevyn (Irish) beautiful.

Keyana, Keyanna (American) forms of Kiana.

Keyara (Irish) a form of Kiara.

Keyona, Keyonna (American) forms of Kiana.

Keysha (American) a form of Keisha.

Keziah (Hebrew) cinnamon-like spice. Bible: one of the daughters of Job.

Khadijah (Arabic) trustworthy. History: Muhammed's first wife.
Khadeeja, Khadeja, Khadejha, Khadija

Khalida (Arabic) immortal, everlasting.

Khrissa (American) a form of Chrissa. (Czech) a form of Krista.
Khryssa, Krissa, Kryssa

Khristina (Russian, Scandinavian) a form of Kristina, Christina.

Ki (Korean) arisen.

Kia (African) season's beginning. (American) a short form of Kiana.
Kiah

Kiana (American) a combination of the prefix Ki + Ana.
Kiahna, Kiani, Kiandra, Kiandria, Kiauna, Kiaundra

Kianna (American) a form of Kiana.
Kianni

Kiara (Irish) little and dark.

Kiaria, Kiarra, Kichi (Japanese) fortunate.

Kiele (Hawaiian) gardenia; fragrant blossom.
Kiela, Kieley, Kielly

Kiera, Kierra (Irish) forms of Kerry.
Kierana, Kieranna, Kierea

Kiersten, Kierstin (Scandanavian) forms of Kirsten.
Keirstan

Kiki (Spanish) a familiar form of names ending in "queta."

Kiku (Japanese) chrysanthemum.

Kiley (Irish) attractive; from the straits.
Kilee, Kilie, Kyli

Kim (Vietnamese) needle. (English) a short form of Kimberly.
Kimette, Kym

Kimana (Shoshone) butterfly.

Kimber (English) a short form of
Kimberly.
Kimbra

Kimberlee, Kimberley (English)
forms of Kimberly.
*Kimbalee, Kimberlea, Kimberlei,
Kimberleigh, Kimbley*

Kimberly ☀ (English) chief, ruler.
*Cymbre, Kimba, Kimbely,
Kimbereley, Kimberely, Kimberli,
Kimberlie, Kimbery, Kimbria,
Kimbrie, Kimbry*

Kimberlyn (English) a form of
Kimberly.

Kimi (Japanese) righteous.
Kimmi, Kimmy

Kimmie (English) a familiar form of
Kimberly.
*Kimee, Kimme, Kimmee, Kimmi,
Kimmy, Kimy*

Kina (Hawaiian) from China.

Kineisha (American) a form of
Keneisha.

Kineta (Greek) energetic.

Kini (Hawaiian) a form of Jean.

Kinsey (English) offspring; relative.
Kinsee, Kinzie

Kinsley (American) a form of Kinsey.

Kioko (Japanese) happy child.

Kiona (Native American) brown hills.
Kionah, Kioni, Kionna

Kira (Persian) sun. (Latin) light.
Kiri, Kiria

Kiran (Hindi) ray of light.

Kirby (Scandinavian) church village.
(English) cottage by the water.

Kirima (Eskimo) hill.

Kirsi (Hindi) amaranth blossoms.

Kirsta (Scandinavian) a form of Kirsten.

Kirsten (Greek) Christian; anointed.
(Scandinavian)
a form of Christine.
*Karsten, Keirstan, Kirsteni, Kirstan,
Kirstene, Kirston, Kjersten, Kursten,
Kyrsten*

Kirstin (Scandinavian) a form of
Kirsten.
Karstin, Kirsteen, Kirstien, Kirstine

Kirstie, Kirsty (Scandinavian) familiar
forms of Kirsten.

Kirstyn (Greek) a form of Kirsten.

Kisa (Russian) kitten.
Kisha

Kishi (Japanese) long and happy life.

Kissa (Ugandan) born after twins.

Kita (Japanese) north.

Kitra (Hebrew) crowned.

Kitty (Greek) a familiar form of
Katherine.

Kiwa (Japanese) borderline.

Kiyana (American) a form of Kiana.

Kizzy (American) a familiar form of
Keziah.

Klara (Hungarian) a form of Clara.

Klarise (German) a form of Klarissa.

Klarissa (German) clear, bright.
   (Italian) a form of Clarissa.

Klaudia (American) a form of Claudia.

Kloe (American) a form of Chloe.

Kodi (American) a form of Codi.

Koffi (Swahili) born on Friday.

Koko (Japanese) stork. See also Coco.

Kolby (American) a form of Colby.

Kolina (Swedish) a form of Katherine.
   See also Colleen.

Kona (Hawaiian) lady. (Hindi) angular.

Konstance (Latin) a form of Constance.

Kora (Greek) a form of Cora.
   Koren

Koral (American) a form of Coral.

Kori (American) a short form of Korina.
   See also Corey, Cori.
   *Koree, Korey, Koria, Korie, Korri,
   Korrie, Korry, Kory*

Korina (Greek) a form of Corina.

Korine (Greek) a form of Korina.

Kornelia (Latin) a form of Cornelia.

Kortney (English) a form of Courtney.
   *Kortnay, Kortnee, Kortni, Kortnie,
   Kortny*

Kosma (Greek) order; universe.

Kosta (Latin) a short form of Constance.

Koto (Japanese) harp.

Kourtney (American) a form of
   Courtney.
   Kourtni, Kourtny, Kourtynie

Kris (American) a short form of Kristine.
   A form of Chris.

Krissy (American) a familiar form of
   Kris.

Krista (Czech) a form of Christina. See
   also Christa.
   *Khrista, Khryssa, Khrysta, Krissa,
   Kryssa*

Kristal (Latin) a form of Crystal.
   Kristale, Kristall, Kristill, Kristl, Kristle

Kristan (Greek) a form of Kristen.

Kristen (Greek) Christian; anointed.
   (Scandinavian)
   a form of Christine.
   Kristene, Kristien

Kristi, Kristie (Scandinavian) short
   forms of Kristine.

Kristian, Kristiana (Greek) Christian;
   anointed. Forms of Christian.
   *Khristian, Kristiane, Kristiann, Kristi-
   Ann, Kristianna, Kristianne, Kristi-
   Anne, Kristienne, Kristyan, Kristyana,
   Kristy-Ann, Kristy-Anne*

Kristin (Scandinavian) a form of
   Kristen. See also Cristen.
   Kristiin

Kristina (Greek) Christian; anointed.
   (Scandinavian) a form of Christina. See
   also Cristina.
   Kristeena, Kristena

Kristine (Scandinavian) a form of
   Christine.
   Kristeen, Kristene, Krystine, Krystyne

Kristy (American) a familiar form of
   Kristine, Krystal. See also Cristy.
   Kristia, Krysia, Krysti

Kristyn (Greek) a form of Kristen.

Krysta (Polish) a form of Krista.
Krystka

Krystal (American) clear, brilliant glass.
Kristabel, Krystalann, Krystalanne,
Krystale, Krystall, Krystil, Krystol

Krystalee (American) a combination of
Krystal + Lee.

Krystalynn (American) a combination
of Krystal + Lynn.
Krystaleen, Krystalina

Krystel (Latin) a form of Krystal.
Kristel, Kristell, Kristelle, Krystelle

Krysten (Greek) a form of Kristen.
Krystyne

Krystian, Krystiana (Greek) forms of
Christian.
Krystianna, Kristyana

Krystin (Czech) a form of Kristin.

Krystina (Greek) a form of Kristina.
Krysteena, Krystena, Krystyna

Krystle (American) a form of Krystal.
Krystl, Krystyl

Kudio (Swahili) born on Monday.

Kuma (Japanese) bear. (Tongan) mouse.

Kumiko (Japanese) girl with braids.

Kumuda (Sanskrit) lotus flower.

Kuniko (Japanese) child from the country.

Kunto (Twi) third-born.

Kuri (Japanese) chestnut.

Kusa (Hindi) God's grass.

Kwanita (Zuni) a form of Juanita.

Kwashi (Swahili) born on Sunday.

Kwau (Swahili) born on Thursday.

Kyana (American) a form of Kiana.

Kyara (Irish) a form of Kiara.

Kyla (Irish) attractive. (Yiddish) crown;
laurel.
Kylea, Kyleah, Kylia

Kyle (Irish) attractive.
Kial

Kylee (Irish) a familiar form of Kyle.
Kylea, Kyleah

Kyleigh (Irish) a form of Kyle.

Kylene (Irish) a form of Kyle.
Kylen, Kylyn, Kylynn

Kylie ☘ (West Australian Aboriginal)
curled stick; boomerang. (Irish) a
familiar form of Kyle.
Keiley, Keilley, Keilly, Keily, Kye, Kyli

Kymberly (English) a form of Kimberly.
Kymberlee, Kymberley, Kymberlie,
Kymberlyn

Kyndal, Kyndall (English) forms of
Kendall.

Kynthia (Greek) a form of Cynthia.

Kyoko (Japanese) mirror.

Kyra (Greek) ladylike. A form of Cyrilla.
Keera, Kyrah, Kyrene, Kyria, Kyriah,
Kyriann, Kyrie

L

Lacey, Lacy (Latin) cheerful. (Greek) familiar forms of Larissa.
Lacee

Lachandra (American) a combination of the prefix La + Chandra.

Laci, Lacie (Latin) forms of Lacey.

Lacrecia (Latin) a form of Lucretia.

Lada (Russian) Mythology: the Slavic goddess of beauty.

Ladasha (American) a combination of the prefix La + Dasha.

Ladeidra (American) a combination of the prefix La + Deidra.

Ladonna (American) a combination of the prefix La + Donna.
Ladon, Ladona, Ladonne, Ladonya

Laela (Arabic, Hebrew) a form of Leila.

Lahela (Hawaiian) a form of Rachel.

Laila (Arabic) a form of Leila.
Laili, Lailie

Laine, Layne (French) short forms of Elaine.
Laina, Lainee

Lainey, Layney (French) familiar forms of Elaine.

Lajila (Hindi) shy, coy.

Lajuana (American) a combination of the prefix La + Juana.

Laka (Hawaiian) attractive; seductive; tame. Mythology: the goddess of the hula.

Lakayla (American) a combination of the prefix La + Kayla.

Lakeisha (American) a combination of the prefix La + Keisha. See also Lekasha.
Lakaiesha, Lakaisha, Lakasha, Lakecia, Lakeesh, Lakeesha, Lakeysha, Lakezia, Lakicia, Lakieshia

Laken, Lakin, Lakyn (American) short forms of Lakendra.

Lakendra (American) a combination of the prefix La + Kendra.
Lakanda, Lakedra

Lakenya (American) a combination of the prefix La + Kenya.

Lakesha, Lakeshia, Lakisha (American) forms of Lakeisha.
Lakecia, Lakeesha, Lakeseia, Lakeshya, Lakesia, Lakeyshia, Lakiesha

Laketa (American) a combination of the prefix La + Keita.
Laketia, Lakita, Lakitia

Lakia (Arabic) found treasure.

Lakota (Dakota) a tribal name.

Lakresha (American) a form of Lucretia.

Lakya (Hindi) born on Thursday.

Lala (Slavic) tulip.

Lalasa (Hindi) love.

Laleh (Persian) tulip.

Lali (Spanish) a form of Lulani.

Lalita (Greek) talkative. (Sanskrit) charming; candid.

Lallie (English) babbler.

Lamesha (American) a combination of the prefix La + Mesha.

Lamia (German) bright land.

Lamis (Arabic) soft to the touch.

Lamonica (American) a combination of the prefix La + Monica.

Lamya (Arabic) dark lipped.

Lan (Vietnamese) flower.

Lana (Latin) woolly. (Irish) attractive, peaceful. A short form of Alana, Elana. (Hawaiian) floating; bouyant.
Lanae, Lanata, Lanay, Laneetra, Lanette, Lanna, Lannah

Landa (Basque) another name for the Virgin Mary.

Landon (English) open, grassy meadow.

Landra (German, Spanish) counselor.

Lane (English) narrow road.
Laina

Laneisha (American) a combination of the prefix La + Keneisha.

Laney (English) a familiar form of Lane.
Lanny

Lani (Hawaiian) sky; heaven. A short form of Atalanta, 'Aulani, Leilani.
Lanita, Lannie

Laporsha (American) a combination of the prefix La + Porsha.

Laqueena (American) a combination of the prefix La + Queenie.

Laquinta (American) a combination of the prefix La + Quintana.

Laquisha (American) a combination of the prefix La + Queisha.
Laquasha, Laquaysha, Laqueisha, Laquesha, Laquiesha

Laquita (American) a combination of the prefix La + Queta.
Laqeita, Laqueta, Laquetta, Laquia, Laquiata, Laquitta

Lara (Greek) cheerful. (Latin) shining; famous. Mythology: a Roman nymph. A short form of Laraine, Larissa, Laura.
Larah, Laretta, Larette

Laraine (Latin) a form of Lorraine.
Lauraine, Laurraine

Larina (Greek) seagull.

Larisa (Greek) a form of Larissa.
Laris

Larissa (Greek) cheerful. See also Lacey.
Laryssa

Lark (English) skylark.

Lashae, Lashay (American) combinations of the prefix La + Shay.

Lashana (American) a combination of the prefix La + Shana.
Lashanay, Lashane, Lashanna, Lashannon, Lashona, Lashonna

Lashanda (American) a combination of the prefix La + Shanda.
Lashandra, Lashanta, Lashante

Lashawna (American) a combination of the prefix La + Shawna.
Lashaun, Lashauna, Lashaune,

Lashaunna, Lashaunta, Lashawn, Lashawnd, Lashawnda, Lashawndra, Lashawne, Lashawnia, Leshawn, Leshawna

Lashonda (American) a combination of the prefix La + Shonda.
Lachonda, Lashaunda, Lashaundra, Lashon, Lashond, Lashonde, Lashondia, Lashondra, Lashonta, Lashunda, Lashundra, Lashunta, Lashunte, Leshande, Leshandra, Leshondra, Leshundra

Latanya (American) a combination of the prefix La + Tanya.
Latana, Latandra, Latania, Latanja, Latanna, Latanua, Latonshia

Latara (American) a combination of the prefix La + Tara.

Latasha (American) a combination of the prefix La + Tasha.
Latacha, Latacia, Latai, Lataisha, Latashia, Lataysha, Letasha, Letashia, Letasiah

Latavia (American) a combination of the prefix La + Tavia.

Lateefah (Arabic) pleasant. (Hebrew) pat, caress.

Latesha (American) a form of Leticia.
Lataeasha, Lateasha, Lateashia, Latecia, Lateicia, Lateisha, Latesa, Lateshia, Latessa, Latisa, Latissa, Leteisha, Leteshia

Latia (American) a combination of the prefix La + Tia.
Latea, Lateia, Lateka

Latika (Hindi) elegant.
Lateka

Latisha (Latin) joy. (American) a combination of the prefix La + Tisha.
Laetitia, Laetizia, Latashia, Lateasha, Lateashia, Latecia, Lateesha, Lateicia, Lateisha, Latice, Laticia, Latiesha, Latishia, Latissha, Latitia

Latona (Latin) Mythology: the powerful goddess who bore Apollo and Diana.
Latonna

Latonya (American) a combination of the prefix La + Tonya. (Latin) a form of Latona.
Latoni, Latonia

Latoria (American) a combination of the prefix La + Tori.
Latoira, Latorio, Latorja, Latorray, Latorreia, Latory, Latorya, Latoyra, Latoyria

Latosha (American) a combination of the prefix La + Tosha.
Latoshia, Latosia

Latoya (American) a combination of the prefix La + Toya.
Latoia, Latoiya, Latoye, Latoyia, Latoyita, Latoyo

Latrice (American) a combination of the prefix La + Trice.
Latrece, Latreece, Latreese, Latresa, Latrese, Latressa, Letreece, Letrice

Latricia (American) a combination of the prefix La + Tricia.
Latrecia, Latresh, Latresha, Latreshia, Latrica, Latrisha, Latrishia

Laura (Latin) crowned with laurel.
Lauralee, Laurelen, Laurella, Lauricia, Laurka, Lavra, Loura

Laurel (Latin) laurel tree.
Laural, Laurell, Laurelle, Lorel

Lauren ☙ (English) a form of Laura.
Laureen, Laurena, Laurene, Laurin

Laurence (Latin) crowned with laurel.

Laurianna (English) a combination of
Laurie + Anna.
*Laureana, Laureen, Lauriana,
Lauriane, Laurina*

Laurie (English) a familiar form of
Laura.
*Lari, Larilia, Laure, Lauré, Lauri,
Lawrie*

Laury (English) a familiar form of
Laura.

Lauryn (English) a familiar form of
Laura.
Laurynn

Laveda (Latin) cleansed, purified.

Lavelle (Latin) cleansing.

Lavena (Irish, French) joy. (Latin) a
form of Lavina.

Laverne (Latin) springtime. (French)
grove of alder trees. See also Verna.

Lavina (Latin) purified; woman of
Rome. See also Vina.

Lavonna (American) a combination of
the prefix La + Yvonne.

Lawan (Tai) pretty.

Lawanda (American) a combination of
the prefix La + Wanda.
Lawynda

Layce (American) a form of Lacey.

Layla (Hebrew, Arabic) a form of Leila.
Layli, Laylie

Le (Vietnamese) pearl.

Lea (Hawaiian) Mythology: the goddess
of canoe makers. (Hebrew) a form of
Leah.

Leah ☙ (Hebrew) weary. Bible: the first
wife of Jacob. See also Lia.
Léa, Leea, Leeah, Leia

Leala (French) faithful, loyal.

Lean, Leann, Leanne (English) forms
of Leeann, Lian.
Leana, Leane

Leandra (Latin) like a lioness.
*Leanda, Leandre, Leandrea,
Leandria, Leeanda, Leeandra*

Leanna, Leeanna (English) forms of
Liana.
Leana, Leianna

Leanore (Greek) a form of Eleanor.
(English) a form of Helen.

Lecia (Latin) a short form of Felecia.
Leshia

Leda (Greek) lady. Mythology: the queen
of Sparta and the mother of Helen of
Troy.

Lee (Chinese) plum. (Irish) poetic.
(English) meadow. A short form of
Ashley, Leah.

Leeann, Leeanne (English) combinations of Lee + Ann. Forms of Lian.
Leane, Leean, Leian, Leiann, Leianne

Leena (Estonian) a form of Helen.
(Greek, Latin, Arabic) a form of Lina.

Leeza (Hebrew) a short form of Aleeza.
(English) a form of Lisa, Liza.
Leesa

Lei (Hawaiian) a familiar form of
Leilani.

Leigh, Leigha (English) forms of Leah.
Leighann, Leighanna, Leighanne

Leiko (Japanese) arrogant.

Leila (Hebrew) dark beauty; night.
(Arabic) born at night. See also Laela,
Layla, Lila.
*Leela, Leelah, Leilah, Leilia, Lela,
Lelah, Leland, Leyla*

Leilani (Hawaiian) heavenly flower;
heavenly child.
Lelani, Lelania

Lekasha (American) a form of
Lakeisha.

Leli (Swiss) a form of Magdalen.

Lelia (Greek) fair speech. (Hebrew,
Arabic) a form of Leila.

Lelya (Russian) a form of Helen.

Lena (Hebrew) dwelling or lodging.
(Latin) temptress. (Norwegian) illustrious. (Greek) a short form of
Eleanor. Music: Lena Horne, a well-
known African American singer and
actress.
Lenah, Lenee, Leni, Lenka, Linah

Lenci (Hungarian) a form of Helen.

Lene (German) a form of Helen.
Leni

Leneisha (American) a combination of
the prefix Le + Keneisha.

Lenia (German) a form of Leona.
Lenea

Lenita (Latin) gentle.
Lenette

Lenore (Greek, Russian) a form of
Eleanor.

Leona (German) brave as a lioness. See
also Lona.
*Leoine, Leola, Leolah, Leone, Leonelle,
Leonia, Leonice, Leonicia, Leonissa,
Liona*

Leonie (German) a familiar form of
Leona.
Léonie

Leonore (Greek) a form of Eleanor. See
also Nora.

Leontine (Latin) like a lioness.
Leonine

Leora (Hebrew) light. (Greek) a familiar
form of Eleanor. See also Liora.

Leotie (Native American) prairie flower.

Lera (Russian) a short form of Valera.

Lesley (Scottish) gray fortress.
Leslea, Leslee, Lezlee, Lezley

Leslie (Scottish) a form of Lesley.
Lesli, Lesslie, Lezli

Lesly (Scottish) a form of Lesley.
Leslye, Lezly

Leta (Latin) glad. (Swahili) bringer.
(Greek) a short form of Aleta.

Leticia (Latin) joy. See also Latisha,
Tisha.
*Laticia, Leisha, Leshia, Let, Leteshia,
Letha, Lethia, Letice, Letichia, Letisha,
Letisia, Letita, Letitia, Letiza, Letizia,
Letycia, Loutitia*

Letty (English) a familiar form of
Leticia.

Levana (Hebrew) moon; white. (Latin)
risen. Mythology: the goddess of newborn babies.

Levani (Fijian) anointed with oil.

Levia (Hebrew) joined, attached.

Levina (Latin) flash of lightning.

Levona (Hebrew) spice; incense.

Lewana (Hebrew) a form of Levana.

Lexandra (Greek) a short form of Alexandra.

Lexi, Lexie (Greek) familiar forms of Alexandra.

Lexia (Greek) a familiar form of Alexandra.

Lexis (Greek) a short form of Alexius, Alexus.

Lexus (Greek) a short form of Alexis.

Leya (Spanish) loyal. (Tamil) the constellation Leo.
Leyla

Lia (Greek) bringer of good news. (Hebrew, Dutch, Italian) dependent. See also Leah.
Liah

Lian (Chinese) graceful willow. (Latin) a short form of Gillian, Lillian.

Liana, Lianna (Latin) youth. (French) bound, wrapped up; tree covered with vines. (English) meadow. (Hebrew) short forms of Eliana.

Liane, Lianne (Hebrew) short forms of Eliane. (English) forms of Lian.

Libby (Hebrew) a familiar form of Elizabeth.

Liberty (Latin) free.

Licia (Greek) a short form of Alicia.
Lycia

Lida (Greek) happy. (Slavic) loved by people. (Latin) a short form of Alida, Elita.

Lide (Latin, Basque) life.

Lidia (Greek) a form of Lydia.
Lidi, Lidija, Lidiya, Lidka

Lien (Chinese) lotus.

Liesabet (German) a short form of Elizabeth.

Liese (German) a familiar form of Elise, Elizabeth.
Liesa

Liesel (German) a familiar form of Elizabeth.
Lisel

Lila (Arabic) night. (Hindi) free will of God. (Persian) lilac. A short form of Dalila, Delilah, Lillian.
Lilah, Lylah

Lilac (Sanskrit) lilac; blue purple.

Lilia (Persian) a form of Lila.
Lili

Lilian (Latin) a form of Lillian.
Liliane

Liliana (Latin) a form of Lillian.
Lileana

Lilibeth (English) a combination of Lily + Beth.

Lilith (Arabic) of the night; night demon. Mythology: the first wife of Adam, according to ancient Jewish legends.

Lillian ☀ (Latin) lily flower.
Lil, Lilas, Lileane, Lilias, Liliha, Lilja, Lilla, Lilli, Lillia, Lillianne, Lis, Liuka

Lillyann (English) a combination of Lily + Ann. (Latin) a form of Lillian.

Lily ☀ (Latin, Arabic) a familiar form of Lilith, Lillian, Lillyann.
Lil, Lîle, Lili, Lilie, Lilijana, Lilika, Lilike, Liliosa, Lilium, Lilka, Lille, Lilli, Lillie, Lilly

Limber (Tiv) joyful.

Lin (Chinese) beautiful jade. (English) a form of Lynn.
Linn

Lina (Greek) light. (Arabic) tender. (Latin) a form of Lena.

Linda (Spanish) pretty.
Lind, Linita

Lindsay (English) a form of Lindsey.
Linsay

Lindsey (English) linden tree island; camp near the stream.
Lind, Lindsea, Lindsee

Lindsi (American) a familiar form of Lindsay, Lindsey.
Lindsie, Lindsy, Lindzy

Lindy (Spanish) a familiar form of Linda.
Lindee, Lindey, Lindi, Lindie

Linette (Welsh) idol. (French) bird.
Lanette, Linet, Linnet, Linnetta, Linnette

Ling (Chinese) delicate, dainty.

Linnea (Scandinavian) lime tree. Botany: the national flower of Sweden.
Linea, Linnaea, Lynea, Lynnea

Linsey (English) a form of Lindsey.
Linsi, Linsie, Linsy, Linzee, Linzey, Linzi, Linzy

Liolya (Russian) a form of Helen.

Liora (Hebrew) light. See also Leora.

Lirit (Hebrew) poetic; lyrical, musical.

Liron (Hebrew) my song.

Lisa (Hebrew) consecrated to God. (English) a short form of Elizabeth.
Liesa, Liisa, Lisa-Marie, Litsa, Lysa

Lisbeth (English) a short form of Elizabeth.

Lise (German) a form of Lisa.

Lisette, Lissette (French) forms of Lisa. (English) familiar forms of Elise, Elizabeth.
Liseta, Lisetta, Lisettina

Lisha (Arabic) darkness before midnight. (Hebrew) a short form of Alisha, Elisha, Ilisha.

Lissa (Greek) honey bee. A short form of Elissa, Elizabeth, Melissa, Millicent.
Lyssa

Lissie (American) a familiar form of Allison, Elise, Elizabeth.

Lita (Latin) a familiar form of names ending in "lita."

Litonya (Moquelumnan) darting hummingbird.

Liv (Latin) a short form of Livia, Olivia.

Livana (Hebrew) a form of Levana.

Livia (Hebrew) crown. A familiar form of Olivia. (Latin) olive.

Liviya (Hebrew) brave lioness; royal crown.

Livona (Hebrew) a form of Levona.

Liz (English) a short form of Elizabeth.

Liza (American) a short form of Elizabeth.
Lizka, Lyza

Lizabeta (Russian) a form of Elizabeth.

Lizabeth (English) a short form of Elizabeth.

Lizbeth (English) a short form of Elizabeth.

Lizet, Lizette (French) forms of Lisette.
Lizete

Lizina (Latvian) a familiar form of Elizabeth.

Lizzy (American) a familiar form of Elizabeth.
Lizzie

Logan (Irish) meadow.

Lois (German) famous warrior.

Lola (Spanish) a familiar form of Carlotta, Dolores, Louise.

Lolita (Spanish) sorrowful. A familiar form of Lola.
Lulita

Lolly (English) sweet; candy. A familiar form of Laura.

Lolotea (Zuni) a form of Dorothy.

Lomasi (Native American) pretty flower.

Lona (Latin) lioness. (English) solitary. (German) a short form of Leona.

London (English) fortress of the moon. Geography: the capital of the United Kingdom.

Loni (American) a form of Lona.
Lonee, Lonie, Lonnie

Lora (Latin) crowned with laurel. (American) a form of Laura.
Lorah, Lorane, Lorann, Lorra, Lorrah, Lorrane

Lore (Basque) flower. (Latin) a short form of Flora.

Lorelei (German) alluring. Mythology: the siren of the Rhine River who lured sailors to their deaths. See also Lurleen.

Lorelle (American) a form of Laurel.

Loren (American) a form of Lauren.
Loreen, Lorne, Lorren, Lorrin, Lorryn, Loryn, Lorynn, Lorynne

Lorena (English) a form of Lauren.
Lorene, Lorenia, Lorenna, Lorina, Lorrina, Lorrine

Lorenza (Latin) a form of Laura.

Loretta (English) a familiar form of Laura.
Larretta, Lauretta, Laurette, Loretah, Lorette, Lorita, Lorretta, Lorrette

Lori (Latin) crowned with laurel. (French) a short form of Lorraine. (American) a familiar form of Laura.
Loree, Lorey, Loria, Lorianna, Lorianne, Lorie, Lorree, Lorrie, Lory

Lorin (American) a form of Loren.
Lorine

Lorinda (Spanish) a form of Laura.

Loris (Latin) thong. (Dutch) clown. (Greek) a short form of Chloris.

Lorna (Latin) crowned with laurel. Literature: probably coined by Richard Blackmore in his novel *Lorna Doone*.
Lorrna

Lorraine (Latin) sorrowful. (French) from Lorraine, a former province of France. See also Rayna.
Lorain, Loraine, Lorayne, Lorein, Loreine, Lorine, Lorrain, Lorraina, Lorrayne, Lorreine

Lotte (German) a short form of Charlotte.

Lotus (Greek) lotus.

Lou (American) a short form of Louise, Luella.
Lu

Louam (Ethiopian) sleep well.

Louisa (English) a familiar form of Louise. Literature: Louisa May Alcott was an American writer and reformer best known for her novel *Little Women*.
Eloisa, Heloisa, Louisian, Louisane, Louisina, Louiza, Luiza, Lujza, Lujzika

Louise (German) famous warrior. See also Alison, Eloise, Heloise, Lois, Lola, Ludovica, Luella, Lulu.
Loise, Louisette, Louisiane, Louisine, Lowise, Loyce, Loyise, Luise

Lourdes (French) from Lourdes, France. Religion: a place where the Virgin Mary was said to have appeared.

Love (English) love, kindness, charity.

Lovisa (German) a form of Louisa.

Luann (Hebrew, German) graceful woman warrior. (Hawaiian) happy; relaxed. (American) a combination of Louise + Ann.
Lu

Luanna (German) a form of Luann.

Lubov (Russian) love.

Lucerne (Latin) lamp; circle of light. Geography: the Lake of Lucerne is in Switzerland.

Lucero (Latin) a form of Lucerne.

Lucetta (English) a familiar form of Lucy.

Lucia (Italian, Spanish) a form of Lucy.
Luciana, Lucianna

Lucie (French) a familiar form of Lucy.

Lucille (English) a familiar form of Lucy.
Lucila, Lucile, Lucilla

Lucinda (Latin) a form of Lucy. See also Cindy.
Lucka, Lucky

Lucine (Arabic) moon. (Basque) a form of Lucy.
Lucienne

Lucita (Spanish) a form of Lucy.

Lucretia (Latin) rich; rewarded.

Lucrezia (Italian) a form of Lucretia. History: Lucrezia Borgia was the Duchess of Ferrara and a patron of learning and the arts.

Lucy (Latin) light; bringer of light.
Luca, Luce, Luci, Lucida, Luciya, Lucya, Luzca, Luzi

Ludmilla (Slavic) loved by the people. See also Mila.

Ludovica (German) a form of Louise.
Ludovika, Ludwiga

Luella (English) elf. (German) a familiar form of Louise.
Lula

Luisa (Spanish) a form of Louisa.

Lulani (Polynesian) highest point of heaven.

Lulu (Arabic) pearl. (English) soothing, comforting. (Native American) hare. (German) a familiar form of Louise, Luella.
Lula

Luna (Latin) moon.

Lupe (Latin) wolf. (Spanish) a short form of Guadalupe.

Lupita (Latin) a form of Lupe.

Lurleen, Lurlene (Scandinavian) war horn. (German) forms of Lorelei.

Lusa (Finnish) a form of Elizabeth.

Lusela (Moquelumnan) like a bear swinging its foot when licking it.

Luvena (Latin, English) little; beloved.

Luyu (Moquelumnan) like a pecking bird.

Luz (Spanish) light. Religion: Nuestra Señora de Luz—Our Lady of the Light—is another name for the Virgin Mary.
Luzi, Luzija

Lycoris (Greek) twilight.

Lyda (Greek) a short form of Lidia, Lydia.

Lydia (Greek) from Lydia, an ancient land in Asia. (Arabic) strife.
Lidija, Lidiya, Lydie, Lydië

Lyla (French) island. (English) a form of Lyle (see Boys' Names). (Arabic, Hindi, Persian) a form of Lila.
Lilah

Lynda (Spanish) pretty. (American) a form of Linda.
Lynde, Lynnda

Lyndell (English) a form of Lynelle.
Lyndall, Lyndel, Lyndella

Lyndi (Spanish) a familiar form of Lynda.
Lyndee, Lindie, Lyndy, Lynndie, Lynndy

Lyndsay (American) a form of Lindsay.
Lyndsaye

Lyndsey (English) linden tree island; camp near the stream. (American) a form of Lindsey.
Lyndsea, Lyndsee, Lyndsi, Lyndsie, Lyndsy, Lynndsie

Lynelle (English) pretty.

Lynette (Welsh) idol. (English) a form of Linette.
Lynett, Lynetta, Lynnet, Lynnette

Lynn, Lynne (English) waterfall; pool below a waterfall.
Linn, Lyn, Lynlee, Lynley, Lynna, Lynnea

Lynnell (English) a form of Lynelle.

Lynsey (American) a form of Lyndsey.
Lynnsey, Lynnzey, Lynsie, Lynsy, Lynzey, Lynzi, Lynzie, Lynzy

Lyra (Greek) lyre player.

Lysandra (Greek) liberator.

Lysanne (American) a combination of Lysandra + Anne.
Lisanne

M

Mab (Irish) joyous. (Welsh) baby. Literature: queen of the fairies.

Mabel (Latin) lovable. A short form of Amabel.
Maybelle

Macawi (Dakota) generous; motherly.

Macayla (American) a form of Michaela.

Macey, Macie, Macy (Polish) familiar forms of Macia.

Machaela (Hebrew) a form of Michaela.

Machiko (Japanese) fortunate child.

Macia (Polish) a form of Miriam.

Mackenna (American) a form of Mackenzie.

Mackenzie ☀ (Irish) child of the wise leader. See also Kenzie.
Macenzie, Mackensi, Mackensie, Mackenzee, Mackenzi, Mackenzia, Mackenzy, Mekenzie, Mykenzie

Mackinsey (Irish) a form of Mackenzie.

Mada (English) a short form of Madaline, Magdalen.
Mahda

Madaline (English) a form of Madeline.
Madailéin, Madaleine

Madalyn (Greek) a form of Madeline.
Madalynn, Madalynne

Maddie (English) a familiar form of Madeline.

Maddison (English) a form of Madison.

Madelaine (French) a form of Madeline.
Madelayne

Madeleine (French) a form of Madeline.

Madelena (English) a form of Madeline.
Madalaina, Madalena, Maddalena, Madelina

Madeline ☀ (Greek) high tower. See also Lena, Lina, Maud.
Madel, Madelene, Madelia, Madella, Madelle, Madelon, Madlen, Madlin, Madline, Madlyn

Madelyn (Greek) a form of Madeline.
Madelynn, Madelynne, Madlyn

Madge (Greek) a familiar form of Madeline, Margaret.

Madilyn (Greek) a form of Madeline.

Madisen (English) a form of Madison.
Madissen

Madison ☀ (English) good; child of Maud.

Madisyn (English) a form of Madison.

Madolyn (Greek) a form of Madeline.
Madoline

Madonna (Latin) my lady.

Madrona (Spanish) mother.

Madyson (English) a form of Madison.
Madysen

Mae (English) a form of May. History:
Mae Jemison was the first African
American woman in space.

Maegan (Irish) a form of Megan.
Maeghan

Maeko (Japanese) honest child.

Maeve (Irish) joyous. Mythology: a
legendary Celtic queen. See also Mavis.

Magali, Magaly (Hebrew) from the
high tower.

Magan, Magen (Greek) forms of
Megan.
Maggen, Maggin

Magda (Czech, Polish, Russian) a form
of Magdalen.
Mahda, Makda

Magdalen (Greek) high tower. Bible:
Magdala was the home of Saint Mary
Magdalen. See also Madeline, Malena,
Marlene.
*Magdala, Magdalene, Magdaline,
Magdalyn, Magdalane, Magdelene,
Magdeline, Magdelyn, Magdlen,
Magdolna, Magola, Maighdlin,
Malaine*

Magdalena (Greek) a form of
Magdalen.
Magdalina, Magdelana, Magdelina

Magena (Native American) coming
moon.

Maggie (Greek) pearl. (English) a
familiar form of Magdalen, Margaret.
*Mag, Magge, Maggee, Maggi, Maggia,
Maggiemae, Mags*

Maggy, Meggy (English) forms of
Maggie.
Maggey

Magnolia (Latin) flowering tree. See
also Nollie.

Mahal (Filipino) love.

Mahala (Arabic) fat, marrow; tender.
(Native American) powerful woman.

Mahalia (American) a form of Mahala.

Maharene (Ethiopian) forgive us.

Mahesa (Hindi) great lord. Religion: a
name for the Hindu god Shiva.

Mahila (Sanskrit) woman.

Mahina (Hawaiian) moon glow.

Mahira (Hebrew) energetic.

Mahogony (Spanish) rich; strong.

Mai (Japanese) brightness. (Vietnamese)
flower. (Navajo) coyote.

Maia (Greek) mother; nurse. (English)
kinswoman; maiden. Mythology: the
loveliest of the Pleiades, the seven
daughters of Atlas, and the mother of
Hermes. See also Maya.
Maiah, Maie

Maida (English) maiden. (Greek) a
short form of Madeline.
Maydena

Maija (Finnish) a form of Mary.

Maika (Hebrew) a familiar form of
Michaela.

Maira, Maire (Irish) forms of Mary.

Maisie (Scottish) familiar forms of
Margaret.

Maita (Spanish) a form of Martha.

Maitlyn (American) a combination of Maita + Lynn.

Maiya (Greek) a form of Maia.

Maja (Arabic) a short form of Majidah.

Majidah (Arabic) splendid.

Makaela, Makaila (American) forms of Michaela.

Makala (Hawaiian) myrtle. (Hebrew) a form of Michaela.

Makana (Hawaiian) gift, present.

Makani (Hawaiian) wind.

Makara (Hindi) Astrology: another name for the zodiac sign Capricorn.

Makayla ❦ (American) a form of Michaela.

Makell (American) a short form of Makaela, Makala, Makayla.

Makenna (American) a form of Mackenna.

Makenzie (Irish) a form of Mackenzie.
Mekenzie, Mykenzie

Mala (Greek) a short form of Magdalen.

Malana (Hawaiian) bouyant, light.

Malaya (Filipino) free.
Malea, Maleah

Malena (Swedish) a familiar form of Magdalen.
Malinna

Malha (Hebrew) queen.

Mali (Tai) jasmine flower. (Tongan) sweet. (Hungarian) a short form of Malika.
Malea

Malia (Hawaiian, Zuni) a form of Mary. (Spanish) a form of Maria.
Malea, Maleah, Maleia, Maliasha, Malie, Maliea, Malli, Mally

Malika (Hungarian) industrious. (Arabic) queen.
Maleeka, Maleka, Maliaka

Malina (Hebrew) tower. (Native American) soothing. (Russian) raspberry.
Malinna

Malinda (Greek) a form of Melinda.
Malinde, Malinna, Malynda

Malini (Hindi) gardener.

Malissa (Greek) a form of Melissa.

Mallalai (Pashto) beautiful.

Malley (American) a familiar form of Mallory.
Malli, Mally

Mallorie (French) a form of Mallory.
Malerie, Mallari, Mallerie, Malloreigh, Mallori

Mallory (German) army counselor. (French) unlucky.
Maliri, Mallary, Mallauri, Mallery, Malloree, Mallorey, Malorym, Malree, Malrie, Mellory

Malorie, Malory (German) forms of Mallory.
Malori, Melorie, Melory

Malva (English) a form of Melba.

Malvina (Scottish) a form of Melvina. Literature: a name created by the eighteenth-century Romantic poet James Macpherson.

Mamie (American) a familiar form of Margaret.

Mamo (Hawaiian) saffron flower; yellow bird.

Mana (Hawaiian) psychic; sensitive.

Manar (Arabic) guiding light.

Manda (Spanish) woman warrior. (Latin) a short form of Amanda.

Mandara (Hindi) calm.

Mandeep (Punjabi) enlightened.

Mandisa (Xhosa) sweet.

Mandy (Latin) lovable. A familiar form of Amanda, Manda, Melinda.
Mandee, Mandi, Mandie

Manette (French) a form of Mary.

Mangena (Hebrew) song, melody.

Mani (Chinese) a mantra repeated in Tibetan Buddhist prayer to impart understanding.

Manka (Polish, Russian) a form of Mary.

Manon (French) a familiar form of Marie.

Manpreet (Punjabi) mind full of love.

Mansi (Hopi) plucked flower.

Manuela (Spanish) a form of Emmanuelle.

Manya (Russian) a form of Mary.

Mara (Hebrew) melody. (Greek) a short form of Amara. (Slavic) a form of Mary.
Mahra, Marah, Maralina, Maraline, Marra

Marabel (English) a form of Mirabel.

Maranda (Latin) a form of Miranda.

Maraya (Hebrew) a form of Mariah.

Marcela (Latin) a form of Marcella.
Marcele, Marcelia

Marcelen (English) a form of Marcella.

Marcella (Latin) martial, warlike. Mythology: Mars was the god of war.
Mairsil, Marca, Marce, Marceil, Marcell, Marcelle, Marcello, Marchella, Marchelle, Marciella, Marcile, Marcilla, Marcille, Marella, Marsella, Marselle, Marsiella

Marcena (Latin) a form of Marcella, Marcia.

Marci, Marcie (English) familiar forms of Marcella, Marcia.
Marca, Marcee, Marcita, Marsi, Marsie

Marcia (Latin) martial, warlike. See also Marquita.
Marchia, Marciale, Marcsa, Martia

Marciann (American) a combination of Marci + Ann.

Marcilynn (American) a combination of Marci + Lynn.

Marcy (English) a form of Marci.
Marsey, Marsy

Mardi (French) born on Tuesday. (Aramaic) a familiar form of Martha.

Mare (Irish) a form of Mary.

Marelda (German) renowned warrior.
Marella

Maren (Latin) sea. (Aramaic) a form of
Mary. See also Marina.
Marin, Marine, Miren

Maresa, Maressa (Latin) forms of
Marisa.

Maretta (English) a familiar form of
Margaret.

Margaret (Greek) pearl. History: Margaret
Hilda Thatcher served as British prime
minister. See also Gita, Greta, Gretchen,
Marjorie, Markita, Meg, Megan, Peggy,
Reet, Rita.
*Maergrethe, Marga, Marganit, Maretha,
Margarett, Margarette, Margarida,
Margaro, Margeret, Margeretta,
Margerette, Margetta, Margisia*

Margarit (Greek) a form of Margaret.
*Margalit, Margalith, Margarid,
Margaritt*

Margarita (Italian, Spanish) a form of
Margaret.
*Margareta, Margaretta, Margarida,
Margaritis, Margaritta, Margeretta,
Margharita, Margherita, Margrieta,
Margrita, Marguarita, Marguerita,
Margurita*

Margaux (French) a form of Margaret.

Marge (English) a short form of
Margaret, Marjorie.

Margery (English) a form of Margaret.
Margerie, Margorie

Margie (English) a familiar form of
Marge, Margaret.
Margey, Margi, Margy

Margit (Hungarian) a form of Margaret.
Marget, Margette

Margo, Margot (French) forms of
Margaret.
Mago, Margaro

Margret (German) a form of Margaret.
Margrieta, Margrita

Marguerite (French) a form of
Margaret.
*Margarete, Margaretha, Margarethe,
Margarite, Margerite, Marguaretta,
Marguarette, Marguarite,
Marguerette, Margurite*

Mari (Japanese) ball. (Spanish) a form
of Mary.

Maria ✿ (Hebrew) bitter; sea of bitter-
ness. (Italian, Spanish) a form of Mary.
*Maie, Marea, Mareah, Mariabella,
Mariae, Mariesa, Mariessa, Mariba,
Marija, Mariya, Mariyah*

Mariah ✿ (Hebrew) a form of Mary.
See also Moriah.
Maraia, Mariyah, Marriah, Meriah

Mariam (Hebrew) a form of Miriam.
Mariame, Mariem, Meryam

Marian (English) a form of Maryann.
*Mariann, Mariene, Marrian,
Marriann*

Mariana, Marianna (Spanish) forms
of Marian.
*Marriana, Marrianna, Maryana,
Maryanna*

Mariane, Marianne (English) forms
of Marian.
Marrianne

Maribel (French) beautiful. (English) a
combination of Maria + Bell.
*Marbelle, Mariabella, Maribella,
Maribelle, Marybel, Marybella,
Marybelle*

Marice (Italian) a form of Mary. See also Maris.
Marica, Marise, Marisse

Maricela (Latin) a form of Marcella.

Maridel (English) a form of Maribel.

Marie (French) a form of Mary.
Maree, Marie-Claude, Marie-Eve, Marie-Pier, Marrie

Mariel, Marielle (German, Dutch) forms of Mary.
Marial, Marieke, Mariele, Marieline, Mariellen, Marielsie, Mariely, Marielys

Mariela, Mariella (German, Dutch) forms of Mary.

Marietta (Italian) a familiar form of Marie.

Marieve (American) a combination of Mary + Eve.

Marigold (English) Mary's gold. Botany: a plant with yellow or orange flowers.

Marika (Dutch, Slavic) a form of Mary.
Marica, Marieke, Marija, Marijke, Marike, Marikia, Mariska, Mariske, Marrika, Maryk, Maryka, Merica, Merika

Mariko (Japanese) circle.

Marilee (American) a combination of Mary + Lee.
Merrili

Marilla (Hebrew, German) a form of Mary.
Marella, Marelle

Marilou (American) a form of Marylou.

Marilyn (Hebrew) Mary's line of descendants. See also Merilyn.
Maralin, Maralyn, Maralyne, Maralynn, Maralynne, Marelyn, Marilin, Marillyn, Marilynn, Marilynne, Marolyn, Marralynn, Marrilin, Marrilyn, Marrilynn, Marrilynne, Marylin, Marylinn, Marylyn, Marylyne, Marylynn, Marylynne

Marina (Latin) sea. See also Maren.
Marena, Marenka, Marinda, Marindi, Marinka, Marrina, Maryna, Merina, Mirena

Marini (Swahili) healthy; pretty.

Marion (French) a form of Mary.
Marrian, Marrion, Maryon, Maryonn

Maris (Latin) sea. (Greek) a short form of Amaris, Damaris. See also Marice.
Marise, Maryse

Marisa (Latin) sea.
Mariesa, Mariessa, Mariza, Marrisa, Marrissa, Marysa, Maryse, Merisa

Marisela (Latin) a form of Marisa.
Mariseli, Marisella, Marishelle

Marisha (Russian) a familiar form of Mary.
Marishenka, Marishka, Mariska

Marisol (Spanish) sunny sea.
Marise, Marizol

Marissa ☀ (Latin) a form of Maris, Marisa.
Marisse, Marrissa, Marrissia, Morissa

Marit (Aramaic) lady.

Marita (Spanish) a form of Marisa. (Aramaic) a form of Marit.
Marité

Maritza (Arabic) blessed.
Maritsa

Mariyan (Arabic) purity.
Mariya, Mariyah

Marja (Finnish) a form of Mary.

Marjan (Persian) coral. (Polish) a form of Mary.

Marjie (Scottish) a familiar form of Marjorie.
Marje

Marjolaine (French) marjoram.

Marjorie (Greek) a familiar form of Margaret. (Scottish) a form of Mary.
Majorie, Margeree, Margerey, Margerie, Margorie, Margory, Marjarie, Marjary, Marjerie, Marjery, Marjorey, Marjori, Marjory

Markayla (American) a combination or Mary + Kayla.
Marka

Markeisha (English) a combination of Mary + Keisha.

Markita (Czech) a form of Margaret.
Marka, Markeda, Markee, Markeeta, Marketa, Marketta, Markia, Markie, Markieta, Markitha, Markketta

Marla (English) a short form of Marlena, Marlene.
Marlah, Marlea, Marleah

Marlana (English) a form of Marlena.
Marlaina, Marlania, Marlanna

Marlee (English) a form of Marlene.
Marlea, Marleah

Marlena (German) a form of Marlene.
Marlaina, Marlanna, Marleena, Marlina, Marlinda, Marlyna, Marna

Marlene (Greek) high tower. (Slavic) a form of Magdalen.
Marlaine, Marlane, Marlayne, Marleen, Marlenne, Marline, Marlyne

Marley (English) a familiar form of Marlene.
Marli, Marlie, Marly

Marlis (English) a combination of Maria + Lisa.

Marlo (English) a form of Mary.

Marlyn (Hebrew) a short form of Marilyn. (Greek, Slavic) a form of Marlene.

Marmara (Greek) sparkling, shining.

Marni (Hebrew) a form of Marnie.

Marnie (Hebrew) a short form of Marnina.
Marna, Marne, Marnee, Marney, Marnja, Marnya

Marnina (Hebrew) rejoice.

Maroula (Greek) a form of Mary.

Marquise (French) noblewoman.

Marquisha (American) a form of Marquise.

Marquita (Spanish) a form of Marcia.
Marqueda, Marquedia, Marquee, Marqueita, Marquet, Marqueta, Marquetta, Marquette, Marquia, Marquida, Marquietta, Marquitra, Marquitia, Marquitta

Marrim (Chinese) tribal name in Manpur state.

Marsala (Italian) from Marseilles, France.

Marsha (English) a form of Marcia.
Marcha, Marshae, Marshay,
Marshayly, Marshel, Marshele,
Marshell, Marshia, Marshiela

Marta (English) a short form of Martha,
Martina.
Martá, Martä, Marte, Martia,
Martitaha, Merta

Martha (Aramaic) lady; sorrowful. Bible:
a friend of Jesus. See also Mardi.
Martaha, Marth, Marthan, Marthe,
Marthy, Marticka, Martita, Martus,
Martuska, Masia

Marti (English) a familiar form of
Martha, Martina.

Martina (Latin) martial, warlike. See
also Tina.
Martel, Martella, Martelle, Martene,
Marthena, Marthina, Marthine,
Martine, Martinia, Martino,
Martisha, Martosia, Martoya,
Martricia, Martrina, Martyna,
Martyne, Martynne

Martiza (Arabic) blessed.

Maru (Japanese) round.

Maruca (Spanish) a form of Mary.

Marvella (French) marvelous.

Mary ✖ (Hebrew) bitter; sea of bitter-
ness. Bible: the mother of Jesus. See also
Maija, Malia, Maren, Mariah, Marjorie,
Maura, Maureen, Miriam, Mitzi, Moira,
Mollie, Muriel.
Maree, Marella, Marelle, Maricara,
Mariquilla, Mariquita, Marye,
Maryla, Marynia, Mavra, Meridel,
Mirja, Morag, Moya

Marya (Arabic) purity; bright whiteness.

Maryam (Hebrew) a form of Miriam.

Maryann, Maryanne (English) combinations of Mary + Ann.
Meryem

Marybeth (American) a combination of
Mary + Beth.
Maribeth, Maribette

Maryellen (American) a combination
of Mary + Ellen.
Mariellen

Maryjane (American) a combination of
Mary + Jane.

Maryjo (American) a combination of
Mary + Jo.

Marykate (American) a combination of
Mary + Kate.

Marylou (American) a combination of
Mary + Lou.

Maryssa (Latin) a form of Marissa.
Maryse, Marysia

Masago (Japanese) sands of time.

Masani (Luganda) gap toothed.

Masha (Russian) a form of Mary.

Mashika (Swahili) born during the
rainy season.

Matana (Hebrew) gift.

Mathena (Hebrew) gift of God.

Mathilde (German) a form of Matilda.

Matilda (German) powerful battler. See
also Maud, Tilda, Tillie.

Matrika (Hindi) mother. Religion: a
name for the Hindu goddess Shakti in
the form of the letters of the alphabet.

Matsuko (Japanese) pine tree.

Mattea (Hebrew) gift of God.
Matte

Mattie, Matty (English) familiar forms of Martha, Matilda.
Matte, Mattey, Matti, Mattye

Matusha (Spanish) a form of Matilda.

Maud, Maude (English) short forms of Madeline, Matilda. See also Madison.
Maudlin

Maura (Irish) dark. A form of Mary, Maureen. See also Moira.
Maure, Maurette, Mauricette, Maurita

Maureen (French) dark. (Irish) a form of Mary.
Maurene, Maurine, Mo, Moreen, Morene, Morine, Morreen, Moureen

Maurelle (French) dark; elfin.

Maurise (French) dark skinned; moor; marshland.
Maurita, Maurizia

Mausi (Native American) plucked flower.

Mauve (French) violet colored.

Mavis (French) thrush, songbird. See also Maeve.
Mavra

Maxie (English) a familiar form of Maxine.
Maxi, Maxy

Maxine (Latin) greatest.
Max, Maxa, Maxeen, Maxena, Maxene, Maxima, Maxime, Maximiliane, Maxina, Maxna, Maxyne

May (Latin) great. (Arabic) discerning. (English) flower; month of May. See also Mae, Maia.
Maj, Mayberry, Maybeth, Mayday, Maydee, Maydena, Maye, Mayela, Mayella, Mayetta, Mayrene

Maya ★ (Hindi) God's creative power. (Greek) mother; grandmother. (Latin) great. A form of Maia.
Mayam

Maybeline (Latin) a familiar form of Mabel.

Maygan, Maygen (Irish) forms of Megan.

Maylyn (American) a combination of May + Lynn.

Mayoree (Tai) beautiful.

Mayra (Tai) a form of Mayoree.

Maysa (Arabic) walks with a proud stride.

Maysun (Arabic) beautiful.

Mazel (Hebrew) lucky.

Mckayla (American) a form of Makayla.

Mckell (American) a form of Makell.

Mckenna (American) a form of Mackenna.

Mckenzie (Scottish) a form of Mackenzie.
McKensi, Mekenzie

Mckinley (Irish) daughter of the learned ruler.

Mckinzie (American) a form of Mackenzie.

Mead, Meade (Greek) honey wine.

Meagan (Irish) a form of Megan.
*Meagain, Meagann, Meagen,
Meagin, Meagnah, Meagon*

Meaghan (Welsh) a form of Megan.
*Maeghan, Meaghann, Meaghen,
Meahgan*

Meara (Irish) mirthful.

Meda (Native American) prophet; priestess.

Medea (Greek) ruling. (Latin) middle.
Mythology: a sorceress who helped
Jason get the Golden Fleece.

Medina (Arabic) History: the site of
Muhammed's tomb.

Medora (Greek) mother's gift.
Literature: a character in Lord Byron's
poem *The Corsair*.

Meena (Hindi) blue semiprecious stone;
bird. (Greek, German, Dutch) a form of
Mena.

Meg (English) a short form of Margaret,
Megan.

Megan ✻ (Greek) pearl; great. (Irish)
a form of Margaret.
*Megean, Megen, Meggan, Meggen,
Megyn, Meygan*

Megane (Irish) a form of Megan.

Megara (Greek) first. Mythology:
Heracles's first wife.

Meggie (English) a familiar form of
Margaret, Megan.

Meghan (Welsh) a form of Megan.
*Meeghan, Meehan, Megha, Meghana,
Meghane, Meghann, Meghanne,
Meghean, Meghen, Mehgan, Mehgen*

Mehadi (Hindi) flower.

Mehira (Hebrew) speedy; energetic.

Mehitabel (Hebrew) benefited by trusting God.

Mehri (Persian) kind; lovable; sunny.

Mei (Hawaiian) great. (Chinese) a short
form of Meiying.

Meira (Hebrew) light.

Meit (Burmese) affectionate.

Meiying (Chinese) beautiful flower.

Meka (Hebrew) a familiar form of
Michaela.

Mekayla (American) a form of
Michaela.
Mekaela

Mel (Portuguese, Spanish) sweet as
honey.

Mela (Hindi) religious service. (Polish)
a form of Melanie.

Melana (Russian) a form of Melanie.

Melanie ✻ (Greek) dark skinned.
*Malania, Malanie, Meila, Meilani,
Meilin, Melaine, Melainie, Melane,
Melanee, Melaney, Melani, Melania,
Mélanie, Melanney, Melannie,
Melany, Melanya, Melasya, Melayne,
Melenia, Mella, Mellanie, Melya,
Milya*

Melantha (Greek) dark flower.

Melba (Greek) soft; slender. (Latin)
mallow flower.

Mele (Hawaiian) song; poem.

Melesse (Ethiopian) eternal.

Melia (German) a short form of Amelia.

Melina (Latin) canary yellow. (Greek) a
short form of Melinda.
*Melaina, Meleana, Meleena, Melena,
Meline, Melinia, Melinna, Melynna*

Melinda (Greek) honey. See also Linda,
Melina, Mindy.
*Maillie, Melinde, Melinder, Mellinda,
Molynda, Milinda, Milynda, Mylenda,
Mylinda, Mylynda*

Meliora (Latin) better.

Melisa (Greek) a form of Melissa.
*Melesa, Mélisa, Melise, Melisha,
Melishia, Melisia, Meliza, Melizah,
Mellisa, Milisa, Mylisa, Mylisia*

Melisande (French) a form of Melissa,
Millicent.

Melissa (Greek) honey bee. See also
Elissa, Lissa, Melisande, Millicent.
*Mallissa, Melessa, Meleta, Mélissa,
Melisse, Melissia, Mellie, Mellissa,
Molissia, Mollissa, Mylissa, Mylissia*

Melita (Greek) a form of Melissa.
(Spanish) a short form of Carmelita
(see Carmelit).

Melly (American) a familiar form of
names beginning with "Mel." See also
Millie.
Mellie

Melody (Greek) melody. See also Elodie.
*Meladia, Melodee, Melodey, Melodi,
Melodia, Melodie, Melodye*

Melonie (American) a form of Melanie.
*Melloney, Mellonie, Mellony, Melonee,
Meloney, Meloni, Melonnie, Melony*

Melosa (Spanish) sweet; tender.

Melvina (Irish) armored chief. See also
Malvina.

Melyne (Greek) a short form of
Melinda.
Melyn, Melynn, Melynne

Melyssa (Greek) a form of Melissa.

Mena (German, Dutch) strong. (Greek)
a short form of Philomena. History:
Menes is believed to be the first king of
Egypt.

Mendi (Basque) a form of Mary.

Meranda (Latin) a form of Miranda.

Mérane (French) a form of Mary.

Mercedes (Latin) reward, payment.
(Spanish) merciful.
Merced, Mercede, Mersade

Mercia (English) a form of Marcia.
History: an ancient British kingdom.

Mercy (English) compassionate, merciful. See also Merry.

Meredith (Welsh) protector of the sea.
*Meredithe, Meredy, Meredyth,
Meredythe, Meridath, Merideth, Meridie,
Meridith, Merridie, Merridith*

Meri (Finnish) sea. (Irish) a short form
of Meriel.

Meriel (Irish) shining sea.

Merilyn (English) a combination of
Merry + Lynn. See also Marilyn.

Merissa (Latin) a form of Marissa.
Merisa

Merle (Latin, French) blackbird.

Merry (English) cheerful, happy. A familiar form of Mercy, Meredith.
Merrili

Meryl (German) famous. (Irish) shining sea. A form of Meriel, Muriel.
Meral, Merel, Merrall, Merrell, Merril, Merrill, Merryl, Meryle, Meryll

Mesha (Hindi) another name for the zodiac sign Aries.

Meta (German) a short form of Margaret.

Mhairie (Scottish) a form of Mary.

Mia ❀ (Italian) mine. A familiar form of Michaela, Michelle.
Mea, Meah, Miah

Micaela (Hebrew) a form of Michaela.

Micah (Hebrew) a short form of Michaela. Bible: one of the Old Testament prophets.
Meecah, Mica, Myca, Mycah

Micayla, Michayla (Hebrew) forms of Michaela.

Michaela (Hebrew) who is like God?
Michael, Michaelann, Michealia, Michaelina, Michaeline, Michaell, Michaella, Michaelyn, Michaila, Michal, Micheal, Micheala, Michelia, Michelina, Michely, Michelyn, Micheyla, Micheline, Miquelle, Mycala, Mychael, Mychal

Michala (Hebrew) a form of Michaela.
Michela

Michele (Italian) a form of Michaela.
Michaelle, Michal, Michela

Michelle ❀ (French) who is like God? See also Shelley.
Macbealle, Machele, Machell, Machella, Machelle, Mechelle, Meichelle, Meschell, Meshell, Meshelle, Michel, Michèle, Michell, Michella, Michellene, Michellyn, Mischel, Mischelle, Mishael, Mishaela, Mishayla, Mishell, Mishelle, Mitchele, Mitchelle

Michi (Japanese) righteous way.

Micki (American) a familiar form of Michaela.

Midori (Japanese) green.

Mieko (Japanese) prosperous.

Mielikki (Finnish) pleasing.

Miette (French) small; sweet.

Migina (Omaha) new moon.

Mignon (French) dainty, petite; graceful.

Miguela (Spanish) a form of Michaela.
Micquel, Miquel, Miquela

Mika (Japanese) new moon. (Russian) God's child. (Native American) wise racoon. (Hebrew) a form of Micah. (Latin) a form of Dominica.
Mikah

Mikaela (Hebrew) a form of Michaela.
Mekaela, Mekala, Mickael, Mickaela, Mickala, Mickalla, Mickeel, Mickell, Mickelle, Mikail, Mikaila, Mikal, Mikalene, Mikalovna, Mikalyn, Mikea, Mikeisha, Mikeita, Mikel, Mikela, Mikele, Mikell, Mikella, Mikesha, Mikeya, Mikie, Mikiela, Mikkel, Mikyla

Mikala (Hebrew) a form of Michaela.
Mickala

Mikayla (American) a form of Mikaela.
Mickayla, Mikayle, Mikyla

Mikhaela (American) a form of Mikaela.

Miki (Japanese) flower stem.
Mikie

Mila (Russian) dear one. (Italian, Slavic) a short form of Camila, Ludmilla.

Milada (Czech) my love.

Milagros (Spanish) miracle.

Milana (Italian) from Milan, Italy. (Russian) a form of Melana.

Mildred (English) gentle counselor.
Mil, Mildrene, Mildrid

Milena (Greek, Hebrew, Russian) a form of Ludmilla, Magdalen, Melanie.

Mileta (German) generous, merciful.

Milia (German) industrious. A short form of Amelia, Emily.
Milya

Miliani (Hawaiian) caress.

Mililani (Hawaiian) heavenly caress.

Milissa (Greek) a form of Melissa.
Milisa

Milka (Czech) a form of Amelia.

Millicent (English) industrious. (Greek) a form of Melissa. See also Lissa, Melisande.

Millie, Milly (English) familiar forms of Amelia, Camille, Emily, Kamila, Melissa, Mildred, Millicent.

Mima (Burmese) woman.

Mimi (French) a familiar form of Miriam.

Mina (German) love. (Persian) blue sky. (Arabic) harbor. (Japanese) south. A short form of names ending in "mina."
Min

Minal (Native American) fruit.

Minda (Hindi) knowledge.

Mindy (Greek) a familiar form of Melinda.
Mindee, Mindi, Mindie, Mindyanne, Mindylee, Myndy

Mine (Japanese) peak; mountain range.

Minerva (Latin) wise. Mythology: the goddess of wisdom.

Minette (French) faithful defender.

Minka (Polish) a short form of Wilhelmina.

Minna (German) a short form of Wilhelmina.

Minnie (American) a familiar form of Mina, Minerva, Minna, Wilhelmina.

Minowa (Native American) singer.

Minta (English) Literature: originally coined by playwright Sir John Vanbrugh in his comedy *The Confederacy*.

Minya (Osage) older sister.

Mio (Japanese) three times as strong.

Mira (Latin) wonderful. (Spanish) look, gaze. A short form of Almira, Amira, Marabel, Mirabel, Miranda.
Mirra

Mirabel (Latin) beautiful.

Miracle (Latin) wonder, marvel.

Miranda (Latin) strange; wonderful; admirable. Literature: the heroine of Shakespeare's *The Tempest.* See also Randi.
Marenda, Miran, Miranada, Mirandia, Mirinda, Mirindé, Mironda, Mirranda, Muranda

Mireille (Hebrew) God spoke. (Latin) wonderful.
Mirella, Mirelle, Mirelys, Mireyda, Mirielle, Mirilla, Myrella, Myrilla

Mireya (Hebrew) a form of Mireille.

Miri (Gypsy) a short form of Miriam.

Miriam (Hebrew) bitter; sea of bitterness. Bible: the original form of Mary. See also Macia, Mimi, Mitzi.
Miram, Mirham, Miriain, Miriama, Miriame, Mirian, Mirit, Mirjam, Mirjana, Mirriam, Mirrian, Miryam, Miryan

Misha (Russian) a form of Michaela.
Mishae

Missy (English) a familiar form of Melissa, Millicent.
Missi, Missie

Misty (English) shrouded by mist.
Missty, Mistee, Mistey, Misti, Mistie, Mistin, Mistina, Mistral, Mistylynn, Mystee, Mysti, Mystie

Mitra (Hindi) Religion: god of daylight. (Persian) angel.

Mituna (Moquelumnan) like a fish wrapped up in leaves.

Mitzi (German) a form of Mary, Miriam.

Miwa (Japanese) wise eyes.

Miya (Japanese) temple.

Miyo (Japanese) beautiful generation.

Miyuki (Japanese) snow.

Moana (Hawaiian) ocean; fragrance.

Mocha (Arabic) chocolate-flavored coffee.

Modesty (Latin) modest.

Moesha (American) a short form of Monisha.

Mohala (Hawaiian) flowers in bloom.

Moira (Irish) great. A form of Mary. See also Maura.
Moirae, Moirah, Moire, Moya, Moyra, Moyrah

Molara (Basque) a form of Mary.

Mollie, Molly (Irish) familiar forms of Mary.
Moll, Mollee, Molley, Molli, Mollissa

Mona (Irish) noble. (Greek) a short form of Monica, Ramona, Rimona.
Moina, Monah, Mone, Monea, Monna, Moyna

Monet (French) Art: Claude Monet was a leading French impressionist remembered for his paintings of water lilies.
Monee

Monica (Greek) solitary. (Latin) advisor.
Monca, Monee, Monia, Monic, Monice, Monicia, Monicka, Monise, Monn, Monnica, Monnie, Monya

Monifa (Yoruba) I have my luck.

Monika (German) a form of Monica.

Monique (French) a form of Monica.
Moniqua, Moniquea, Moniquie, Munique

Monisha (American) a combination of Monica + Aisha.

Montana (Spanish) mountain. Geography: a U. S. state.

Mora (Spanish) blueberry.
Moria

Morela (Polish) apricot.

Morena (Irish) a form of Maureen.

Morgan ☀ (Welsh) seashore. Literature: Morgan le Fay was the half-sister of King Arthur.
Morgana, Morgance, Morgane, Morganetta, Morganette, Morganica, Morgann, Morganna, Morganne, Morgen, Morgyn, Morrigan

Morghan (Welsh) a form of Morgan.

Moriah (Hebrew) God is my teacher. (French) dark skinned. Bible: the mountain on which the Temple of Solomon was built. See also Mariah.
Moria, Moriel, Morit, Morria, Morriah

Morie (Japanese) bay.

Morowa (Akan) queen.

Morrisa (Latin) dark skinned; moor; marshland.
Morissa

Moselle (Hebrew) drawn from the water. (French) a white wine.

Mosi (Swahili) first-born.

Moswen (Tswana) white.

Mouna (Arabic) wish, desire.

Mrena (Slavic) white eyes.

Mumtaz (Arabic) distinguished.

Mura (Japanese) village.

Muriel (Arabic) myrrh. (Irish) shining sea. A form of Mary. See also Meryl.
Muire, Murial, Muriell, Murielle

Musetta (French) little bagpipe.

Muslimah (Arabic) devout believer.

Mya ☀ (Burmese) emerald. (Italian) a form of Mia.

Myesha (American) a form of Moesha.

Mykaela, Mykayla (American) forms of Mikaela.

Myla (English) merciful.

Mylene (Greek) dark.
Mylaine, Mylana, Mylee, Myleen

Myra (Latin) fragrant ointment.
Myrena, Myria

Myranda (Latin) a form of Miranda.

Myriam (American) a form of Miriam.
Myriame, Myryam

Myrna (Irish) beloved.

Myrtle (Greek) dark green shrub.

N

Nabila (Arabic) born to nobility.

Nadda (Arabic) generous; dewy.
Nada

Nadette (French) a short form of Bernadette.

Nadia (French, Slavic) hopeful.
Nadea, Nadezhda, Nadie, Nadiya,
Nadja, Nady, Nadya

Nadine (French, Slavic) a form of
Nadia.
Nadean, Nadeana, Nadeen, Nadena,
Nadene, Nadien, Nadina, Nadyne,
Naidene, Naidine

Nadira (Arabic) rare, precious.

Naeva (French) a form of Eve.

Nafuna (Luganda) born feet first.

Nagida (Hebrew) noble; prosperous.

Nahid (Persian) Mythology: another
name for Venus, the goddess of love and
beauty.

Nahimana (Dakota) mystic.

Naida (Greek) water nymph.

Naila (Arabic) successful.

Nairi (Armenian) land of rivers. History:
a name for ancient Armenia.

Naiya (Greek) a form of Naida.

Najam (Arabic) star.

Najila (Arabic) brilliant eyes.

Nakeisha (American) a combination of
the prefix Na + Keisha.

Nakeita (American) a form of Nikita.

Nakia (Arabic) pure.
Nakea, Nakeia

Nakita (American) a form of Nikita.
Nakkita, Naquita

Nalani (Hawaiian) calm as the heavens.

Nami (Japanese) wave.

Nan (German) a short form of
Fernanda. (English) a form of Ann.
Nanice, Nanine

Nana (Hawaiian) spring.

Nanci (English) a form of Nancy.
Nancie, Nancsi

Nancy (English) gracious. A familiar
form of Nan.
Nainsi, Nance, Nancee, Nancey,
Nancine, Nancye, Nanice, Nanncey,
Nanncy, Nanouk, Nansee, Nansey,
Nanuk

Nanette (French) a form of Nancy.
Nineta, Ninete, Ninetta, Ninette,
Ninita, Ninnetta, Ninnette, Nynette

Nani (Greek) charming. (Hawaiian)
beautiful.

Naomi (Hebrew) pleasant, beautiful.
Bible: Ruth's mother-in-law.
Naoma, Naomia, Naomy, Navit,
Neoma, Neomi, Noami, Nomi

Naomie (Hebrew) a form of Naomi.

Nara (Greek) happy. (English) north.
(Japanese) oak.

Narcissa (Greek) daffodil. Mythology:
Narcissus was the youth who fell in love
with his own reflection.

Narelle (Australian) woman from the
sea.

Nari (Japanese) thunder.

Narmada (Hindi) pleasure giver.

Nashawna (American) a combination
of the prefix Na + Shawna.

Nashota (Native American) double;
second-born twin.

Nastasia (Greek) a form of Anastasia.

Nasya (Hebrew) miracle.

Nata (Sanskrit) dancer. (Latin) swimmer. (Native American) speaker; creator. (Polish, Russian) a form of Natalie. See also Nadia.

Natacha (Russian) a form of Natasha.
Natachia, Natacia, Naticha

Natalee, Natali (Latin) forms of Natalie.
Nattlee

Natalia (Russian) a form of Natalie. See also Talia.
Nacia, Natala, Natalea, Nataliia, Natalija, Natalina, Natalja, Natalya, Nathalia

Natalie ☙ (Latin) born on Christmas day. See also Nata, Natasha, Noel, Talia.
Nat, Natalène, Natelie, Natilie, Natlie, Nattalie, Nattilie

Nataline (Latin) a form of Natalie.
Natalene, Natalyn

Natalle (French) a form of Natalie.

Nataly (Latin) a form of Natalie.

Natane (Arapaho) daughter.

Natania (Hebrew) gift of God.

Natara (Arabic) sacrifice.

Natasha (Russian) a form of Natalie. See also Stacey, Tasha.
Nahtasha, Natasa, Natascha, Natashah, Natashea, Natashia, Natashiea, Natashja, Natasia, Natassija, Natassja, Natasza, Natausha, Natawsha, Nathasha, Nathassha, Natisha, Natishia, Netasha, Notasha, Notosha

Natesa (Hindi) cosmic dancer. Religion: another name for the Hindu god Shiva.

Nathalie, Nathaly (Latin) forms of Natalie.
Nathalia

Natie (English) a familiar form of Natalie.
Nati, Natti, Nattie, Natty

Natosha (Russian) a form of Natasha.
Natoshia, Netosha, Notosha

Nava (Hebrew) beautiful; pleasant.
Navit

Nayely (Irish) a form of Neila.

Neala (Irish) a form of Neila.

Necha (Spanish) a form of Agnes.

Neci (Hungarian) fiery, intense.

Neda (Slavic) born on Sunday.

Nedda (English) prosperous guardian.

Neely (Irish) a familiar form of Neila, Nelia.

Neema (Swahili) born during prosperous times.

Neena (Spanish) a form of Nina.
Nena

Neila (Irish) champion. See also Neala, Neely.

Nekeisha (American) a form of Nakeisha.

Nekia (Arabic) a form of Nakia.

Nelia (Spanish) yellow. (Latin) a familiar form of Cornelia.
Neli

Nelle (Greek) stone.

Nellie, Nelly (English) familiar forms of Cornelia, Eleanor, Helen, Prunella. *Nel, Neli, Nell, Nella, Nelley, Nelli, Nellianne, Nellice, Nellis, Nelma*

Nenet (Egyptian) born near the sea. Mythology: Nunet was the goddess of the sea.

Neola (Greek) youthful.

Neona (Greek) new moon.

Nereida (Greek) a form of Nerine.

Nerine (Greek) sea nymph.

Nerissa (Greek) sea nymph. See also Rissa.

Nessa (Scandinavian) promontory. (Greek) a short form of Agnes. See also Nessie. *Nesha, Neshia, Nessia*

Nessie (Greek) a familiar form of Agnes, Nessa, Vanessa.

Neta (Hebrew) plant, shrub. See also Nettie.

Netis (Native American) trustworthy.

Nettie (French) a familiar form of Annette, Nanette, Antoinette.

Neva (Spanish) snow. (English) new. Geography: a river in Russia.

Nevada (Spanish) snow. Geography: a western U. S. state.

Nevaeh ☙ (American) the word *heaven* spelled backward.

Nevina (Irish) worshipper of the saint.

Neylan (Turkish) fulfilled wish.

Neza (Slavic) a form of Agnes.

Nia (Irish) a familiar form of Neila. Mythology: Nia Ben Aur was a legendary Welsh woman. *Niah*

Niabi (Osage) fawn.

Nichelle (American) a combination of Nicole + Michelle. Culture: Nichelle Nichols was the first African American woman featured in a television drama (*Star Trek*). *Nichele, Nishelle*

Nichole (French) a form of Nicole. *Nichol, Nichola, Nicholle*

Nicki (French) a familiar form of Nicole. *Nicci, Nickey, Nickeya, Nickia, Nickie, Nickiya, Nicky*

Nickole (French) a form of Nicole. *Nickol*

Nicola (Italian) a form of Nicole. *Nacola, Necola, Nichola, Nickola, Nicolea, Nicolla, Nikkola, Nikola, Nikolia, Nykola*

Nicole ☙ (French) a form of Nicholas. See also Colette, Cosette, Nikita. *Nacole, Necole, Nica, Nicia, Nicol, Nicoli, Nicolie, Niquole, Nocole*

Nicolette (French) a form of Nicole. *Nicholette, Nicoletta, Nikkolette, Nikoleta, Nikoletta, Nikolette*

Nicoline (French) a familiar form of Nicole.

Nicolle (French) a form of Nicole. *Nicholle*

Nida (Omaha) Mythology: an elflike creature.

Nidia (Latin) nest.

Niesha (American) pure.
(Scandinavian) a form of Nissa.
*Neisha, Neishia, Neissia, Nesha,
Neshia, Nesia, Nessia, Niessia*

Nige (Latin) dark night.

Nika (Russian) belonging to God.
Nikka

Nikayla, Nikelle (American) forms of
Nicole.

Nike (Greek) victorious. Mythology: the
goddess of victory.

Niki (Russian) a short form of Nikita.
(American) a familiar form of Nicole.
Nikia

Nikita (Russian) victorious people.
Nikkita, Niquita, Niquitta

Nikki (American) a familiar form of
Nicole, Nikita.
Nikia, Nikkey, Nikkia, Nikkie, Nikky

Nikole (French) a form of Nicole.
Nikkole, Nikola, Nikolle

Nila (Latin) Geography: the Nile River is
in Africa. (Irish) a form of Neila.

Nili (Hebrew) Botany: a pea plant that
yields indigo.

Nima (Hebrew) thread. (Arabic) blessing.

Nina (Hebrew) a familiar form of
Hannah. (Spanish) girl. (Native
American) mighty. (Hebrew) a familiar
form of Hannah.
Ninacska, Ninja, Ninosca, Ninoshka

Ninon (French) a form of Nina.

Nirel (Hebrew) light of God.

Nirveli (Hindi) water child.

Nisa (Arabic) woman.

Nisha (American) a form of Niesha,
Nissa.

Nishi (Japanese) west.

Nissa (Hebrew) sign, emblem.
(Scandinavian) friendly elf; brownie.
See also Nyssa.
Nissy

Nita (Hebrew) planter. (Choctaw) bear.
(Spanish) a short form of Anita,
Juanita.
Nitika

Nitara (Hindi) deeply rooted.

Nitasha (American) a form of Natasha.

Nitsa (Greek) a form of Helen.

Nituna (Native American) daughter.

Nitza (Hebrew) flower bud.

Nixie (German) water sprite.

Niya (Irish) a form of Nia.

Nizana (Hebrew) a form of Nitza.

Noel (Latin) Christmas. See also Natalie.
*Noël, Noela, Noeleen, Noelene,
Noelia, Noeline, Noelyn, Noelynn,
Noleen, Novelenn, Novelia, Nowel,
Noweleen, Nowell*

Noelani (Hawaiian) beautiful one from
heaven.
Noela

Noelle (French) Christmas.
Noell, Noella, Noelleen, Noellyn

Noemi (Hebrew) a form of Naomi.
Nohemi, Nomi

Noemie (Hebrew) a form of Noemi.

Noemy (Hebrew) a form of Noemi.

Noga (Hebrew) morning light.

Nohely (Latin) a form of Noel.

Nokomis (Dakota) moon daughter.

Nola (Latin) small bell. (Irish) famous; noble. A short form of Fionnula.

Noleta (Latin) unwilling.

Nollie (English) a familiar form of Magnolia.

Noma (Hawaiian) a form of Norma.

Nona (Latin) ninth.
Noni, Nonie

Noor (Aramaic) a form of Nura.

Nora (Greek) light. A familiar form of Eleanor, Honora, Leonore.
Norah

Noreen (Irish) a form of Eleanor, Nora. (Latin) a familiar form of Norma.
Noorin, Noreena, Noren, Norene, Norina, Norine, Nureen

Norell (Scandinavian) from the north.

Nori (Japanese) law, tradition.

Norma (Latin) rule, precept.
Normi, Normie

Nova (Latin) new. A short form of Novella, Novia. (Hopi) butterfly chaser. Astronomy: a star that releases bright bursts of energy.

Novella (Latin) newcomer.

Novia (Spanish) sweetheart.

Nu (Burmese) tender. (Vietnamese) girl.

Nuala (Irish) a short form of Fionnula.

Nuela (Spanish) a form of Amelia.

Nuna (Native American) land.

Nunciata (Latin) messenger.

Nura (Aramaic) light.

Nuria (Aramaic) the Lord's light.

Nurita (Hebrew) Botany: a flower with red and yellow blossoms.

Nuru (Swahili) daylight.

Nusi (Hungarian) a form of Hannah.

Nuwa (Chinese) mother goddess. Mythology: another name for Nü-gua, the creator of mankind.

Nya (Irish) a form of Nia.
Nyah

Nycole (French) a form of Nicole.

Nydia (Latin) nest.

Nyesha (American) a form of Niesha.

Nyla (Latin, Irish) a form of Nila.

Nyoko (Japanese) gem, treasure.

Nyomi (Hebrew) a form of Naomi.
Nyome

Nyree (Maori) sea.

Nyssa (Greek) beginning. See also Nissa.
Nissi, Nissy, Nysa

Nyusha (Russian) a form of Agnes.

O

Oba (Yoruba) chief, ruler.

Obelia (Greek) needle.

Oceana (Greek) ocean. Mythology: Oceanus was the god of the ocean.

Octavia (Latin) eighth. See also Tavia.
Octavice, Octavie, Octavienne, Octavise, Octivia, Ottavia

Odeda (Hebrew) strong; courageous.

Odele (Greek) melody, song.

Odelia (Greek) ode; melodic. (Hebrew) I will praise God. (French) wealthy. See also Odetta.

Odella (English) wood hill.

Odera (Hebrew) plough.

Odessa (Greek) odyssey, long voyage.

Odetta (German, French) a form of Odelia.

Odina (Algonquin) mountain.

Ofelia (Greek) a form of Ophelia.

Ofira (Hebrew) gold.

Ofra (Hebrew) a form of Aphra.

Ogin (Native American) wild rose.

Ohanna (Hebrew) God's gracious gift.

Okalani (Hawaiian) heaven.

Oki (Japanese) middle of the ocean.

Oksana (Latin) a form of Osanna.

Ola (Greek) a short form of Olesia.(Scandinavian) ancestor.

Olathe (Native American) beautiful.

Oleda (Spanish) a form of Alida. See also Leda.

Olena (Russian) a form of Helen.
Olenka

Olesia (Greek) a form of Alexandra.
Cesya

Oletha (Scandinavian) nimble.

Olethea (Latin) truthful. See also Alethea.

Olga (Scandinavian) holy. See also Helga, Olivia.
Olenka, Olia, Olva

Oliana (Polynesian) oleander.

Olina (Hawaiian) filled with happiness.

Olinda (Latin) scented. (Spanish) protector of property. (Greek) a form of Yolanda.

Olisa (Ibo) God.

Olive (Latin) olive tree.

Olivia ★ (Latin) a form of Olive. (English) a form of Olga. See also Liv, Livia.
Oliva, Olivea, Olivetta, Olivianne, Oliwia, Olva

Ollie (English) a familiar form of Olivia.
Olly, Ollye

Olwen (Welsh) white footprint.

Olympia (Greek) heavenly.

Olyvia (Latin) a form of Olivia.

Oma (Hebrew) reverent. (German) grandmother. (Arabic) highest.

Omaira (Arabic) red.

Omega (Greek) last, final, end. Linguistics: the last letter in the Greek alphabet.

Ona (Latin, Irish) a form of Oona, Una. (English) river.

Onatah (Iroquois) daughter of the earth and the corn spirit.

Onawa (Native American) wide awake.

Ondine (Latin) a form of Undine. *Ondina, Ondyne*

Ondrea (Czech) a form of Andrea.

Oneida (Native American) eagerly awaited.

Onella (Hungarian) a form of Helen.

Onesha (American) a combination of Ondrea + Aisha.

Oni (Yoruba) born on holy ground.

Onora (Latin) a form of Honora.

Oona (Latin, Irish) a form of Una.

Opa (Choctaw) owl. (German) grandfather.

Opal (Hindi) precious stone.

Ophelia (Greek) helper. Literature: Hamlet's love interest in the Shakespearean play *Hamlet*.

Oprah (Hebrew) a form of Orpah. *Ophra, Ophrah, Opra*

Ora (Latin) prayer. (Spanish) gold. (English) seacoast. (Greek) a form of Aura.

Orabella (Latin) a form of Arabella.

Oralee (Hebrew) the Lord is my light. See also Yareli.

Oralia (French) a form of Aurelia. See also Oriana.

Orea (Greek) mountains.

Orela (Latin) announcement from the gods; oracle.

Orenda (Iroquois) magical power.

Oretha (Greek) a form of Aretha.

Oriana (Latin) dawn, sunrise. (Irish) golden. *Ori*

Orina (Russian) a form of Irene.

Orinda (Hebrew) pine tree. (Irish) light skinned, white.

Orino (Japanese) worker's field. *Ori*

Oriole (Latin) golden; black-and-orange bird.

Orla (Irish) golden woman.

Orlanda (German) famous throughout the land.

Orlenda (Russian) eagle.

Orli (Hebrew) light.

Ormanda (Latin) noble. (German) mariner.

Ornice (Hebrew) cedar tree. (Irish) pale; olive colored.

Orpah (Hebrew) runaway. See also Oprah.

Orquidea (Spanish) orchid.

Orsa (Latin) a short form of Orseline. See also Ursa.

Ortensia (Italian) a form of Hortense.

Orva (French) golden; worthy. (English) brave friend.

Osanna (Latin) praise the Lord.

Osen (Japanese) one thousand.

Oseye (Benin) merry.

Osma (English) divine protector.

Otilie (Czech) lucky heroine.

Ovia (Latin, Danish) egg.

Owena (Welsh) born to nobility; young warrior.

Oya (Moquelumnan) called forth.

Oz (Hebrew) strength.

Ozara (Hebrew) treasure, wealth.

Paca (Spanish) a short form of Pancha. See also Paka.

Padget (French) a form of Page.

Padma (Hindi) lotus.

Page (French) young assistant.

Paige `*` (English) young child.

Paisley (Scottish) patterned fabric first made in Paisley, Scotland.

Paiton (English) warrior's town.

Paka (Swahili) kitten. See also Paca.

Pakuna (Moquelumnan) deer bounding while running downhill.

Palila (Polynesian) bird.

Pallas (Greek) wise. Mythology: another name for Athena, the goddess of wisdom.

Palma (Latin) palm tree.

Palmira (Spanish) a form of Palma.

Paloma (Spanish) dove. See also Aloma.

Pamela (Greek) honey.
Pam, Pama, Pamala, Pamalla, Pamelia, Pamelina, Pamella, Pamilla, Pammela, Pammi, Pammie, Pammy, Pamula

Pancha (Spanish) free; from France.

Pandita (Hindi) scholar.

Pandora (Greek) all-gifted. Mythology: a woman who opened a box out of curiosity and released evil into the world. See also Dora.

Pansy (Greek) flower; fragrant. (French) thoughtful.

Panthea (Greek) all the gods.

Panya (Swahili) mouse; tiny baby. (Russian) a familiar form of Stephanie.

Panyin (Fante) older twin.

Paola (Italian) a form of Paula.
Paolina

Papina (Moquelumnan) vine growing on an oak tree.

Paquita (Spanish) a form of Frances.

Pari (Persian) fairy eagle.

Paris (French) Geography: the capital of France. Mythology: the Trojan prince who started the Trojan War by abducting Helen.
Parice, Paries, Parisa, Pariss, Parissa

Parker (English) park keeper.

Parris (French) a form of Paris.

Parthenia (Greek) virginal.

Parveneh (Persian) butterfly.

Pascale (French) born on Easter or Passover.

Pasha (Greek) sea.

Passion (Latin) passion.

Pasua (Swahili) born by cesarean section.

Pat (Latin) a short form of Patricia, Patsy.

Pati (Moquelumnan) fish baskets made of willow branches.

Patia (Gypsy, Spanish) leaf. (Latin, English) a familiar form of Patience, Patricia.

Patience (English) patient.
Paciencia

Patra (Greek, Latin) a form of Petra.

Patrice (French) a form of Patricia.
Patrease, Patrece, Patreece, Patreice, Patriece, Patryce, Pattrice

Patricia (Latin) noblewoman. See also Payton, Peyton, Tricia, Trisha, Trissa.
Patresa, Patrica, Patriceia, Patricja, Patricka, Patrickia, Patrisha, Patrishia, Patrizia, Patrizzia

Patsy (Latin) a familiar form of Patricia.

Patty (English) a familiar form of Patricia.

Paula (Latin) small. See also Pavla, Polly.
Paliki, Paulane, Paulann, Paule, Paulla, Pavia

Paulette (Latin) a familiar form of Paula.
Pauletta, Paulita, Paullette

Paulina (Slavic) a form of Paula.
Paulene, Pawlina

Pauline (French) a form of Paula.
Pauleen, Paulene, Paulyne

Pausha (Hindi) lunar month of Capricorn.

Pavla (Czech, Russian) a form of Paula.

Paxton (Latin) peaceful town.

Payge (English) a form of Paige.

Payton (Irish) a form of Patricia.

Paz (Spanish) peace.

Pazi (Ponca) yellow bird.

Pazia (Hebrew) golden.

Peace (English) peaceful.

Pearl (Latin) jewel.
Pearle, Pearleen, Pearlena, Pearlene, Pearlette, Pearline, Perlette, Perline, Perlline

Peggy (Greek) a familiar form of
Margaret.
Peg, Pegeen, Pegg, Peggey, Peggi,
Peggie, Pegi

Peke (Hawaiian) a form of Bertha.

Pela (Polish) a short form of Penelope.

Pelagia (Greek) sea.

Pelipa (Zuni) a form of Philippa.

Pemba (Bambara) the power that con-
trols all life.

Penda (Swahili) loved.

Penelope (Greek) weaver. Mythology:
the clever and loyal wife of Odysseus, a
Greek hero.

Peni (Carrier) mind.

Peninah (Hebrew) pearl.

Penny (Greek) a familiar form of
Penelope, Peninah.
Penee, Penney, Penni, Pennie

Peony (Greek) flower.

Pepita (Spanish) a familiar form of
Josephine.

Pepper (Latin) condiment from the
pepper plant.

Perah (Hebrew) flower.

Perdita (Latin) lost. Literature: a character in Shakespeare's play *The Winter's*
Tale.

Perfecta (Spanish) flawless.

Peri (Greek) mountain dweller.
(Persian) fairy or elf.

Perla (Latin) a form of Pearl.
Pearla

Perlie (Latin) a familiar form of Pearl.
Pearlie

Pernella (Greek, French) rock. (Latin) a
short form of Petronella.

Perri (Greek, Latin) small rock; traveler.
(French) pear tree. (Welsh) child of
Harry.
Perry

Persephone (Greek) Mythology: the
goddess of the underworld.

Persis (Latin) from Persia.

Peta (Blackfoot) golden eagle.

Petra (Greek, Latin) small rock. A short
form of Petronella.
Pet, Petena, Peterina, Petrice, Petrina,
Petrine, Pietra

Petronella (Greek) small rock. (Latin)
of the Roman clan Petronius.

Petula (Latin) seeker.

Petunia (Native American) flower.

Peyton (Irish) a form of Patricia.

Phaedra (Greek) bright.

Phallon (Irish) a form of Fallon.

Phebe (Greek) a form of Phoebe.
Pheba, Pheby

Pheodora (Greek, Russian) a form of
Feodora.

Philana (Greek) lover of mankind.

Philantha (Greek) lover of flowers.

Philicia (Latin) a form of Phylicia.
Philica, Philycia

Philippa (Greek) lover of horses. See
also Filippa.
*Phil, Philipa, Philippe, Phillipina,
Phillippine, Phillie, Philly, Pippy*

Philomena (Greek) love song; loved
one. Bible: a first-century saint. See also
Filomena, Mena.

Phoebe (Greek) shining.
Phaebe, Phoebey

Phylicia (Latin) fortunate; happy.
(Greek) a form of Felicia.
*Phylecia, Phylesia, Phylisha, Phylisia,
Phyllecia, Phyllicia, Phyllisia*

Phyllida (Greek) a form of Phyllis.

Phyllis (Greek) green bough.
*Filise, Fillys, Fyllis, Philis, Phillis,
Philliss, Philys, Philyss, Phylis, Phylliss,
Phyllys*

Pia (Italian) devout.

Piedad (Spanish) devoted; pious.

Pier (French) a form of Petra.
Pierette, Pierrette

Pierce (English) a form of Petra.

Pilar (Spanish) pillar, column.

Ping (Chinese) duckweed. (Vietnamese)
peaceful.

Pinga (Eskimo) Mythology: the goddess
of game and the hunt.

Piper (English) pipe player.

Pippa (English) a short form of Phillipa.

Pippi (French) rosy cheeked.
Pippy

Pita (African) fourth daughter.

Placidia (Latin) serene.

Pleasance (French) pleasant.

Polla (Arabic) poppy.

Polly (Latin) a familiar form of Paula.
Pali, Pauli, Paulie, Pauly

Pollyam (Hindi) goddess of the plague.
Religion: the Hindu name invoked to
ward off bad spirits.

Pollyanna (English) a combination of
Polly + Anna. Literature: an overly
optimistic heroine created by Eleanor
Porter.

Poloma (Choctaw) bow.

Pomona (Latin) apple. Mythology: the
goddess of fruit and fruit trees.

Poni (African) second daughter.

Poppy (Latin) poppy flower.

Pora, Poria (Hebrew) fruitful.

Porcha (Latin) a form of Portia.
Porchai

Porscha, Porsche (German) forms of
Portia.
*Porcsha, Porcshe, Porsché, Porschea,
Porschia, Pourche*

Porsha (Latin) a form of Portia.
Porshai, Porshay, Porshe, Porshia

Portia (Latin) offering. Literature: the
heroine of Shakespeare's play *The
Merchant of Venice*.
Portiea

Precious (French) precious; dear.

Presley (English) priest's meadow.

Prima (Latin) first, beginning; first child.

Primavera (Italian, Spanish) spring.

Primrose (English) primrose flower.

Princess (English) daughter of royalty.
Princcess, Princetta, Princie, Princilla

Priscilla (Latin) ancient.
*Cilla, Piri, Precilla, Prescilla, Pricila,
Pricilla, Pris, Prisca, Priscella,
Priscila, Priscill, Priscille, Prisella,
Prisila, Prisilla, Prissilla, Prysilla*

Prissy (Latin) a familiar form of
Priscilla.

Priya (Hindi) beloved; sweet natured.

Procopia (Latin) declared leader.

Promise (Latin) promise, pledge.

Pru (Latin) a short form of Prudence.

Prudence (Latin) cautious; discreet.

Prudy (Latin) a familiar form of
Prudence.

Prunella (Latin) brown; little plum. See
also Nellie.

Psyche (Greek) soul. Mythology: a
beautiful mortal loved by Eros, the
Greek god of love.

Pua (Hawaiian) flower.

Pualani (Hawaiian) heavenly flower.

Purity (English) purity.

Pyralis (Greek) fire.

Qadira (Arabic) powerful.

Qamra (Arabic) moon.

Qitarah (Arabic) fragrant.

Quaashie (Ewe) born on Sunday.

Quadeisha (American) a combination
of Qadira + Aisha.

Quaneisha (American) a combination of
the prefix Qu + Niesha.

Quanesha (American) a form of
Quaneisha.

Quanika (American) a combination of
the prefix Qu + Nika.

Quanisha (American) a form of
Quaneisha.

Quartilla (Latin) fourth.

Qubilah (Arabic) agreeable.

Queen (English) queen. See also Quinn.

Queenie (English) a form of Queen.

Queisha (American) a short form of
Quaneisha.
Qeysha, Queshia

Quenby (Scandinavian) feminine.

Quenisha (American) a combination of
Queen + Aisha.

Quenna (English) a form of Queen.

Querida (Spanish) dear; beloved.

R

Questa (French) searcher.

Queta (Spanish) a short form of names ending in "queta" or "quetta."

Quiana (American) a combination of the prefix Qu + Anna.
Quian, Quianna

Quinby (Scandinavian) queen's estate.

Quincy (Irish) fifth.

Quinella (Latin) a form of Quintana.

Quinesha, Quinisha (American) forms of Quenisha.

Quinetta (Latin) a form of Quintana.

Quinn (German, English) queen. See also Queen.
Quin, Quinna

Quinshawna (American) a combination of Quinn + Shauna.

Quintana (Latin) fifth. (English) queen's lawn. See also Quinella, Quinetta.
Quinntina, Quinta, Quintanna, Quintara, Quintarah, Quintia, Quintila, Quintilla, Quintina, Quintona, Quintonice

Quintessa (Latin) essence. See also Tess.

Quintrell (American) a combination of Quinn + Trella.

Quiterie (Latin, French) tranquil.

Qwanisha (American) a form of Quaneisha.

Rabecca (Hebrew) a form of Rebecca.
Rabecka

Rabi (Arabic) breeze.

Rachael (Hebrew) a form of Rachel.
Rachaele, Rachalle

Racheal (Hebrew) a form of Rachel.

Rachel ✌ (Hebrew) female sheep. Bible: the second wife of Jacob. See also Lahela, Rae, Rochelle.
Racha, Rachal, Rachela, Rachelann, Rachele, Rahel, Rahela, Rahil, Ray, Raycene, Rey, Ruchel

Rachelle (French) a form of Rachel. See also Shelley.
Rachalle, Rachell, Rachella, Raechell, Raechelle, Raeshelle, Rashele, Rashell, Raychell, Rayshell, Ruchelle

Racquel (French) a form of Rachel.
Rackel, Racquell, Racquella, Racquelle

Radella (German) counselor.

Radeyah (Arabic) content, satisfied.

Radinka (Slavic) full of life; happy, glad.

Radmilla (Slavic) worker for the people.

Rae (English) doe. (Hebrew) a short form of Rachel.
Raeh, Raeneice, Raeneisha, Raesha, Ray, Raye, Rayetta, Rayette, Rayma, Rey

Raeann (American) a combination of Rae + Ann. See also Rayanne.
Raea, Raeanna, Raeanne

Raechel (Hebrew) a form of Rachel.
Raechele, Raechell

Raeden (Japanese) Mythology: Raiden
was the god of thunder and lightning.
Raeda, Raedeen

Raegan (Irish) a form of Reagan.

Raelene (American) a combination of
Rae + Lee.

Raelyn, Raelynn (American) forms of
Raelene.

Raena (German) a form of Raina.
Raenah

Raeven (English) a form of Raven.
Raewyn

Rafa (Arabic) happy; prosperous.

Rafaela (Hebrew) a form of Raphaela.

Ragan (Irish) a form of Reagan.

Ragine (English) a form of Regina.
Ragina

Ragnild (Scandinavian) battle counsel.

Raheem (Punjabi) compassionate God.

Ráidah (Arabic) leader.

Raina (German) mighty. (English) a
short form of Regina. See also Rayna.
Raheena, Rainna

Rainbow (English) rainbow.

Raine (Latin) a short form of Regina. A
form of Raina, Rane.
Reyne

Raisa (Russian) a form of Rose.

Raizel (Yiddish) a form of Rose.

Raja (Arabic) hopeful.

Raku (Japanese) pleasure.

Raleigh (Irish) a form of Riley.

Rama (Hebrew) lofty, exalted. (Hindi)
godlike. Religion: an incarnation of the
Hindu god Vishnu.

Raman (Spanish) a form of Ramona.

Ramandeep (Sikh) covered by the light
of the Lord's love.

Ramla (Swahili) fortuneteller.

Ramona (Spanish) mighty; wise protec-
tor. See also Mona.
*Ramonda, Raymona, Romona,
Romonda*

Ramsey (English) ram's island.

Ran (Japanese) water lily.
(Scandinavian) destroyer. Mythology:
the Norse sea goddess who destroys.

Rana (Sanskrit) royal. (Arabic) gaze,
look.

Ranait (Irish) graceful; prosperous.

Randall (English) protected.
*Randa, Randah, Randal, Randalee,
Randel, Randell, Randelle, Randilee,
Randilynn, Randlyn, Randyl*

Randi, Randy (English) familiar forms
of Miranda, Randall.
*Rande, Randee, Randeen, Randene,
Randey, Randie, Randii*

Rane (Scandinavian) queen.

Rani (Sanskrit) queen. (Hebrew) joyful.
A short form of Kerani.

Ranita (Hebrew) song; joyful.
Ranata

Raniyah (Arabic) gazing.

Rapa (Hawaiian) moonbeam.

Raphaela (Hebrew) healed by God.

Raphaelle (French) a form of
Raphaela.

Raquel (French) a form of Rachel.
*Rakel, Rakhil, Rakhila, Raqueal,
Raquela, Raquella, Raquelle,
Rickquel, Ricquelle, Rikell, Rikelle,
Rockell*

Rasha (Arabic) young gazelle.
Rahshea

Rashawna (American) a combination
of the prefix Ra + Shawna.

Rashel, Rashelle (American) forms of
Rachel.
Rashele, Rashell

Rashida (Swahili, Turkish) righteous.
*Rahshea, Rahsheda, Rahsheita,
Rashdah, Rasheda, Rashedah,
Rasheeda, Rasheeta, Rasheida,
Rashidi*

Rashieka (Arabic) descended from
royalty.

Rasia (Greek) rose.

Ratana (Tai) crystal.

Ratri (Hindi) night. Religion: the goddess of the night.

Raula (French) wolf counselor.

Raven (English) blackbird.
*Raveen, Raveena, Ravena,
Ravennah*

Ravin (English) a form of Raven.
Ravi, Ravine

Ravyn (English) a form of Raven.

Rawnie (Gypsy) fine lady.

Raya (Hebrew) friend.
Ray

Rayanne (American) a form of Raeann.
Rayona, Rayonna

Raychel, Raychelle (Hebrew) forms of
Rachel.
Raychell

Raylene (American) a form of Raylyn.
Ralina

Raymonde (German) wise protector.
Rayma

Rayna (Scandinavian) mighty. (Yiddish)
pure, clean. (English) king's advisor.
(French) a familiar form of Lorraine.
See also Raina.
*Rayne, Raynell, Raynelle, Raynette,
Rayona, Rayonna*

Rayven (English) a form of Raven.
Rayvin

Rayya (Arabic) thirsty no longer.

Razi (Aramaic) secretive.

Raziya (Swahili) agreeable.

Rea (Greek) poppy flower.

Reagan (Irish) little ruler.

Reanna (German, English) a form of
Raina. (American) a form of Raeann.
Reannah

Reanne (American) a form of Raeann,
Reanna.

Reba (Hebrew) fourth-born child. A
short form of Rebecca. See also Reva,
Riva.
Rabah, Reeba, Rheba

Rebeca (Hebrew) an alernate form of
Rebecca.

Rebecca ☝ (Hebrew) tied, bound.
Bible: the wife of Isaac. See also Becca,
Becky.
*Rebbecca, Rebeccah, Rebeccea,
Rebeccka, Rebecha, Rebecka,
Rebeckah, Rebeckia, Rebecky,
Rebeque*

Rebekah (Hebrew) a form of Rebecca.
*Rebeka, Rebekha, Rebekka,
Rebekkah, Rebekke, Revecca,
Revekka, Rifka*

Rebi (Hebrew) a familiar form of
Rebecca.
Ree

Reena (Greek) peaceful. (English) a
form of Rina. (Hebrew) a form of
Rinah.
Reen, Reenie

Reet (Estonian) a form of Margaret.
Reatha

Regan (Irish) a form of Reagan.

Reganne (Irish) a form of Reagan.
Regin

Reggie (English) a familiar form of
Regina.
Reggi, Reggy, Regi, Regia, Regie

Regina (Latin) queen. (English) king's
advisor. Geography: the capital of
Saskatchewan. See also Gina.
*Rega, Regena, Regennia, Regiena,
Reginia, Regis*

Regine (Latin) a form of Regina.
Regin

Rei (Japanese) polite, well behaved.

Reilly (Irish) a form of Riley.

Reina (Spanish) a short form of Regina.
See also Reyna.
Reine, Reinette, Reiny, Reiona, Renia

Rekha (Hindi) thin line.

Remedios (Spanish) remedy.

Remi (French) from Rheims, France.

Remington (English) raven estate.

Ren (Japanese) arranger; water lily;
lotus.

Rena (Hebrew) song; joy. A familiar form
of Irene, Regina, Renata, Sabrina,
Serena.
Rinna, Rinnah

Renae (French) a form of Renée.
Renay

Renata (French) a form of Renée.
*Ranata, Renada, Renyatta, Rinada,
Rinata*

Rene (Greek) a short form of Irene,
Renée.
Reen, Reenie, Reney

Renée (French) born again.
Renay, Renee, Renell, Renelle

Renita (French) a form of Renata.
Reneeta, Renetta, Renitza

Rennie (English) a familiar form of
Renata.

Reseda (Spanish) fragrant mignonette
blossom.

Reshawna (American) a combination
of the prefix Re + Shawna.

Resi (German) a familiar form of
Theresa.

Reta (African) shaken.
Reeta, Rheta

Reubena (Hebrew) behold a child.

Reva (Latin) revived. (Hebrew) rain;
one-fourth. A form of Reba, Riva.
Ree, Reeva, Revia, Revida

Reveca, Reveka (Slavic) forms of
Rebecca, Rebekah.
Revecca, Revekka

Rexanne (American) queen.

Reyhan (Turkish) sweet-smelling flower.

Reyna (Greek) peaceful. (English) a
form of Reina.

Reynalda (German) king's advisor.

Réz (Latin, Hungarian) copper-colored
hair.

Reza (Czech) a form of Theresa.

Rhea (Greek) brook, stream. Mythology:
the mother of Zeus.
Rheá, Rhéa, Rhealyn

Rheanna, Rhianna (Greek) forms of
Rhea.
*Rheana, Rheann, Rheanne, Rhiana,
Rhiauna*

Rhian (Welsh) a short form of
Rhiannon.
*Rhianne, Rhyan, Rhyann, Rian,
Riane, Riann, Rianne, Riayn*

Rhiannon (Welsh) witch; nymph; god-
dess.
*Rheannan, Rheannon, Rhianen,
Rhiannen, Rhianon, Rhianwen,
Rhinnon, Rhyanna, Riannon,
Rianon*

Rhoda (Greek) from Rhodes, Greece.
*Rhode, Rhodeia, Rhodie, Rhody,
Roda, Rodi, Rodie, Rodina*

Rhona (Scottish) powerful, mighty.
(English) king's advisor.
Rhonnie

Rhonda (Welsh) grand.
Rhondene, Rhondiesha

Ria (Spanish) river.

Riana, Rianna (Irish) short forms of
Briana. (Arabic) forms of Rihana.
Rhyanna

Rica (Spanish) a short form of Erica,
Frederica, Ricarda. See also Enrica,
Sandrica, Terrica, Ulrica.

Ricarda (Spanish) rich and powerful
ruler.

Richael (Irish) saint.

Richelle (German, French) a form of
Ricarda.
*Richel, Richela, Richele, Richell,
Richella, Richia*

Rickelle (American) a form of Raquel.

Ricki, Rikki (American) familiar forms
of Erica, Frederica, Ricarda.
*Rici, Rickia, Rickie, Rickilee, Rickina,
Rickita, Ricky, Ricquie, Riki, Rikia,
Rikita, Rikky*

Ricquel (American) a form of Raquel.
Ricquelle, Rikell, Rikelle

Rida (Arabic) favored by God.

Rihana (Arabic) sweet basil.
Rhiana

Rika (Swedish) ruler.
Ricka

Rilee (Irish) a form of Riley.

Riley ꙰ (Irish) valiant.
Rileigh, Rilie

Rilla (German) small brook.

Rima (Arabic) white antelope.

Rimona (Hebrew) pomegranate. See also
Mona.

Rin (Japanese) park. Geography: a
Japanese village.

Rina (English) a short form of names
ending in "rina." (Hebrew) a form of
Rena, Rinah.

Rinah (Hebrew) joyful.

Riona (Irish) saint.

Risa (Latin) laughter.

Risha (Hindi) born during the lunar
month of Taurus.

Rishona (Hebrew) first.

Rissa (Greek) a short form of Nerissa.

Rita (Sanskrit) brave; honest. (Greek) a
short form of Margarita.
*Reatha, Reda, Reeta, Reida, Reitha,
Rheta, Riet, Ritamae, Ritamarie*

Ritsa (Greek) a familiar form of
Alexandra.

Riva (French) river bank. (Hebrew) a
short form of Rebecca. See also Reba,
Reva.

River (Latin, French) stream, water.

Rivka (Hebrew) a short form of Rebecca.

Riza (Greek) a form of Theresa.

Roanna (American) a form of Rosanna.
Ranna, Roanne

Robbi, Robbie (English) familiar forms
of Roberta.
Robby

Roberta (English) famous brilliance.
Roba, Robena, Robertena, Robertina

Robin (English) robin. A form of
Roberta.
*Robann, Robbin, Robena, Robina,
Robine, Robinia, Robinn, Robinta*

Robinette (English) a familiar form of
Robin.

Robyn (English) a form of Robin.
Robbyn, Robyne, Robynn, Robynne

Rochelle (French) large stone.
(Hebrew) a form of Rachel. See also
Shelley.
*Roch, Rochele, Rochell, Rochella,
Rochette, Rockelle, Roshele, Roshell,
Roshelle*

Rocio (Spanish) dewdrops.
Rocío

Roderica (German) famous ruler.

Rodnae (English) island clearing.

Rodneisha (American) a combination
of Rodnae + Aisha.

Rohana (Hindi) sandalwood.
(American) a combination of Rose +
Hannah.

Rohini (Hindi) woman.

Rolanda (German) famous throughout
the land.

Rolene (German) a form of Rolanda.

Roma (Latin) from Rome.

Romaine (French) from Rome.
Romona

Romy (French) a familiar form of
Romaine. (English) a familiar form of
Rosemary.
Romi

Rona (Scandinavian) a short form of
Ronalda.

Ronaele (Greek) the name Eleanor
spelled backwards.

Ronda (Welsh) a form of Rhonda.
Rondai, Rondesia, Rondi

Rondelle (French) short poem.
Rhondelle, Rondel, Ronndelle

Roneisha (American) a combination of
Rhonda + Aisha.

Ronelle (Welsh) a form of Rhonda,
Ronda.

Ronisha (American) a form of Roneisha.

Ronli (Hebrew) joyful.

Ronnette (Welsh) a familiar form of
Rhonda, Ronda.

Ronni, Ronnie, Ronny (American)
familiar forms of Veronica and names
beginning with "Ron."

Rori, Rory (Irish) famous brilliance;
famous ruler.

Ros, Roz (English) short forms of
Rosalind, Rosalyn.

Rosa (Italian, Spanish) a form of Rose.
History: Rosa Parks inspired the
American Civil Rights movement by
refusing to give up her bus seat to a
white man in Montgomery, Alabama.
See also Charo, Roza.

Rosabel (French) beautiful rose.

Rosalba (Latin) white rose.

Rosalie (English) a form of Rosalind.
*Rosalea, Rosalee, Rosaleen, Rosalene,
Rosalia, Roselia, Rosilee, Rosli,
Rozali, Rozália, Rozalie, Rozele*

Rosalind (Spanish) fair rose.
*Rosalinde, Rosalynd, Rosalynde,
Roselind, Rozalind, Rozland*

Rosalinda (Spanish) a form of
Rosalind.
Rosalina

Rosalyn (Spanish) a form of Rosalind.
*Rosaleen, Rosalin, Rosaline,
Rosalyne, Rosalynn, Rosalynne,
Rosilyn, Roslin, Roslyne, Roslynn,
Rozalyn, Rozlyn*

Rosamond (German) famous guardian.

Rosanna, Roseanna (English) combi-
nations of Rose + Anna.
*Ranna, Rosana, Rosannah,
Roseana, Roseannah, Rosehanah,
Rosehannah, Rossana, Rossanna,
Rozana, Rozanna*

Rosanne, Roseanne (English) combi-
nations of Rose + Ann.
*Roanne, Rosan, Rosann, Roseann,
Rose Ann, Rose Anne, Rossann,
Rossanne, Rozann, Rozanne*

Rosario (Filipino, Spanish) rosary.

Rose (Latin) rose. See also Chalina,
Raisa, Raizel, Roza.
*Rada, Rasine, Rois, Róise, Rosella,
Roselle, Rosse*

Roselani (Hawaiian) heavenly rose.

Roselyn (Spanish) a form of Rosalind.
*Roseleen, Roselin, Roseline, Roselynn,
Roselynne*

Rosemarie (English) a combination of
Rose + Marie.
Rosemaria, Rose Marie

Rosemary (English) a combination of
Rose + Mary.
Romi

Rosetta (Italian) a form of Rose.
Roseta, Rosette

Roshan (Sanskrit) shining light.

Roshawna (American) a combination
of Rose + Shawna.

Rosie (English) a familiar form of
Rosalind, Rosanna, Rose.
Rosse

Rosina (English) a familiar form of
Rose.

Rosita (Spanish) a familiar form of
Rose.
Roseta

Roslyn (Scottish) a form of Rossalyn.
Roslin, Roslynn

Rossalyn (Scottish) cape; promontory.

Rowan (English) tree with red berries.
(Welsh) a form of Rowena.

Rowena (Welsh) fair-haired. (English)
famous friend. Literature: Ivanhoe's
love interest in Sir Walter Scott's novel
Ivanhoe.
Ranna

Roxana, Roxanna (Persian) forms of
Roxann.
Rocsana

Roxann, Roxanne (Persian) sunrise.
Literature: Roxanne is the heroine of
Edmond Rostand's play *Cyrano de
Bergerac.*
Rocxann, Roxianne

Roxy (Persian) a familiar form of
Roxann.

Royale (English) royal.

Royanna (English) queenly, royal.

Roza (Slavic) a form of Rosa.
Rozele

Rozene (Native American) rose blossom.

Ruana (Hindi) stringed musical instrument.

Rubena (Hebrew) a form of Reubena.

Rubi (French) a form of Ruby.
Rubia, Rubie

Ruby (French) precious stone.
*Rubetta, Rubette, Rubey, Rubiann,
Rubyann, Rubye*

Ruchi (Hindi) one who wishes to please.

Rudee (German) famous wolf.

Rudra (Hindi) seeds of the rudraksha
plant.

Rue (German) famous. (French) street.
(English) regretful; strong-scented
herbs.

Ruffina (Italian) redhead.

Rui (Japanese) affectionate.

Rukan (Arabic) steady; confident.

Rula (Latin, English) ruler.

Runa (Norwegian) secret; flowing.

Ruperta (Spanish) a form of Roberta.

Rupinder (Sanskrit) beautiful.

Ruri (Japanese) emerald.

Rusalka (Czech) wood nymph. (Russian) mermaid.

Russhell (French) redhead; fox colored.

Rusti (English) redhead.

Ruth (Hebrew) friendship. Bible: daughter-in-law of Naomi.
Rutha, Ruthalma, Ruthe, Ruthella, Ruthetta, Ruthven

Ruthann (American) a combination of Ruth + Ann.
Ruthina, Ruthine

Ruthie (Hebrew) a familiar form of Ruth.
Ruthi, Ruthy

Ruza (Czech) rose.

Ryan, Ryann (Irish) little ruler.
Raiann, Raianne, Rhyann, Riane, Ryana, Ryanna, Ryanne, Rye, Ryen, Ryenne

Ryba (Czech) fish.

Rylee (Irish) valiant.
Rye

Ryleigh, Rylie (Irish) forms of Rylee.

Ryley (Irish) a form of Rylee.

Ryo (Japanese) dragon.

S

Saarah (Arabic) princess.

Saba (Arabic) morning. (Greek) a form of Sheba.

Sabi (Arabic) young girl.

Sabina (Latin) History: the Sabine were a tribe in ancient Italy. See also Bina.
Sabienne, Sabine, Sabinka, Sabinna, Sabiny, Saby, Sabyne, Savina, Sebina, Sebinah

Sabiya (Arabic) morning; eastern wind.

Sable (English) sable; sleek.
Sabel, Sabela, Sabella

Sabra (Hebrew) thorny cactus fruit. (Arabic) resting. History: a name for native-born Israelis, who were said to be hard on the outside and soft and sweet on the inside.
Sabira, Sabrah, Sabre, Sabriya, Sebra

Sabreena (English) a form of Sabrina.

Sabrina (Latin) boundary line. (English) princess. (Hebrew) a familiar form of Sabra. See also Bree, Brina, Rena, Zabrina.
Sabre, Sabrinia, Sabrinna, Sebree

Sabryna (English) a form of Sabrina.

Sacha (Russian) a form of Sasha.

Sachi (Japanese) blessed; lucky.

Sada (Japanese) chaste. (English) a form of Sadie.
Sadah

Sade (Hebrew) a form of Chadee, Sarah, Shardae, Sharday.
Sáde, Sadé, Sadee

Sadella (American) a combination of Sade + Ella.
Sadelle, Sydel, Sydell, Sydella, Sydelle

Sadhana (Hindi) devoted.

Sadie (Hebrew) a familiar form of Sarah. See also Sada.
Sadee, Sady, Sadye, Saidee

Sadira (Persian) lotus tree. (Arabic) star.

Sadiya (Arabic) lucky, fortunate.

Sadzi (Carrier) sunny disposition.

Saffron (English) Botany: a plant with purple or white flowers whose orange stigmas are used as a spice.

Safiya (Arabic) pure; serene; best friend.
Safa, Safeya, Saffa, Safia, Safiyah

Sagara (Hindi) ocean.

Sage (English) wise. Botany: an herb used as a seasoning.

Sahara (Arabic) desert; wilderness.
Sabra

Sai (Japanese) talented.

Saida (Hebrew) a form of Sarah. (Arabic) happy; fortunate.

Saige (English) a form of Sage.

Saira (Hebrew) a form of Sara.

Sakaë (Japanese) prosperous.

Sakari (Hindi) sweet.

Saki (Japanese) cloak; rice wine.

Sakti (Hindi) energy, power.

Sakuna (Native American) bird.

Sakura (Japanese) cherry blossom; wealthy; prosperous.

Sala (Hindi) sala tree. Religion: the sacred tree under which Buddha died.

Salali (Cherokee) squirrel.

Salama (Arabic) peaceful. See also Zulima.

Salena (French) a form of Salina.
Saleena

Salima (Arabic) safe and sound; healthy.

Salina (French) solemn, dignified.
Salinda

Salliann (English) a combination of Sally + Ann.

Sally (English) princess. History: Sally Ride, an American astronaut, became the first U. S. woman in space.
Sal, Salaid, Sallee, Salletta, Sallette, Salley, Salli, Sallie

Salome (Hebrew) peaceful. History: Salome Alexandra was a ruler of ancient Judea. Bible: the niece of King Herod.

Salvadora (Spanish) savior.

Salvia (Spanish) healthy; saved. (Latin) a form of Sage.

Samala (Hebrew) asked of God.

Samanta (Hebrew) a form of Samantha.
Smanta

Samantha ☀ (Aramaic) listener.
(Hebrew) told by God.
*Sam, Samana, Samanath,
Samanatha, Samanitha, Samanithia,
Samanth, Samanthe, Samanthi,
Samanthia, Sammanth,
Sammantha, Semantha, Simantha,
Smantha, Symantha*

Samara (Latin) elm-tree seed.
*Samaria, Samarie, Samarra,
Samera, Sameria, Sammar,
Sammara, Samora*

Samatha (Hebrew) a form of Samantha.
Sammatha

Sameh (Hebrew) listener. (Arabic) forgiving.

Sami (Arabic) praised. (Hebrew) a short
form of Samantha, Samuela.

Samira (Arabic) entertaining.

Samone (Hebrew) a form of Simone.

Samuela (Hebrew) heard God, asked of
God.

Samuelle (Hebrew) a form of Samuela.

Sana (Arabic) mountaintop; splendid;
brilliant.
Sanaa, Sanáa

Sancia (Spanish) holy, sacred.

Sandeep (Punjabi) enlightened.

Sandi (Greek) a familiar form of
Sandra.
*Sandee, Sandia, Sandie, Sandiey,
Sandine, Sanndie*

Sandra (Greek) defender of mankind. A
short form of Cassandra. History:
Sandra Day O'Connor was the first
woman appointed to the U.S. Supreme

Court. See also Zandra.
Sahndra, Sandira, Sandría

Sandrea (Greek) a form of Sandra.
Sandria

Sandrica (Greek) a form of Sandra. See
also Rica.

Sandrine (Greek) a form of Alexandra.

Sandy (Greek) a familiar form of
Cassandra, Sandra.
Sandya, Sandye

Sanne (Hebrew, Dutch) lily.

Santana (Spanish) saint.
*Santa, Santaniata, Santanna,
Santanne, Santena, Santenna*

Santina (Spanish) little saint.

Sanura (Swahili) kitten.

Sanuye (Moquelumnan) red clouds at
sunset.

Sanya (Sanskrit) born on Saturday.

Sanyu (Luganda) happiness.

Sapata (Native American) dancing bear.

Sapphira (Hebrew) a form of Sapphire.

Sapphire (Greek) blue gemstone.

Sara ☀ (Hebrew) a form of Sarah.
Saralee, Sarra

Sarah ☀ (Hebrew) princess. Bible: the
wife of Abraham and mother of Isaac.
See also Sadie, Saida, Sally, Saree,
Sharai, Shari, Zara, Zarita.
*Sahra, Saraha, Sarahann, Sarann,
Sorcha*

Sarai, Saray (Hebrew) forms of Sarah.

Saralyn (American) a combination of Sarah + Lynn.

Saree (Arabic) noble. (Hebrew) a familiar form of Sarah.
Sareeka, Sari, Sarika, Sarka, Sarri, Sarrie, Sary

Sariah (Hebrew) forms of Sarah.

Sarila (Turkish) waterfall.

Sarina (Hebrew) a familiar form of Sarah.
Sareen, Sarena, Sarene, Sarinna, Sarinne

Sarita (Hebrew) a familiar form of Sarah.
Saretta, Sarette, Saritia

Sarolta (Hungarian) a form of Sarah.

Sarotte (French) a form of Sarah.

Sarrah (Hebrew) a form of Sarah.
Sarra

Sasa (Japanese) assistant. (Hungarian) a form of Sarah, Sasha.

Sasha (Russian) defender of mankind. See also Zasha.
Sahsha, Sascha, Saschae, Sashah, Sashana, Sashel, Sashia, Sashira, Sashsha, Sasjara, Sasshali, Sausha, Shasha, Shashi, Shashia

Sass (Irish) Saxon.

Satara (American) a combination of Sarah + Tara.

Satin (French) smooth, shiny.

Satinka (Native American) sacred dancer.

Sato (Japanese) sugar.

Saundra (English) a form of Sandra, Sondra.
Saundee, Saundi, Saundie, Saundy

Saura (Hindi) sun worshiper.

Savana, Savanna (Spanish) forms of Savannah.
Savina

Savanah (Spanish) a form of Savannah.

Savannah ✻ (Spanish) treeless plain.
Sahvannah, Savanha, Savannha, Savauna, Sevan, Sevanah, Sevanh, Sevann, Sevanna, Svannah

Sawa (Japanese) swamp. (Moquelumnan) stone.

Sawyer (English) wood worker.

Sayde, Saydee (Hebrew) forms of Sadie.
Saydie

Sayo (Japanese) born at night.

Sayra (Hebrew) a form of Sarah.
Sayre

Scarlett (English) bright red. Literature: Scarlett O'Hara is the heroine of Margaret Mitchell's novel *Gone with the Wind*.
Scarlet, Scarlette, Scarlotte, Skarlette

Schyler (Dutch) sheltering.

Scotti (Scottish) from Scotland.

Seana, Seanna (Irish) forms of Jane. See also Shauna, Shawna.

Sebastiane (Greek) venerable. (Latin) revered. (French) a form of Sebastian (see Boys' Names).

Seble (Ethiopian) autumn.

Sebrina (English) a form of Sabrina.

Secilia (Latin) a form of Cecilia.

Secunda (Latin) second.

Seda (Armenian) forest voices.

Sedna (Eskimo) well-fed. Mythology: the
goddess of sea animals.

Seelia (English) a form of Sheila.

Seema (Greek) sprout. (Afghan) sky;
profile.

Sefa (Swiss) a familiar form of Josefina.

Seirra (Irish) a form of Sierra.
Seiarra, Seira

Seki (Japanese) wonderful.

Sela (English) a short form of Selena.

Selam (Ethiopian) peaceful.

Selda (German) a short form of
Griselda. (Yiddish) a form of Zelda.

Selena (Greek) moon. Mythology:
Selene was the goddess of the moon.
See also Celena.
*Saleena, Selen, Séléné, Selenia, Sena,
Syleena, Sylena*

Selene (Greek) a form of Selena.

Selia (Latin) a short form of Cecilia.

Selima (Hebrew) peaceful.

Selina (Greek) a form of Celina, Selena.
*Selie, Selinda, Seline, Selinka, Selyna,
Selyne, Sylina*

Selma (German) divine protector.
(Irish) fair, just. (Scandinavian)
divinely protected. (Arabic) secure. See
also Zelma.

Sema (Turkish) heaven; divine omen.

Sen (Japanese) Mythology: a magical
forest elf that lives for thousands of
years.

Senalda (Spanish) sign.
Sena

Seneca (Iroquoian) a tribal name.

Septima (Latin) seventh.

Sequoia (Cherokee) giant redwood tree.

Serafina (Hebrew) burning; ardent.
Bible: seraphim are an order of angels.

Serena (Latin) peaceful. See also Rena.
*Saryna, Serenah, Serene, Serenna,
Serrena*

Serenity (Latin) peaceful.

Serilda (Greek) armed warrior woman.

Serina (Latin) a form of Serena.
Sereena, Serrin, Serrina, Seryna

Sevilla (Spanish) from Seville.

Shaba (Spanish) rose.

Shada (Native American) pelican.
Shadae

Shaday (American) a form of Sade.

Shadrika (American) a combination of
the prefix Sha + Rika.

Shae (Irish) a form of Shea.
Shaenel, Shaeya, Shaia

Shaelee (Irish) a form of Shea.
Shaeleigh, Shaelie, Shaely

Shaelyn (Irish) a form of Shea.

Shafira (Swahili) distinguished.

Shahar (Arabic) moonlit.

Shahina (Arabic) falcon.

Shahla (Afghani) beautiful eyes.

Shaianne (Cheyenne) a form of Cheyenne.
Shaeen, Shaeine

Shaila (Latin) a form of Sheila.
Shaela, Shaelea

Shaina (Yiddish) beautiful.
Shaena, Shainah, Shaine, Shainna, Shajna, Shanie, Shayndel, Sheina, Sheindel

Shajuana (American) a combination of the prefix Sha + Juanita. See also Shawanna.

Shaka (Hindi) a form of Shakti. A short form of names beginning with "Shak." See also Chaka.

Shakarah (American) a combination of the prefix Sha + Kara.

Shakayla (Arabic) a form of Shakila.

Shakeena (American) a combination of the prefix Sha + Keena.

Shakeita (American) a combination of the prefix Sha + Keita. See also Shaqueita.
Shakeeta, Shaketa, Shaketha, Shakethia, Shaketia, Shakita, Sheketa, Shekita

Shakera (Arabic) a form of Shakira.
Shakerah, Shakeria, Shakeriay, Shakeyra

Shakia (American) a combination of the prefix Sha + Kia.
Shakeeia, Shakeeyah, Shakeia,
Shakeya, Shakiya, Shekeia, Shekia, Shekiah, Shikia

Shakila (Arabic) pretty.

Shakira (Arabic) thankful.
Shaakira, Shakir, Shakirah, Shakirat, Shakirra, Shekiera, Shekira, Shikira

Shakti (Hindi) energy, power. Religion: a form of the Hindu goddess Devi.

Shakyra (Arabic) a form of Shakira.

Shalana (American) a combination of the prefix Sha + Lana.
Shalaina, Shalaine, Shalane, Shalann

Shaleah (American) a combination of the prefix Sha + Leah.

Shaleisha (American) a combination of the prefix Sha + Aisha.

Shalena (American) a combination of the prefix Sha + Lena.

Shalisa (American) a combination of the prefix Sha + Lisa.

Shalita (American) a combination of the prefix Sha + Lita.

Shalona (American) a combination of the prefix Sha + Lona.

Shalonda (American) a combination of the prefix Sha + Ondine.
Shalonde, Shalondine

Shalyn (American) a combination of the prefix Sha + Lynn.

Shamara (Arabic) ready for battle.

Shameka (American) a combination of the prefix Sha + Meka.
Shameca, Shamecca, Shamecha, Shameika, Shameke, Shamekia

Shamika (American) a combination of the prefix Sha + Mika.
Shameeka, Shamica, Shamicia, Shamicka, Shamieka, Shamikia

Shamira (Hebrew) precious stone.
Shamir, Shamiran, Shamiria

Shamiya (American) a combination of the prefix Sha + Mia.

Shana (Hebrew) God is gracious. (Irish) a form of Jane.
Shaana, Shan, Shannah

Shanae (Irish) a form of Shana.
Shanay, Shanea

Shanda (American) a form of Chanda, Shana.
Shandah, Shannda

Shandi (English) a familiar form of Shana.
Shandee, Shandeigh, Shandey, Shandice, Shandie

Shandra (American) a form of Shanda. See also Chandra.
Shandrea, Shandreka, Shandri, Shandria, Shandriah, Shandrice, Shandrie, Shandry

Shane (Irish) a form of Shana.
Shanea, Shanie

Shaneisha (American) a combination of the prefix Sha + Aisha.

Shaneka (American) a form of Shanika.
Shanecka, Shaneikah, Shanekia, Shanequa, Shaneyka, Shonneka

Shanel, Shanell, Shanelle (American) forms of Chanel.
Schanel, Schanell, Shanella, Shannel, Shenel, Shenela, Shenell, Shenelle, Shonelle, Shynelle

Shaneta (American) a combination of the prefix Sha + Neta.
Shonetta

Shani (Swahili) a form of Shany.

Shania (American) a form of Shana.

Shanice (American) a form of Janice. See also Chanise.

Shanida (American) a combination of the prefix Sha + Ida.

Shanika (American) a combination of the prefix Sha + Nika.
Shanica, Shanicca, Shanicka, Shanieka, Shanike, Shanikia, Shanikka, Shanikqua, Shanikwa, Shenika, Shonnika

Shaniqua (American) a form of Shanika.
Shanique, Sheniqua

Shanise (American) a form of Shanice.

Shanita (American) a combination of the prefix Sha + Nita.
Shanitha, Shanitra, Shanitta

Shanley (Irish) hero's child.

Shanna (Irish) a form of Shana, Shannon.
Shanea, Shannah, Shannea

Shannen (Irish) a form of Shannon.

Shannon (Irish) small and wise.
Shanan, Shann, Shannan, Shanneen, Shannie, Shannin, Shannyn, Shanon

Shanta, Shantae, Shante (French) forms of Chantal.
Shantai, Shantay, Shantaya, Shantaye, Shantea, Shantee, Shantée

Shantal (American) a form of Shantel.
Shontal

Shantana (American) a form of
Santana.

Shantara (American) a combination of
the prefix Sha + Tara.

Shanteca (American) a combination of
the prefix Sha + Teca.

Shantel, Shantell (American) song.
_Shanntell, Shantale, Shanteal,
Shanteil, Shantele, Shantella,
Shantelle, Shantrell, Shantyl, Shantyle,
Shauntel, Shauntell, Shauntelle,
Shauntrel, Shauntrell, Shauntrella,
Shentel, Shentelle, Shontal, Shontalla,
Shontalle_

Shanteria (American) a form of
Shantara.

Shantesa (American) a combination of
the prefix Sha + Tess.

Shantia (American) a combination of
the prefix Sha + Tia.

Shantille (American) a form of
Chantilly.
Shanteil, Shantyl, Shantyle

Shantina (American) a combination of
the prefix Sha + Tina.

Shantora (American) a combination of
the prefix Sha + Tory.

Shantrice (American) a combination of
the prefix Sha + Trice. See also
Chantrice.

Shany (Swahili) marvelous, wonderful.
Shannea, Shannie

Shappa (Native American) red thunder.

Shaquanda (American) a combination of
the prefix Sha + Wanda.

Shaqueita, Shaquita (American)
forms of Shakeita.
Shaqueta, Shaquetta

Shaquila, Shaquilla (American) forms
of Shakila.

Shaquira (American) a form of Shakira.

Shara (Hebrew) a short form of Sharon.
_Shaara, Sharah, Sharal, Sharala,
Sharalee, Sharlyn, Sharlynn, Sharra_

Sharai (Hebrew) princess. See also
Sharon.
_Sharae, Sharaé, Sharah, Sharaiah,
Sharay, Sharaya_

Sharan (Hindi) protector.

Shardae, Sharday (Punjabi) charity.
(Yoruba) honored by royalty. (Arabic)
runaway. A form of Chardae.
_Shadae, Sharda, Shar-Dae, Shardai,
Shar-Day, Sharde, Shardea, Shardee,
Shardée, Shardei, Shardeia, Shardey_

Sharee (English) a form of Shari.
Shareen, Shareena, Sharine

Shari (French) beloved, dearest.
(Hungarian) a form of Sarah. See also
Sharita, Sheree, Sherry.
_Sharian, Shariann, Sharianne,
Sharie, Sharra, Sharree, Sharrie,
Sharry, Shary_

Sharice (French) a form of Cherise.

Sharik (African) child of God.

Sharissa (American) a form of Sharice.
Shericia

Sharita (French) a familiar form of Shari. (American) a form of Charity. See also Sherita.
Shareeta, Sharrita

Sharla (French) a short form of Sharlene, Sharlotte.

Sharlene (French) little and strong.
Scharlane, Scharlene, Shar, Sharlaina, Sharlaine, Sharlane, Sharlanna, Sharlee, Sharleen, Sharleine, Sharlena, Sharleyne, Sharline, Sharlyn, Sharlynn, Sharlynne, Sherlean, Sherlene, Sherline

Sharlotte (American) a form of Charlotte.

Sharma (American) a short form of Sharmaine.

Sharmaine (American) a form of Charmaine.

Sharna (Hebrew) a form of Sharon.

Sharon (Hebrew) desert plain. A form of Sharai.
Shaaron, Shareen, Sharen, Sharin, Sharran, Sharren, Sharrin, Sharron, Sharyn, Sharyon, Sheren, Sheron, Sherryn

Sharonda (Hebrew) a form of Sharon.

Sharrona (Hebrew) a form of Sharon.
Sheron

Shatara (Hindi) umbrella. (Arabic) good; industrious. (American) a combination of Sharon + Tara.
Shataria, Shatarra, Shataura, Shateira, Shaterah, Shateria, Shatherian, Shatierra, Shatiria

Shatoria (American) a combination of the prefix Sha + Tory.

Shauna (Hebrew) God is gracious. (Irish) a form of Shana. See also Seana, Shona.
Shaun, Shaunah, Shaune, Shaunee, Shauneen, Shaunelle, Shaunette, Shauni, Shaunice, Shaunicy, Shaunie, Shaunika, Shaunisha, Shaunna, Shaunnea, Shaunua, Shaunya

Shaunda (Irish) a form of Shauna. See also Shanda, Shawnda, Shonda.
Shaundal, Shaundala, Shaundel, Shaundela, Shaundell, Shaundelle, Shaundra, Shaundrea, Shaundree, Shaundria, Shaundrice

Shaunta (Irish) a form of Shauna. See also Shawnta, Shonta.
Shauntrel, Shauntrell, Shauntrella

Shavon (American) a form of Shavonne.
Schavon, Schevon, Shavan, Shavana, Shavaun, Shavonda, Shavone

Shavonne (American) a combination of the prefix Sha + Yvonne. See also Siobhan.
Shavanna, Shavondra, Shavonn, Shavonna, Shavonni, Shavontae, Shavonte, Shavonté, Shavoun, Shivaun, Shivawn, Shivonne, Shyvon, Shyvonne

Shawanna (American) a combination of the prefix Sha + Wanda. See also Shajuana, Shawna.

Shawna (Hebrew) God is gracious. (Irish) a form of Jane. A form of Shana, Shauna. See also Seana, Shona.
Shawn, Shawnai, Shawneen, Shawneena, Shawnell, Shawnette, Shawnna, Shawnra, Sheona, Siân, Siana

Shawnda (Irish) a form of Shawna. See
also Shanda, Shaunda, Shonda.
*Shawndal, Shawndala, Shawndan,
Shawndel, Shawndra, Shawndrea,
Shawndree, Shawndreel, Shawndrell,
Shawndria*

Shawnee (Irish) a form of Shawna.
Shawne, Shawni, Shawnie

Shawnika (American) a combination
of Shawna + Nika.
Shawneika, Shawnicka

Shawnta (Irish) a form of Shawna. See
also Shaunta, Shonta.

Shay, Shaye (Irish) forms of Shea.
*Shaya, Shayda, Shayha, Shayia, Shey,
Sheye*

Shayla (Irish) a form of Shay.
*Shaylagh, Shaylah, Shaylain, Shaylan,
Shaylea, Shaylla, Sheyla*

Shaylee (Irish) a form of Shea.
Shayley, Shayli, Shaylie, Shayly, Shealy

Shaylyn (Irish) a form of Shea.
Shaylin, Shaylynn, Shealyn, Sheylyn

Shayna (Hebrew) beautiful.
*Shaynae, Shayne, Shaynee, Shayney,
Shayni, Shaynie, Shayny, Sheana,
Sheanna*

Shea (Irish) fairy palace.
*Shealy, Shealyn, Sheann, Sheannon,
Sheanta, Sheaon, Shearra, Sheatara,
Sheaunna, Sheavon*

Sheba (Hebrew) a short form of
Bathsheba. Geography: an ancient
country of south Arabia.

Sheena (Hebrew) God is gracious.
(Irish) a form of Jane.
Sheenagh, Sheenah, Sheenan,

*Sheeneal, Sheenika, Sheenna, Sheina,
Shiona*

Sheila (Latin) blind. (Irish) a form of
Cecelia. See also Cheyla, Zelizi.
*Seila, Sheela, Sheelagh, Sheelah,
Sheilagh, Sheilah, Sheileen, Sheiletta,
Sheilia, Sheillynn, Sheilya, Shela,
Shelagh, Shelah, Shelia, Shiela, Shila,
Shilah, Shilea*

Shelbi, Shelbie (English) forms of
Shelby.

Shelby ☀ (English) ledge estate.
*Schelby, Shel, Shelbe, Shelbee, Shelbey,
Shellby*

Sheldon (English) farm on the ledge.

Shelee (English) a form of Shelley.
Shelia

Shelisa (American) a combination of
Shelley + Lisa.

Shelley, Shelly (English) meadow on
the ledge. (French) familiar forms of
Michelle. See also Rochelle.
*Shell, Shella, Shellaine, Shellana,
Shellary, Shellee, Shellene, Shelli,
Shellian, Shellie, Shellina*

Shelsea (American) a form of Chelsea.

Shena (Irish) a form of Sheena.
*Shenada, Shenae, Shenay, Shenda,
Shene, Shenea, Sheneda, Shenee,
Sheneena, Shenica, Shenika, Shenina,
Sheniqua, Shenita, Shenna*

Shera (Aramaic) light.
*Sheera, Sheerah, Sherae, Sherah,
Sheralee, Sheralle, Sheralyn,
Sheralynn, Sheralynne, Sheray,
Sheraya*

Sheree (French) beloved, dearest.
*Scherie, Sheeree, Shere, Shereé,
Sherrelle, Shereen, Shereena*

Sherelle (French) a form of Cherelle,
Sheryl.
*Sherell, Sheriel, Sherrel, Sherrell,
Sherrelle, Shirelle*

Sheri, Sherri (French) forms of Sherry.
Sheria, Sheriah, Sherie, Sherrie

Sherian (American) a combination of
Sheri + Ann.
Sherianne, Sherrina

Sherice (French) a form of Cherise.
Shericia

Sheridan (Irish) wild.

Sherika (Punjabi) relative. (Arabic)
easterner.
*Shereka, Sherica, Shericka, Sherrica,
Sherricka, Sherrika*

Sherissa (French) a form of Sherry,
Sheryl.
Shericia

Sherita (French) a form of Sherry,
Sheryl. See also Sharita.
Shereta, Sheretta, Sherette, Sherrita

Sherleen (French, English) a form of
Sheryl, Shirley.
*Sherlene, Sherline, Shirlena, Shirlina,
Shirlyn*

Sherry (French) beloved, dearest. A
familiar form of Sheryl. See also Sheree.
*Sherey, Sherrey, Sherria, Sherriah,
Sherrie, Sherye, Sheryy*

Sheryl (French) beloved. A familiar form
of Shirley. See also Sherry.
*Sharel, Sharil, Sharilyn, Sharyl,
Sharyll, Sheral, Sherell, Sheriel, Sheril,
Sherill, Sherily, Sherilyn, Sherral,*

*Sherrelle, Sherril, Sherrill, Sherryl,
Sherylly*

Sherylyn (American) a combination of
Sheryl + Lynn. See also Cherilyn.
Sheralyn, Sherilyn, Sherryn

Shevonne (American) a combination of
the prefix She + Yvonne.

Sheyenne (Cheyenne) a form of
Cheyenne. See also Shyann, Shyanne.

Shianne (Cheyenne) a form of
Cheyenne.

Shifra (Hebrew) beautiful.

Shika (Japanese) gentle deer.

Shilo (Hebrew) God's gift. Bible: a sanctuary for the Israelites where the Ark of
the Covenant was kept.
Shiloh

Shina (Japanese) virtuous, good;
wealthy. (Chinese) a form of China.

Shino (Japanese) bamboo stalk.

Shiquita (American) a form of Chiquita.

Shira (Hebrew) song.
*Shirah, Shiray, Shire, Shiree, Shiri,
Shirit*

Shirlene (English) a form of Shirley.

Shirley (English) bright meadow. See
also Sheryl.
*Sherlee, Sherley, Sherli, Sherlie, Shir,
Shirl, Shirlee, Shirlie, Shirly, Shirlly,
Shurlee, Shurley*

Shivani (Hindi) life and death.

Shizu (Japanese) silent.

Shona (Irish) a form of Jane. A form of
Shana, Shauna, Shawna.
*Shiona, Shonagh, Shonah, Shonalee,
Shone, Shonee, Shonette, Shoni,
Shonna*

Shonda (Irish) a form of Shona. See
also Shanda, Shaunda, Shawnda.
*Shondalette, Shondalyn, Shondel,
Shondelle, Shondi, Shondia, Shondie,
Shondra, Shondreka, Shounda*

Shonta (Irish) a form of Shona. See also
Shaunta, Shawnta.

Shoshana (Hebrew) a form of Susan.
*Shosha, Shoshan, Shoshanah,
Shoshane, Shoshanha, Shoshann,
Shoshanna, Shoshannah, Shoshauna,
Shoushan, Sosha, Soshana*

Shu (Chinese) kind, gentle.

Shug (American) a short form of Sugar.

Shula (Arabic) flaming, bright.

Shulamith (Hebrew) peaceful. See also
Sula.

Shunta (Irish) a form of Shonta.

Shura (Russian) a form of Alexandra.

Shyann, Shyanne (Cheyenne) forms of
Cheyenne. See also Sheyenne.

Shyla (English) a form of Sheila.

Shyra (Hebrew) a form of Shira.

Siara (Irish) a form of Sierra.
Siarah, Siarra, Sieara

Sianna (Irish) a form of Seana.
Siana

Sibeta (Moquelumnan) finding a fish
under a rock.

Sibley (English) sibling; friendly.
(Greek) a form of Sybil.

Sidney (French) a form of Sydney.

Sidonia (Hebrew) enticing.
Sydania, Syndonia

Sidonie (French) from Saint-Denis,
France. See also Sydney.

Sidra (Latin) star child.

Sienna (American) a form of Ciana.

Siera (Irish) a form of Sierra.
Sieria

Sierra (Irish) black. (Spanish) saw
toothed. Geography: any rugged range
of mountains that, when viewed from a
distance, has a jagged profile. See also
Ciara.
*Seara, Searria, Seera, Siearra,
Sierrah, Sierre*

Sigfreda (German) victorious peace. See
also Freda.

Sigmunda (German) victorious protector.

Signe (Latin) sign, signal.
(Scandinavian) a short form of
Sigourney.

Sigourney (English) victorious con-
querer.

Sigrid (Scandinavian) victorious counselor.

Sihu (Native American) flower; bush.

Siko (African) crying baby.

Silvia (Latin) a form of Sylvia.
Silivia, Silva

Simcha (Hebrew) joyful.

Simone (Hebrew) she heard. (French) a form of Simon (see Boys' Names). *Siminie, Simmi, Sinmie, Simmona, Simmone, Simoane, Simona, Simonetta, Simonette, Simonia, Simonina, Simonne, Somone*

Simran (Sikh) absorbed in God.

Sina (Irish) a form of Seana.

Sinclaire (French) prayer.

Sindy (American) a form of Cindy.

Sinead (Irish) a form of Jane.

Siobhan (Irish) a form of Joan. See also Shavonne.
Shibahn, Shibani, Shibhan, Shioban, Shobana, Shobha, Shobhana, Siobahn, Siobhana, Siobhann, Siobhon, Siovaun, Siovhan

Sirena (Greek) enchanter. Mythology: Sirens were sea nymphs whose singing enchanted sailors and made them crash their ships into nearby rocks.

Sisika (Native American) songbird.

Sissy (American) a familiar form of Cecelia.

Sita (Hindi) a form of Shakti.

Siti (Swahili) respected woman.

Skye (Arabic) water giver. (Dutch) a short form of Skyler. Geography: an island in the Hebrides, Scotland.
Sky

Skylar (Dutch) a form of Skyler.

Skyler (Dutch) sheltering.

Sloane (Irish) warrior.

Socorro (Spanish) helper.

Sofia ☀ (Greek) a form of Sophia. See also Zofia, Zsofia.
Sofeea, Sofeeia, Soffi, Sofi, Soficita, Sofie, Sofija, Sofiya, Sofya

Solada (Tai) listener.

Solana (Spanish) sunshine.

Solange (French) dignified.

Soledad (Spanish) solitary.

Solenne (French) solemn, dignified.

Soma (Hindi) lunar.

Sommer (English) summer; summoner. (Arabic) black. See also Summer.
Sommar, Sommara

Sondra (Greek) defender of mankind.
Sondre, Sonndra, Sonndre

Sonia (Russian, Slavic) a form of Sonya.
Sonica, Sonida, Sonita, Sonni, Sonnie, Sonny

Sonja (Scandinavian) a form of Sonya.
Sonjae, Sonjia

Sonya (Greek) wise. (Russian, Slavic) a form of Sophia.
Sunya

Sook (Korean) pure.

Sopheary (Cambodian) beautiful girl.

Sophia ☀ (Greek) wise. See also Sonya, Zofia.

Sophie (Greek) a familiar form of Sophia. See also Zocha.
Sophey, Sophi, Sophy

Sophronia (Greek) wise; sensible.

Sora (Native American) chirping songbird.

Soraya (Persian) princess.

Sorrel (French) reddish brown. Botany: a plant whose leaves are used as salad greens.

Soso (Native American) tree squirrel dining on pine nuts; chubby-cheeked baby.

Souzan (Persian) burning fire.

Spencer (English) dispenser of provisions.

Speranza (Italian) a form of Esperanza.

Spring (English) springtime.

Stacey, Stacy (Greek) resurrection. (Irish) a short form of Anastasia, Eustacia, Natasha.
Stace, Stacee, Staceyan, Staceyann, Staicy, Stayce, Staycee

Staci, Stacie (Greek) forms of Stacey.
Stacci, Stayci

Stacia (English) a short form of Anastasia.
Stasia, Staysha

Starla (English) a form of Starr.

Starleen (English) a form of Starr.

Starley (English) a familiar form of Starr.
Starle, Starlee

Starling (English) bird.

Starr (English) star.
Star, Staria, Starlet, Starlette, Starlight, Starly, Starri, Starria, Starrika, Starrsha, Starsha, Starshanna

Stasya (Greek) a familiar form of Anastasia. (Russian) a form of Stacey.
Stasia

Stefani, Steffani (Greek) forms of Stephanie.
Stafani, Steffane

Stefanie (Greek) a form of Stephanie.
Stafanie, Staffany, Stefaney, Stefania, Stefanié, Stefanija, Stefannie, Stefcia, Stefenie, Steffanie, Stefka

Stefany, Steffany (Greek) forms of Stephanie.

Steffi (Greek) a familiar form of Stefanie, Stephanie.
Stefcia, Steffie, Stefka

Stella (Latin) star. (French) a familiar form of Estelle.
Steile, Stellina

Stepania (Russian) a form of Stephanie.
Stephana

Stephani (Greek) a form of Stephanie.
Stephania

Stephanie ☼ (Greek) crowned. See also Estefani, Estephanie, Panya, Stevie, Zephania.
Stamatios, Steffie, Stephaija, Stephaine, Stephanas, Stephane, Stephanee, Stephanida, Stéphanie, Stephanine, Stephann, Stephannie, Stephianie, Stesha, Stevanee

Stephany (Greek) a form of Stephanie.
Stephaney

Stephene (Greek) a form of Stephanie.

Stephenie (Greek) a form of Stephanie.
Stephena

Stephney (Greek) a form of Stephanie.

Sterling (English) valuable; silver penny.

Stevie (Greek) a familiar form of
Stephanie.
*Steva, Stevana, Stevanee, Stevee,
Stevena, Stevey, Stevi, Stevy, Stevye*

Stina (German) a short form of
Christina.

Stockard (English) stockyard.

Stormie (English) a form of Stormy.
Stormi

Stormy (English) impetuous by nature.
Storm, Storme

Suchin (Tai) beautiful thought.

Sue (Hebrew) a short form of Susan,
Susanna.
Suetta

Sueann, Sueanna (American) combinations of Sue + Ann, Sue + Anna.
Suann, Suanna, Suanne, Sueanne

Suela (Spanish) consolation.

Sugar (American) sweet as sugar.

Sugi (Japanese) cedar tree.

Suke (Hawaiian) a form of Susan.

Sukey (Hawaiian) a familiar form of
Susan.

Sukhdeep (Sikh) light of peace and
bliss.

Suki (Japanese) loved one.
(Moquelumnan) eagle-eyed.

Sula (Icelandic) large sea bird. (Greek,
Hebrew) a short form of Shulamith,
Ursula.

Suletu (Moquelumnan) soaring bird.

Sulia (Latin) a form of Julia.

Sulwen (Welsh) bright as the sun.

Sumalee (Tai) beautiful flower.

Sumati (Hindi) unity.

Sumaya (American) a combination of
Sue + Maya.

Sumi (Japanese) elegant, refined.

Summer (English) summertime. See
also Sommer.
*Sumer, Summar, Summerbreeze,
Summerhaze, Summerlee*

Sun (Korean) obedient.
Sunya

Sunee (Tai) good.

Sun-Hi (Korean) good; joyful.

Suni (Zuni) native; member of our tribe.
Sunni, Sunnie

Sunki (Hopi) swift.

Sunny (English) bright, cheerful.
Sunni, Sunnie

Sunshine (English) sunshine.

Surata (Pakistani) blessed joy.

Suri (Todas) pointy nose.

Surya (Sanskrit) Mythology: a sun god.

Susammi (French) a combination of
Susan + Aimee.

Susan (Hebrew) lily. See also Shoshana,
Sukey, Zsa Zsa, Zusa.
*Sawsan, Siusan, Sosana, Sosanna,
Suesan, Sueva, Suisan, Susann,
Susen, Suson, Suzan*

Susana (Hebrew) a form of Susan.
Susanah

Susanna, Susannah (Hebrew) forms of Susan. See also Xuxa, Zanna, Zsuzsanna.
Sonel, Sosana, Suesanna, Susanah

Suse (Hawaiian) a form of Susan.

Susette (French) a familiar form of Susan, Susanna.
Susetta

Susie, Suzie (American) familiar forms of Susan, Susanna.
Susey, Susi, Sussi, Sussy, Susy, Suze, Suzi, Suzy

Suzanna, Suzannah (Hebrew) forms of Susan.
Suzana

Suzanne (English) a form of Susan.
Susanne, Suszanne, Suzane, Suzann, Suzzane, Suzzann, Suzzanne

Suzette (French) a form of Susan.
Suzetta

Suzu (Japanese) little bell.

Suzuki (Japanese) bell tree.

Svetlana (Russian) bright light.

Syá (Chinese) summer.

Sybella (English) a form of Sybil.

Sybil (Greek) prophet. Mythology: sibyls were oracles who relayed the messages of the gods. See also Cybele, Sibley.

Sydnee (French) a form of Sydney.

Sydney ✹ (French) from Saint-Denis, France. See also Sidonie.
Sy, Syd, Sydel, Sydelle, Sydna, Sydny, Sydnye, Syndona, Syndonah

Sydni, Sydnie (French) forms of Sydney.

Sying (Chinese) star.

Sylvana (Latin) forest.
Silvaine, Silvanna, Silviane, Sylva, Sylvaine, Sylvanna, Sylvina, Sylvinnia, Sylvonna

Sylvia (Latin) forest. Literature: Sylvia Plath was a well-known American poet. See also Silvia, Xylia.
Sylvette, Sylwia

Sylvianne (American) a combination of Sylvia + Anne.

Sylvie (Latin) a familiar form of Sylvia.
Silvi, Silvy, Sylvi

Symone (Hebrew) a form of Simone.
Symona

Symphony (Greek) symphony, harmonious sound.

Syreeta (Hindi) good traditions. (Arabic) companion.

T

Tabatha (Greek, Aramaic) a form of Tabitha.
Tabathe, Tabathia, Tabbatha

Tabby (English) a familiar form of Tabitha.
Tabbi

Tabia (Swahili) talented.

Tabetha (Greek, Aramaic) a form of Tabitha.

Tabina (Arabic) follower of Muhammad.

Tabitha (Greek, Aramaic) gazelle. *Tabbee, Tabbetha, Tabbey, Tabbi, Tabbie, Tabbitha, Tabithia, Tabotha, Tabtha*

Tabytha (Greek, Aramaic) a form of Tabitha.

Tacey (English) a familiar form of Tacita.

Taci (Zuni) washtub. (English) a form of Tacey.

Tacita (Latin) silent.

Tadita (Omaha) runner.

Taelor (English) a form of Taylor.

Taesha (Latin) a form of Tisha. (American) a combination of the prefix Ta + Aisha. *Teisha, Tesha*

Taffy (Welsh) beloved.

Tahira (Arabic) virginal, pure.

Tahlia (Greek, Hebrew) a form of Talia.

Tailor (English) a form of Taylor.

Taima (Native American) clash of thunder.

Taipa (Moquelumnan) flying quail.

Taite (English) cheerful.

Taja (Hindi) crown.

Taka (Japanese) honored.

Takala (Hopi) corn tassel.

Takara (Japanese) treasure.

Takayla (American) a combination of the prefix Ta + Kayla.

Takeisha (American) a combination of the prefix Ta + Keisha.

Takenya (Hebrew) animal horn. (Moquelumnan) falcon. (American) a combination of the prefix Ta + Kenya.

Takeria (American) a form of Takira.

Taki (Japanese) waterfall.

Takia (Arabic) worshiper. *Takeiyah, Takeya, Takija, Takiya, Takiyah, Takkia, Taqiyya, Taquaia, Taquaya, Taquiia, Tekeyia, Tekiya, Tikia, Tykeia, Tykia*

Takila (American) a form of Tequila.

Takira (American) a combination of the prefix Ta + Kira.

Tala (Native American) stalking wolf.

Talasi (Hopi) corn tassel.

Taleah (American) a form of Talia.

Taleisha (American) a combination of Talia + Aisha.

Talena (American) a combination of the prefix Ta + Lena.

Talesha (American) a form of Taleisha.

Talia (Greek) blooming. (Hebrew) dew from heaven. (Latin, French) birthday. A short form of Natalie. See also Thalia. *Taliah, Taliatha, Tallia, Tallya, Talya, Tylia*

Talina (American) a combination of Talia + Lina.

Talisa (English) a form of Tallis.

Talitha (Arabic) young girl. *Taliatha, Taliya*

Taliyah (Greek) a form of Talia.
Talieya, Talya, Talyah

Talley (French) a familiar form of Talia.
Tali, Tallie, Tally

Tallis (French, English) forest.

Tallulah (Choctaw) leaping water.

Tam (Vietnamese) heart.

Tama (Japanese) jewel.
Tamala

Tamaka (Japanese) bracelet.

Tamar (Hebrew) a short form of Tamara.
(Russian) History: a twelfth-century
Georgian queen. (Hebrew) a short form
of Tamara.
Tamer, Tamor, Tamour

Tamara (Hebrew) palm tree. See also
Tammy.
*Tamará, Tamarah, Tamaria,
Tamarin, Tamarla, Tamarra,
Tamarria, Tamarrian, Tamarsha,
Tamary, Tameriás, Tamma,
Tammara, Tamora, Tamoya, Tamura,
Tamyra, Temara, Temarian, Thama,
Thamar, Thamara, Thamarra,
Timara, Tomara, Tymara*

Tamassa (Hebrew) a form of
Thomasina.

Tameka (Aramaic) twin.
*Tameca, Tamecia, Tamecka,
Tameeka, Tamekia, Tamiecka,
Tamieka, Temeka, Timeeka, Timeka,
Tomeka, Tomekia, Trameika,
Tymeka, Tymmeeka, Tymmeka*

Tamera (Hebrew) a form of Tamara.
*Tamer, Tamerai, Tameria, Tammera,
Thamer, Timera*

Tamesha (American) a combination of
the prefix Ta + Mesha.

Tamika (Japanese) a form of Tamiko.
*Tamica, Tamieka, Tamikia, Tamikka,
Timika, Timikia, Tomika, Tymika,
Tymmicka*

Tamiko (Japanese) child of the people.
Tami, Tamike, Tamiqua, Tamiyo

Tamila (American) a combination of the
prefix Ta + Mila.
*Tamala, Tamela, Tamelia, Tamilla,
Tamille, Tamillia, Tamilya*

Tamira (Hebrew) a form of Tamara.
Tamyra

Tammi, Tammie (English) forms of
Tammy.
*Tami, Tamia, Tamiah, Tamie,
Tamijo, Tamiya*

Tammy (English) twin. (Hebrew) a
familiar form of Tamara.
*Tamilyn, Tamlyn, Tammee, Tammey,
Tamy, Tamya*

Tamra (Hebrew) a short form of Tamara.
Tammra, Tamrah

Tamsin (English) a short form of
Thomasina.

Tana (Slavic) a short form of Tanya.
*Taina, Tanae, Tanaeah, Tanah,
Tanairi, Tanairy, Tanalia, Tanara,
Tanavia, Tanaya, Tanaz, Tanna,
Tannah*

Tandy (English) team.

Taneisha, Tanesha (American) combinations of the prefix Ta + Niesha. *Tahniesha, Tanasha, Tanashia, Taneesha, Taneshea, Taneshia, Tanesia, Tanesian, Tanessa, Tanessia, Taniesha, Tanneshia, Tanniecia, Tanniesha, Tantashea*

Taneya (Russian, Slavic) a form of Tanya. *Tanea*

Tangia (American) a combination of the prefix Ta + Angela.

Tani (Japanese) valley. (Slavic) stand of glory. A familiar form of Tania. *Tahnee, Tany*

Tania (Russian, Slavic) fairy queen. *Taneea, Tanija, Taniya, Tannia, Tanniya, Tannya, Tarnia*

Taniel (American) a combination of Tania + Danielle. *Teniel*

Tanika (American) a form of Tania. *Tannica, Tianeka, Tianika*

Tanis, Tannis (Slavic) forms of Tania, Tanya. *Tanas, Tanese, Taniese, Tanka, Tannese, Tanniece, Tanniese, Tannise, Tannus, Tannyce, Tenice, Tenise, Tonise, Tranice, Tranise, Tynice, Tyniece, Tyniese, Tynise*

Tanisha (American) a combination of the prefix Ta + Nisha. *Tahniscia, Tahnisha, Tanasha, Tanashea, Tanicha, Taniesha, Tanish*

Tanissa (American) a combination of the prefix Tania + Nissa. *Tanesa, Tanisa, Tannesa, Tannisa, Tennessa, Tranissa*

Tanita (American) a combination of the prefix Ta + Nita.

Tanith (Phoenician) Mythology: Tanit is the goddess of love.

Tanner (English) leather worker, tanner.

Tansy (Greek) immortal. (Latin) tenacious, persistent.

Tanya (Russian, Slavic) fairy queen. *Tahnee, Tahnya, Tanaya, Taniya, Tanka, Tannya, Tanoya, Tany, Tanyia, Taunya, Thanya*

Tao (Chinese, Vietnamese) peach.

Tara (Aramaic) throw; carry. (Irish) rocky hill. (Arabic) a measurement. *Taira, Tairra, Taraea, Tarah, Taráh, Tarai, Taralee, Tarali, Tarasa, Tarasha, Taraya, Tarha, Tayra, Tebra*

Taraneh (Persian) melody.

Taree (Japanese) arching branch.

Tari (Irish) a familiar form of Tara. *Tarin, Tarina*

Tarissa (American) a combination of Tara + Rissa. *Taris, Tarisa, Tarise*

Tarra (Irish) a form of Tara. *Tarrah*

Taryn (Irish) a form of Tara. *Taran, Tareen, Tareena, Taren, Tarene, Tarin, Tarina, Tarren, Tarrena, Tarrin, Tarron, Tarryn, Taryna*

Tasarla (Gypsy) dawn.

Tasha (Greek) born on Christmas day.
(Russian) a short form of Natasha. See
also Tashi, Tosha.
*Tacha, Tachiana, Tachika, Tahsha,
Tasenka, Taska, Thasha, Tiaisha,
Tysha*

Tashana (American) a combination of
the prefix Ta + Shana.
Tashiana, Tashina

Tashara (American) a combination of
the prefix Ta + Shara.

Tashawna (American) a combination
of the prefix Ta + Shawna.
Tiashauna

Tasheena (American) a combination of
the prefix Ta + Sheena.
Tashina

Tashelle (American) a combination of
the prefix Ta + Shelley.

Tashi (Hausa) a bird in flight. (Slavic) a
form of Tasha.
Tashia

Tasia (Slavic) a familiar form of Tasha.
*Tachia, Tasiya, Tassi, Tassia, Tassiana,
Tassie, Tasya*

Tassos (Greek) a form of Theresa.

Tata (Russian) a familiar form of
Tatiana.
Tatia

Tate (English) a short form of Tatum. A
form of Taite, Tata.

Tatiana (Slavic) fairy queen. See also
Tanya, Tiana.
*Tatania, Tatanya, Tati, Tatia, Tatie,
Tatihana, Tatjana, Tiatiana*

Tatianna (Slavic) a form of Tatiana.
Taitiann, Taitianna

Tatiyana (Slavic) a form of Tatiana.

Tatum (English) cheerful.
Tatumn

Tatyana (Slavic) a form of Tatiana.
Tatyanah, Tatyanna

Taura (Latin) bull. Astrology: Taurus is a
sign of the zodiac.

Tauri (English) a form of Tory.

Tavia (Latin) a short form of Octavia.
See also Tawia.
Taiva, Tauvia, Tava, Tavah, Tavita

Tavie (Scottish) twin.

Tawanna (American) a combination of
the prefix Ta + Wanda.

Tawia (African) born after twins.
(Polish) a form of Tavia.

Tawni (English) a form of Tawny.
*Tauni, Taunia, Tawnia, Tawnie,
Tiawni*

Tawny (Gypsy) little one. (English)
brownish yellow, tan.
*Tahnee, Tany, Tauna, Tauné,
Taunisha, Tawnee, Tawnesha,
Tawney, Tawnyell, Tiawna*

Tawnya (American) a combination of
Tawny + Tonya.
Tawna

Taya, Taye (English) short forms of
Taylor.
Tayra

Tayla (English) a short form of Taylor.

Taylar (English) a form of Taylor.

Tayler (English) a form of Taylor.

Taylor ✿ (English) tailor.
Taiylor, Talor, Talora, Tayllor, Taylore

Tazu (Japanese) stork; longevity.

Teagan (Welsh) beautiful, attractive.
*Taegen, Teaghen, Teegan, Teeghan,
Tegwen, Teigan, Tejan, Tiegan, Tigan,
Tijan, Tijana*

Teaira (Latin) a form of Tiara.
*Teairra, Teara, Tearia, Tearra,
Tearria*

Teal (English) river duck; blue green.

Teanna (American) a combination of
the prefix Te + Anna. A form of Tiana.
Teana, Teena

Teca (Hungarian) a form of Theresa.

Tecla (Greek) God's fame.

Teddi (Greek) a familiar form of
Theodora.

Tedra (Greek) a short form of Theodora.

Tegan (Welsh) a form of Teagan.
Tega, Teghan, Tegin

Telisha (American) a form of Taleisha.

Temira (Hebrew) tall.

Tempest (French) stormy.

Tenesha, Tenisha (American) combi-
nations of the prefix Te + Niesha.
*Tenecia, Teneesha, Teneisha, Teneshia,
Tenesia, Tenessa, Teneusa, Tenezya,
Teniesha*

Tennille (American) a combination of
the prefix Te + Nellie.
*Tanille, Teneal, Teneil, Teneille, Teniel,
Tenille, Tenneal, Tenneill, Tenneille,
Tennia, Tennie, Tennielle, Tennile,
Tineal, Tiniel, Tonielle, Tonille*

Teodora (Czech) a form of Theodora.

Teona, Teonna (Greek) forms of Tiana,
Tianna.

Tequila (Spanish) a kind of liquor. See
also Takila.

Tera, Terra (Latin) earth. (Japanese)
swift arrow. (American) forms of Tara.
Teria, Terria

Teralyn (American) a combination of
Terri + Lynn.
Taralyn

Teresa (Greek) a form of Theresa. See
also Tressa.
*Taresa, Taressa, Terasa, Tercza,
Tereasa, Tereatha, Teresea, Teresha,
Teresia, Teresina, Teresita, Tereska,
Tereson, Teressa, Teretha, Tereza,
Terezia, Terezie, Terezilya, Terezinha,
Terezka, Terezsa, Terisa, Terisha,
Teriza, Terrasa, Terresa, Terresia,
Terrosina, Tersa, Teruska, Terza, Teté,
Tyresa, Tyresia*

Terese (Greek) a form of Teresa.
*Tarese, Taress, Taris, Tarise, Tereese,
Teress, Terez, Teris, Terrise*

Teri (Greek) reaper. A familiar form of
Theresa.
Terie

Terrelle (Greek) a form of Theresa.
Tyrell, Tyrelle

Terrene (Latin) smooth.
Tareena, Terene, Terrosina, Tyrene

Terri (Greek) reaper. A familiar form of
Theresa.
Terree, Terria, Terrie

Terriann (American) a combination of
Terri + Ann.
Terria

Terrianna (American) a combination of Terri + Anna.
Tyrina

Terrica (American) a combination of Terri + Erica. See also Rica.
Tereka, Tyrica, Tyricka, Tyrikka, Tyronica

Terry (Greek) a short form of Theresa.
Tere, Teree, Terelle, Terene, Terie, Terrey, Terrie, Terrye, Tery

Terry-Lynn (American) a combination of Terry + Lynn.
Terelyn, Terelynn, Terri-Lynn, Terrilynn, Terrylynn

Tertia (Latin) third.
Terza

Tess (Greek) a short form of Quintessa, Theresa.

Tessa (Greek) reaper.
Tesa, Tesha, Tesia, Tessia, Tezia

Tessie (Greek) a familiar form of Theresa.

Tetsu (Japanese) strong as iron.

Tetty (English) a familiar form of Elizabeth.

Tevy (Cambodian) angel.

Teylor (English) a form of Taylor.

Thaddea (Greek) courageous. (Latin) praiser.

Thalassa (Greek) sea, ocean.

Thalia (Greek) a form of Talia. Mythology: the Muse of comedy.

Thana (Arabic) happy occasion.

Thanh (Vietnamese) bright blue. (Punjabi) good place.
Thantra, Thanya

Thao (Vietnamese) respectful of parents.

Thea (Greek) goddess. A short form of Althea.
Theo

Thelma (Greek) willful.

Thema (African) queen.

Theodora (Greek) gift of God. See also Dora, Dorothy, Feodora.
Theo

Theone (Greek) gift of God.

Theophania (Greek) God's appearance. See also Tiffany.
Theo

Theophila (Greek) loved by God.
Theo

Theresa (Greek) reaper. See also Resi, Reza, Riza, Tassos, Teca, Terrelle, Tracey, Tracy, Zilya.
Thérèse, Theresia, Theresina, Theresita, Theressa, Thereza, Thersa, Thersea

Therese (Greek) a form of Theresa.
Terise, Theresia, Theressa, Therra, Therressa, Thersa

Theta (Greek) Linguistics: a letter in the Greek alphabet.

Thetis (Greek) disposed. Mythology: the mother of Achilles.

Thi (Vietnamese) poem.
Thia, Thy, Thya

Thirza (Hebrew) pleasant.

Thomasina (Hebrew) twin. See also Tamassa.

Thora (Scandinavian) thunder.

Thuy (Vietnamese) gentle.

Tia (Greek) princess. (Spanish) aunt.
Téa, Teah, Teeya, Teia, Ti, Tiakeisha, Tialeigh, Tiamarie, Tianda, Tiandria, Tiante, Tiia

Tiana, Tianna (Greek) princess. (Latin) short forms of Tatiana.
Teana, Tiahna, Tiaon

Tiara (Latin) crowned.
Teair, Teara, Téare, Tearia, Tearria, Teearia, Teira, Teirra, Tiaira, Tyara

Tiarra (Latin) a form of Tiara.
Tiairra, Tyarra

Tiauna (Greek) a form of Tiana.

Tiberia (Latin) Geography: the Tiber River in Italy.

Tichina (American) a combination of the prefix Ti + China.

Tida (Tai) daughter.

Tiera, Tierra (Latin) forms of Tiara.
Tiéra, Tierre, Tierrea, Tierria

Tierney (Irish) noble.
Tiernan

Tiff (Latin) a short form of Tiffani, Tiffanie, Tiffany.

Tiffani, Tiffanie (Latin) forms of Tiffany.
Tephanie, Tifanee, Tifani, Tifanie, Tiffanee, Tiffayne, Tiffeni, Tiffenie, Tiffennie, Tiffiani, Tiffianie, Tiffine, Tiffini, Tiffinie, Tiffni, Tiffynie, Tifni

Tiffany (Latin) trinity. (Greek) a short form of Theophania. See also Tyfany.
Taffanay, Taffany, Tifaney, Tifany,

Tiffaney, Tiffanny, Tiffeney, Tiffiany, Tiffiney, Tiffiry, Tiffnay, Tiffney, Tiffry, Triffany

Tiffy (Latin) a familiar form of Tiffani, Tiffany.

Tijuana (Spanish) Geography: a border town in Mexico.
Tiajuanna, Tiawanna

Tilda (German) a short form of Matilda.

Tillie (German) a familiar form of Matilda.

Timi (English) a familiar form of Timothea.

Timothea (English) honoring God.

Tina (Spanish, American) a short form of Augustine, Martina, Christina, Valentina.
Teena, Teina, Tena, Tenae, Tine, Tinnia, Tynka

Tinble (English) sound bells make.

Tinesha (American) a combination of the prefix Ti + Niesha.

Tinisha (American) a form of Tenisha.

Tiona, Tionna (American) forms of Tiana.

Tiphanie (Latin) a form of Tiffany.
Tiphani, Tiphany

Tiponya (Native American) great horned owl.

Tipper (Irish) water pourer. (Native American) a short form of Tiponya.

Tira (Hindi) arrow.

Tirtha (Hindi) ford.

Tirza (Hebrew) pleasant.
Thersa

Tisa (Swahili) ninth-born.

Tish (Latin) a short form of Tisha.

Tisha (Latin) joy. A short form of Leticia.
Tesha, Teisha, Tiesha, Tieshia, Tishal, Tishia, Tysha, Tyshia

Tita (Greek) giant. (Spanish) a short form of names ending in "tita." A form of Titus (see Boys' Names).

Titania (Greek) giant. Mythology: the Titans were a race of giants.

Titiana (Greek) a form of Titania.

Tivona (Hebrew) nature lover.

Tiwa (Zuni) onion.

Tiyana (Greek) a form of Tiana.

Tobi (Hebrew) God is good.

Tocarra (American) a combination of the prefix To + Cara.

Toinette (French) a short form of Antoinette.

Toki (Japanese) hopeful.

Tola (Polish) a form of Toinette.

Tomi (Japanese) rich.

Tommie (Hebrew) a short form of Thomasina.

Tomo (Japanese) intelligent.

Tonesha (American) a combination of the prefix To + Niesha.

Toni (Greek) flourishing. (Latin) praise-worthy.
Tonee, Toney, Tonie, Tonni, Tonnie, Tony

Tonia (Latin, Slavic) a form of Toni, Tonya.
Tonja, Tonje, Tonna, Tonni, Tonnia, Tonnie, Tonnja

Tonisha (American) a form of Toneisha.
Tonise

Tonya (Slavic) fairy queen.
Tonnya, Tonyetta

Topaz (Latin) golden yellow gem.

Topsy (English) on top. Literature: a slave in Harriet Beecher Stowe's novel *Uncle Tom's Cabin.*

Tora (Japanese) tiger.

Tori (Japanese) bird. (English) a form of Tory.
Torrita

Toria (English) a form of Tori, Tory.
Torria

Toriana (English) a form of Tori.

Torie, Torrie (English) forms of Tori.

Torilyn (English) a combination of Tori + Lynn.

Torri (English) a form of Tori.

Tory (English) victorious. (Latin) a short form of Victoria.
Torey, Torrey, Torreya, Torrye, Torya, Torye

Tosha (Punjabi) armaments. (Polish) a familiar form of Antonia. (Russian) a form of Tasha.
Toshea, Toshia, Toshiea, Toshke, Tosia, Toska

Toshi (Japanese) mirror image.

Toski (Hopi) squashed bug.

Totsi (Hopi) moccasins.

Tottie (English) a familiar form of Charlotte.

Tovah (Hebrew) good.

Toya (Spanish) a form of Tory.
Toia, Toyanika, Toyanna, Toyea, Toylea, Toyleah, Toylenn, Toylin, Toylyn

Tracey (Greek) a familiar form of Theresa. (Latin) warrior.
Trace, Tracee, Tracell, Traice, Trasey, Treesy

Traci, Tracie (Latin) forms of Tracey.
Tracia, Tracilee, Tracilyn, Tracilynn, Tracina, Traeci

Tracy (Greek) a familiar form of Theresa. (Latin) warrior.
Treacy

Tralena (Latin) a combination of Tracy + Lena.

Tranesha (American) a combination of the prefix Tra + Niesha.
Tranice

Trashawn (American) a combination of the prefix Tra + Shawn (see Shawna).

Trava (Czech) spring grasses.

Treasure (Latin) treasure, wealth; valuable.

Trella (Spanish) a familiar form of Estelle.

Tresha (Greek) a form of Theresa.

Tressa (Greek) a short form of Theresa. See also Teresa.
Treaser, Tresa, Tresca, Trese, Treska, Tressia, Tressie, Trez, Treza, Trisa

Trevina (Irish) prudent. (Welsh) homestead.

Trevona (Irish) a form of Trevina.

Triana (Latin) third. (Greek) a form of Trina.

Trice (Greek) a short form of Theresa.
Treece

Tricia (Latin) a form of Trisha.
Trica, Tricha, Trichelle, Tricina, Trickia

Trilby (English) soft hat.

Trina (Greek) pure.
Treena, Treina, Trenna, Trinia, Trinchen, Trind, Trinda, Trine, Trinette, Trinica, Trinice, Triniece, Trinika, Trinique, Trinisa

Trini (Greek) a form of Trina.
Trinia

Trinity ❋ (Latin) triad. Religion: the Father, the Son, and the Holy Spirit.
Trinnette

Trish (Latin) a short form of Beatrice, Trisha.

Trisha (Latin) noblewoman. (Hindi) thirsty. See also Tricia.
Treasha, Trishann, Trishanna, Trishanne, Trishara, Trishia, Trishna, Trissha

Trissa (Latin) a familiar form of
Patricia.
Trisa

Trista (Latin) a short form of Tristen.
Trisatal, Tristess, Tristia, Trysta,
Trystia

Tristan (Latin) bold.
Tristian, Tristiana, Trystan

Tristen (Latin) a form of Tristan.

Tristin (Latin) a form of Tristan.
Tristina, Tristine

Triston, Trystyn (Latin) forms of
Tristan.

Trixie (American) a familiar form of
Beatrice.

Troya (Irish) foot soldier.

Trudel (Dutch) a form of Trudy.

Trudy (German) a familiar form of
Gertrude.
Truda, Trude, Trudessa, Trudey,
Trudi, Trudie

Trycia (Latin) a form of Trisha.

Tryna (Greek) a form of Trina.

Tryne (Dutch) pure.
Trine

Tsigana (Hungarian) a form of Zigana.

Tu (Chinese) jade.

Tuesday (English) born on the third day
of the week.

Tula (Hindi) born in the lunar month of
Capricorn.

Tullia (Irish) peaceful, quiet.

Tulsi (Hindi) basil, a sacred Hindi herb.

Turquoise (French) blue-green semiprecious stone.

Tusa (Zuni) prairie dog.

Tuyen (Vietnamese) angel.

Tuyet (Vietnamese) snow.

Twyla (English) woven of double thread.
Twila, Twilla

Tyanna (American) a combination of
the prefix Ty + Anna.

Tyeisha (American) a form of Tyesha.
Tyisha

Tyesha (American) a combination of Ty
+ Aisha.
Tyisha

Tyfany (American) a short form of
Tiffany.

Tykeisha (American) a form of
Takeisha.

Tykera (American) a form of Takira.

Tyler (English) tailor.
Tyller, Tylor

Tyna (Czech) a short form of Kristina.

Tyne (English) river.
Tine

Tynesha (American) a combination of
Ty + Niesha.

Tynisha (American) a form of Tynesha.
Tynise

Tyra (Scandinavian) battler. Mythology: Tyr was the god of war. A form of Thora. (Hindi) a form of Tira.
Tyraa, Tyrah, Tyran, Tyree, Tyrena, Tyria

Tyshanna (American) a combination of Ty + Shawna.

Tytiana (Greek) a form of Titania.

U

U (Korean) gentle.

Udele (English) prosperous.

Ula (Irish) sea jewel. (Scandinavian) wealthy. (Spanish) a short form of Eulalia.

Ulani (Polynesian) cheerful.

Ulima (Arabic) astute; wise.

Ulla (German, Swedish) willful. (Latin) a short form of Ursula.
Ulli

Ulrica (German) wolf ruler; ruler of all. See also Rica.
Ulka, Ullrica, Ullricka, Ullrika, Ulrika, Ulrike

Ultima (Latin) last, endmost, farthest.

Ululani (Hawaiian) heavenly inspiration.

Ulva (German) wolf.

Uma (Hindi) mother. Religion: another name for the Hindu goddess Devi.

Umay (Turkish) hopeful.

Umeko (Japanese) plum-blossom child; patient.

Una (Latin) one; united. (Hopi) good memory. (Irish) a form of Agnes. See also Oona.

Undine (Latin) little wave. Mythology: the undines were water spirits. See also Ondine.

Unice (English) a form of Eunice.

Unika (American) a form of Unique.

Unique (Latin) only one.

Unity (English) unity.

Unn (Norwegian) she who is loved.

Unna (German) woman.

Urania (Greek) heavenly. Myth-ology: the Muse of astronomy.

Urbana (Latin) city dweller.

Urika (Omaha) useful to everyone.

Urit (Hebrew) bright.
Urice

Ursa (Greek) a short form of Ursula. (Latin) a form of Orsa.

Ursula (Greek) little bear. See also Sula, Ulla, Vorsila.
Ursala, Ursel, Ursela, Ursella, Ursely, Ursilla, Ursillane, Ursola, Ursule, Ursulina, Ursuline, Urszula, Urszuli, Urzula

Usha (Hindi) sunrise.

Ushi (Chinese) ox. Astrology: a sign of the Chinese zodiac.

Uta (German) rich. (Japanese) poem.

Utina (Native American) woman of my country.

V

Vail (English) valley.
Vale

Val (Latin) a short form of Valentina, Valerie.

Vala (German) singled out.

Valarie (Latin) a form of Valerie.
Valarae, Valaree, Valarey, Valari, Valaria, Vallarie

Valda (German) famous ruler.
Valida

Valencia (Spanish) strong. Geography: a region in eastern Spain.
Valecia, Valence, Valenica, Valentia, Valenzia

Valene (Latin) a short form of Valentina.
Valaine, Valean, Valeda, Valeen, Valen, Valena, Valeney, Valien, Valina, Valine, Vallan, Vallen

Valentina (Latin) strong. History: Valentina Tereshkova, a Soviet cosmonaut, was the first woman in space. See also Tina, Valene, Valli.
Valantina, Vale, Valentijn, Valentin, Valentine, Valtina, Valyn, Valynn

Valera (Russian) a form of Valerie. See also Lera.

Valeria (Latin) a form of Valerie.
Valaria, Valeriana, Valeriane, Veleria

Valerie (Latin) strong.
Vairy, Vale, Valeree, Valeri, Valérie,
Valka, Valleree, Valleri, Vallerie, Vallirie, Valry, Valya, Velerie

Valery (Latin) a form of Valerie.
Valerye, Vallery

Valeska (Slavic) glorious ruler.

Valli (Latin) a familiar form of Valentina, Valerie. Botany: a plant native to India.

Valma (Finnish) loyal defender.

Valonia (Latin) shadow valley.

Valora (Latin) a form of Valerie.
Velora

Valorie (Latin) a form of Valerie.

Vanda (German) a form of Wanda.

Vanesa (Greek) a form of Vanessa.
Vanesha, Vanesia, Vanisa

Vanessa ☙ (Greek) butterfly. Literature: a name invented by Jonathan Swift as a nickname for Esther Vanhomrigh. See also Nessie.
Van, Vanassa, Vaneshia, Vanesse, Vanessia, Vanessica, Vaneza, Vaniece, Vaniessa, Vanija, Vanika, Vanissa, Vanita, Vanni, Vannie, Vanny, Varnessa

Vanetta (English) a form of Vanessa.
Vanita

Vania, Vanya (Russian) familiar forms of Anna.
Vanija

Vanity (English) vain.

Vanna (Cambodian) golden. (Greek) a short form of Vanessa.
Vana, Vanae, Vannah, Vannalee, Vannaleigh, Vannie, Vanny

Vannesa, Vannessa (Greek) forms of
Vanessa.
Vanneza

Vanora (Welsh) white wave.

Vantrice (American) a combination of
the prefix Van + Trice.

Varda (Hebrew) rose.

Varvara (Slavic) a form of Barbara.
Vara

Vashti (Persian) lovely. Bible: the wife of
Ahasuerus, king of Persia.

Veanna (American) a combination of
the prefix Ve + Anna.

Veda (Sanskrit) sacred lore; knowledge.
Religion: the Vedas are the sacred writ-
ings of Hinduism.

Vedette (Italian) sentry; scout. (French)
movie star.

Vega (Arabic) falling star.

Velda (German) a form of Valda.

Velika (Slavic) great, wondrous.

Velma (German) a familiar form of
Vilhelmina.

Velvet (English) velvety.

Venecia (Italian) from Venice, Italy.

Venessa (Latin) a form of Vanessa.

Venus (Latin) love. Mythology: the
goddess of love and beauty.

Vera (Latin) true. (Slavic) faith. A short
form of Elvera, Veronica. See also
Verena, Wera.
*Vara, Veera, Veira, Veradis, Vere,
Verla, Viera, Vira*

Verbena (Latin) sacred plants.

Verda (Latin) young, fresh.

Verdad (Spanish) truthful.

Verena (Latin) truthful. A familiar form
of Vera, Verna.
Verusya, Virna

Verenice (Latin) a form of Veronica.

Verity (Latin) truthful.

Verlene (Latin) a combination of
Veronica + Lena.

Verna (Latin) springtime. (French) a
familiar form of Laverne. See also
Verena, Wera.
*Verla, Verne, Vernetia, Vernetta,
Vernette, Vernia, Vernita, Verusya,
Viera, Virida, Virna, Virnell*

Vernice (Latin) a form of Bernice,
Verna.
*Vernese, Vernesha, Verneshia,
Vernessa, Vernis, Vernisha, Vernisheia*

Veronica (Latin) true image. See also
Ronni, Weronika.
*Varonica, Veranique, Verhonica,
Verinica, Verohnica, Veron, Verona,
Veronic, Véronic, Veronice, Veronne,
Veronnica, Vironica, Vron, Vronica*

Veronika (Latin) a form of Veronica.

Veronique, Véronique (French) forms
of Veronica.
(Latin) evening star.

Vesta (Latin) keeper of the house.
Mythology: the goddess of the home.

Veta (Slavic) a familiar form of
Elizabeth.

Vi (Latin, French) a short form of Viola, Violet.

Vianca (Spanish) a form of Bianca.

Vianey (American) a familiar form of Vianna.

Vianna (American) a combination of Vi + Anna.

Vica (Hungarian) a form of Eve.

Vicki, Vickie (Latin) familiar forms of Victoria.
Vic, Vicci, Vicke, Vickee, Vickiana, Vickilyn, Vickki, Vika, Viki, Vikie, Vikki, Vikky

Vicky (Latin) a familiar form of Victoria.
Viccy, Vickey, Viky, Vikkey, Vikky

Victoria ❧ (Latin) victorious. See also Tory, Wicktoria, Wisia.
Victoire, Victoriana, Victorie, Victorina, Victorine, Victory, Vyctoria

Vida (Sanskrit) a form of Veda. (Hebrew) a short form of Davida.

Vidonia (Portuguese) branch of a vine.

Vienna (Latin) Geography: the capital of Austria.

Viktoria (Latin) a form of Victoria.

Vilhelmina (German) a form of Wilhelmina.

Villette (French) small town.

Vilma (German) a short form of Vilhemina.

Vina (Hindi) Mythology: a musical instrument played by the Hindu goddess of wisdom. (Spanish) vineyard. (Hebrew) a short form of Davina.

(English) a short form of Alvina. See also Lavina.

Vincentia (Latin) victor, conqueror.

Viñita (Spanish) a form of Vina.

Viola (Latin) violet; stringed instrument in the violin family. Literature: the heroine of Shakespeare's play *Twelfth Night*.

Violet (French) Botany: a plant with purplish blue flowers.
Violette, Vyolet, Vyoletta, Vyolette

Violeta (French) a form of Violet.
Violetta

Virgilia (Latin) rod bearer, staff bearer.

Virginia (Latin) pure, virginal. Literature: Virginia Woolf was a well-known British writer. See also Gina, Ginger, Ginny, Jinny.
Verginia, Verginya, Virge, Virgen, Virgenia, Virgenya, Virgie, Virgine, Virginië, Virginio, Virginnia, Virgy, Virjeana

Virginie (French) a form of Virginia.

Viridiana (Latin) a form of Viridis.

Viridis (Latin) green.
Virida

Virtue (Latin) virtuous.

Vita (Latin) life.

Vitoria (Spanish) a form of Victoria.

Viv (Latin) a short form of Vivian.

Viva (Latin) a short form of Aviva, Vivian.

Viveca (Scandinavian) a form of Vivian.

Vivian (Latin) full of life.
Vevay, Vevey, Vivee, Vivi, Vivia,
Viviane, Viviann, Vivianne, Vivie,
Vivien, Vivienne, Vivina, Vivion,
Vivyan, Vivyann, Vivyanne, Vyvyan,
Vyvyann, Vyvyanne

Viviana (Latin) a form of Vivian.
Vivianna, Vivyana, Vyvyana

Vondra (Czech) loving woman.

Voneisha (American) a combination of
Yvonne + Aisha.

Vonna (French) a form of Yvonne.

Vonny (French) a familiar form of
Yvonne.
Vonni, Vonnie

Vontricia (American) a combination of
Yvonne + Tricia.

Vorsila (Greek) a form of Ursula.

W

Wadd (Arabic) beloved.

Waheeda (Arabic) one and only.

Wainani (Hawaiian) beautiful water.

Wakana (Japanese) plant.

Wakanda (Dakota) magical power.

Wakeisha (American) a combination
of the prefix Wa + Keisha.

Walad (Arabic) newborn.

Walda (German) powerful; famous.

Waleria (Polish) a form of Valerie.

Walker (English) cloth; walker.

Wallis (English) from Wales.

Wanda (German) wanderer. See also
Wendy.
Wahnda, Wandah, Wandely, Wandis,
Wandja, Wandzia, Wannda, Wonda,
Wonnda

Wandie (German) a familiar form of
Wanda.
Wandi, Wandy

Waneta (Native American) charger. See
also Juanita.

Wanetta (English) pale face.

Wanika (Hawaiian) a form of Juanita.

Warda (German) guardian.

Washi (Japanese) eagle.

Wattan (Japanese) homeland.

Wauna (Moquelumnan) snow geese
honking.

Wava (Slavic) a form of Barbara.

Waverly (English) quaking aspen-tree
meadow.

Waynesha (American) a combination
of Waynette + Niesha.

Waynette (English) wagon maker.

Weeko (Dakota) pretty girl.

Wehilani (Hawaiian) heavenly adorn-
ment.

Wenda (Welsh) a form of Wendy.

Wendelle (English) wanderer.

Wendi (Welsh) a form of Wendy.
Wendie

Wendy (Welsh) white; light skinned. A familiar form of Gwendolyn, Wanda. *Wende, Wendee, Wendey, Wendye*

Wera (Polish) a form of Vera. See also Verna.

Weronika (Polish) a form of Veronica.

Wesisa (Musoga) foolish.

Weslee (English) western meadow.

Whitley (English) white field.

Whitney (English) white island. *Whiteney, Whitne, Whitné, Whitnee, Whitneigh, Whitny, Whitnye, Whytne, Whytney, Witney*

Whitnie (English) a form of Whitney.

Whittney (English) a form of Whitney. *Whittany, Whitteny*

Whoopi (English) happy; excited.

Wicktoria (Polish) a form of Victoria.

Wilda (German) untamed. (English) willow.

Wileen (English) a short form of Wilhelmina.

Wilhelmina (German) a form of Wilhelm (see Boys' Names). See also Billie, Guillerma, Helma, Minka, Minna, Minnie.

Wilikinia (Hawaiian) a form of Virginia.

Willa (German) a short form of Wilhelmina.

Willette (English) a familiar form of Wilhelmina, Willa.

Willie (English) a familiar form of Wilhelmina.

Willow (English) willow tree.

Wilma (German) a short form of Wilhelmina.

Wilona (English) desired.

Win (German) a short form of Winifred. See also Edwina.

Winda (Swahili) hunter.

Windy (English) windy.

Winema (Moquelumnan) woman chief.

Winifred (German) peaceful friend. (Welsh) a form of Guinevere. See also Freddi, Una, Winnie.

Winna (African) friend.

Winnie (English) a familiar form of Edwina, Gwyneth, Winnifred, Winona, Wynne. History: Winnie Mandela kept the anti-apartheid movement alive in South Africa while her then-husband, Nelson Mandela, was imprisoned. Literature: the lovable bear in A. A. Milne's children's story *Winnie-the-Pooh*.

Winola (German) charming friend.

Winona (Lakota) oldest daughter. *Wanona, Wenona, Wenonah, Winonah*

Winter (English) winter. *Wintr*

Wira (Polish) a form of Elvira.

Wisia (Polish) a form of Victoria.

Wren (English) wren, songbird.

Wyanet (Native American) legendary beauty.

Wynne (Welsh) white, light skinned. A short form of Blodwyn, Guinivere, Gwyneth.

Wynonna (Lakota) a form of Winona. *Wynnona, Wynona*

Wynter (English) a form of Winter.

Wyoming (Native American) Geography: a western U. S. state.

Xandra (Greek) a form of Zandra. (Spanish) a short form of Alexandra.

Xanthe (Greek) yellow, blond. See also Zanthe.

Xanthippe (Greek) a form of Xanthe. History: Socrates's wife.

Xaviera (Basque) owner of the new house. (Arabic) bright. See also Javiera, Zaviera. *Xavia*

Xela (Quiché) my mountain home.

Xena (Greek) a form of Xenia.

Xenia (Greek) hospitable. See also Zena, Zina. *Xeenia*

Xiang (Chinese) fragrant.

Xiomara (Teutonic) glorious forest.

Xiu Mei (Chinese) beautiful plum.

Xochitl (Aztec) place of many flowers.

Xuan (Vietnamese) spring.

Xuxa (Portuguese) a familiar form of Susanna.

Xylia (Greek) a form of Sylvia.

Yachne (Hebrew) hospitable.

Yadira (Hebrew) friend.

Yael (Hebrew) strength of God. See also Jael.

Yaffa (Hebrew) beautiful. See also Jaffa.

Yahaira (Hebrew) a form of Yakira.

Yajaira (Hebrew) a form of Yakira.

Yakira (Hebrew) precious; dear.

Yalanda (Greek) a form of Yolanda.

Yalena (Greek, Russian) a form of Helen. See also Lena, Yelena.

Yaletha (American) a form of Oletha.

Yamary (American) a combination of the prefix Ya + Mary.

Yamelia (American) a form of Amelia.

Yamila (Arabic) a form of Jamila.

Yaminah (Arabic) right, proper.

Yamka (Hopi) blossom.

Yamuna (Hindi) sacred river.

Yana (Slavic) a form of Jana.

Yanaba (Navajo) brave.

Yaneli (American) a combination of the prefix Ya + Nellie.

Yanet (American) a form of Janet.

Yáng (Chinese) sun.

Yareli (American) a form of Oralee.

Yarina (Slavic) a form of Irene.

Yaritza (American) a combination of Yana + Ritsa.

Yarkona (Hebrew) green.

Yarmilla (Slavic) market trader.

Yashira (Afghan) humble; takes it easy. (Arabic) wealthy.

Yasmeen (Persian) a form of Yasmin.
Yasmene

Yasmin, Yasmine (Persian) jasmine flower.
Yashmine, Yasiman, Yasimine, Yasma, Yasmain, Yasmaine, Yasmina, Yasminda, Yasmon, Yasmyn, Yesmean, Yesmeen, Yesmin, Yesmina, Yesmine, Yesmyn

Yasu (Japanese) resting, calm.

Yazmin (Persian) a form of Yasmin.
Yazmen, Yazmina, Yazmine

Yecenia (Arabic) a form of Yesenia.

Yehudit (Hebrew) a form of Judith.

Yei (Japanese) flourishing.

Yeira (Hebrew) light.

Yekaterina (Russian) a form of Katherine.

Yelena (Russian) a form of Helen, Jelena. See also Lena, Yalena.

Yelisabeta (Russian) a form of Elizabeth.

Yemena (Arabic) from Yemen.

Yen (Chinese) yearning; desirous.

Yenene (Native American) shaman.

Yenifer (Welsh) a form of Jennifer.

Yeo (Korean) mild.

Yepa (Native American) snow girl.

Yesenia (Arabic) flower.
Yesnia

Yesica (Hebrew) a form of Jessica.

Yessenia (Arabic) a form of Yesenia.
Yessena, Yissenia

Yessica (Hebrew) a form of Jessica.

Yetta (English) a short form of Henrietta.

Yeva (Ukrainian) a form of Eve.

Yiesha (Arabic, Swahili) a form of Aisha.

Yín (Chinese) silver.

Ynez (Spanish) a form of Agnes. See also Inez.

Yoanna (Hebrew) a form of Joanna.

Yocelin, Yocelyn (Latin) forms of Jocelyn.

Yoi (Japanese) born in the evening.

Yoki (Hopi) bluebird.

Yoko (Japanese) good girl.
Yo

Yolie (Greek) a familiar form of Yolanda.
Yola

Yolanda (Greek) violet flower. See also Iolanthe, Jolanda, Olinda.
Yolaine, Yolana, Yoland, Yolande, Yolane, Yolanna, Yolantha, Yolanthe, Yolette, Yolonda, Yorlanda, Youlanda, Yulanda, Yulonda

Yoluta (Native American) summer flower.

Yomara (American) a combination of Yolanda + Tamara.

Yon (Burmese) rabbit. (Korean) lotus blossom.

Yoné (Japanese) wealth; rice.

Yonina (Hebrew) a form of Jonina.

Yonita (Hebrew) a form of Jonita.

Yoomee (Coos) star.

Yordana (Basque) descendant. See also Jordana.

Yori (Japanese) reliable.

Yoselin (Latin) a form of Jocelyn.

Yosepha (Hebrew) a form of Josephine.

Yoshi (Japanese) good; respectful.

Yovela (Hebrew) joyful heart; rejoicer.

Ysabel (Spanish) a form of Isabel.

Ysanne (American) a combination of Ysabel + Ann.

Yseult (German) ice rule. (Irish) fair; light skinned. (Welsh) a form of Isolde.

Yuana (Spanish) a form of Juana.

Yudelle (English) a form of Udele.

Yudita (Russian) a form of Judith.

Yuki (Japanese) snow.

Yulene (Basque) a form of Julia.

Yulia (Russian) a form of Julia.

Yuliana (Spanish) a form of Juliana.

Yuri (Japanese) lily.
Yuriko, Yuriyo

Yvanna (Slavic) a form of Ivana.

Yvette (French) a familiar form of Yvonne. See also Evette, Ivette.
Yavette, Yevett, Yevette, Yevetta, Yvetta

Yvonne (French) young archer. (Scandinavian) yew wood; bow wood. See also Evonne, Ivonne, Vonna, Vonny, Yvette.
Yavanda, Yavanna, Yavanne, Yavonda, Yavonna, Yavonne, Yveline, Yvon, Yvone, Yvonna, Yvonny

Z

Zabrina (American) a form of Sabrina.

Zacharie (Hebrew) God remembered.
Zacari, Zacceaus, Zacchaea, Zachoia, Zackeisha, Zakaria, Zakaya, Zakeshia, Zakiah, Zakiyah, Zechari

Zachary (Hebrew) a form of Zacharie.
Zackery

Zada (Arabic) fortunate, prosperous.

Zafina (Arabic) victorious.

Zafirah (Arabic) successful; victorious.

Zahar (Hebrew) daybreak; dawn.

Zahavah (Hebrew) golden.

Zahra (Swahili) flower. (Arabic) white.

Zaira (Hebrew) a form of Zara.

Zakia (Swahili) smart. (Arabic) chaste.
Zakiah

Zakira (Hebrew) a form of Zacharie.
Zakir

Zakiya (Arabic) a form of Zakia.
Zakiyah

Zalika (Swahili) born to royalty.

Zaltana (Native American) high mountain.

Zandra (Greek) a form of Sandra.

Zaneta (Spanish) a form of Jane.

Zanna (Spanish) a form of Jane.
(English) a short form of Susanna.

Zanthe (Greek) a form of Xanthe.

Zara (Hebrew) a form of Sarah, Zora.
Zarah, Zaree, Zareen, Zareena, Zaria

Zarifa (Arabic) successful.

Zarita (Spanish) a form of Sarah.

Zasha (Russian) a form of Sasha.

Zaviera (Spanish) a form of Xaviera.

Zawati (Swahili) gift.

Zayit (Hebrew) olive.

Zaynah (Arabic) beautiful.

Zea (Latin) grain.

Zelda (Yiddish) gray haired. (German) a
short form of Griselda. See also Selda.

Zelene (English) sunshine.
Zeleen, Zelena, Zeline

Zelia (Spanish) sunshine.
Zele, Zelie, Zélie, Zelina

Zelizi (Basque) a form of Sheila.

Zelma (German) a form of Selma.

Zemirah (Hebrew) song of joy.

Zena (Greek) a form of Xenia.
(Ethiopian) news. (Persian) woman.
See also Zina.
*Zeena, Zeenat, Zeenet, Zeenia,
Zeenya, Zein, Zeina, Zenah, Zenana,
Zenea, Zenia, Zenya*

Zenaida (Greek) white-winged dove.

Zenda (Persian) sacred; feminine.

Zenobia (Greek) sign, symbol. History: a
queen who ruled the city of Palmyra in
ancient Syria.

Zephania, Zephanie (Greek) forms of
Stephanie.

Zephyr (Greek) west wind.

Zera (Hebrew) seeds.

Zerdali (Turkish) wild apricot.

Zerlina (Latin, Spanish) beautiful dawn.
Music: a character in Mozart's opera
Don Giovanni.

Zerrin (Turkish) golden.

Zeta (English) rose. Linguistics: a letter
in the Greek alphabet.

Zetta (Portuguese) rose.

Zhana, Zhane (Slavic) forms of Jane.

Zhen (Chinese) chaste.

Zia (Latin) grain. (Arabic) light.

Zigana (Hungarian) gypsy girl. See also Tsigana.

Zihna (Hopi) one who spins tops.

Zilla (Hebrew) shadow.

Zilpah (Hebrew) dignified. Bible: Jacob's wife.

Zilya (Russian) a form of Theresa.

Zimra (Hebrew) song of praise.

Zina (African) secret spirit. (English) hospitable. (Greek) a form of Zena.
Zinah, Zine

Zinnia (Latin) Botany: a plant with beautiful, rayed, colorful flowers.

Zipporah (Hebrew) bird. Bible: Moses' wife.

Zita (Spanish) rose. (Arabic) mistress. A short form of names ending in "sita" or "zita."

Ziva (Hebrew) bright; radiant.

Zizi (Hungarian) a familiar form of Elizabeth.

Zocha (Polish) a form of Sophie.

Zoe ✹ (Greek) life.
Zoé, Zoë, Zoee, Zoelie, Zoeline, Zoelle, Zoie

Zoey (Greek) a form of Zoe.
Zooey

Zofia (Slavic) a form of Sophia. See also Sofia.

Zohar (Hebrew) shining, brilliant.

Zohra (Hebrew) blossom.

Zohreh (Persian) happy.

Zola (Italian) piece of earth.

Zona (Latin) belt, sash.

Zondra (Greek) a form of Zandra.

Zora (Slavic) aurora; dawn. See also Zara.
Zorah, Zorana, Zoreen, Zoreena, Zorna, Zorra, Zorrah, Zorya

Zorina (Slavic) golden.
Zorana, Zorna

Zoya (Slavic) a form of Zoe.

Zsa Zsa (Hungarian) a familiar form of Susan.

Zsofia (Hungarian) a form of Sofia.

Zsuzsanna (Hungarian) a form of Susanna.

Zudora (Sanskrit) laborer.

Zuleika (Arabic) brilliant.

Zulima (Arabic) a form of Salama.

Zurafa (Arabic) lovely.

Zuri (Basque) white; light skinned. (Swahili) beautiful.
Zuria, Zurisha

Zusa (Czech, Polish) a form of Susan.

Zuwena (Swahili) good.

Zytka (Polish) rose.

Aakash (Hindi) a form of Akash.

Aaron ❦ (Hebrew) enlightened. (Arabic) messenger. Bible: the brother of Moses and the first high priest. See also Ron.
Aahron, Aaran, Aaren, Aareon, Aarin, Aaronn, Aarron, Aaryn, Aeron, Abaron, Ahran, Ahren, Aranne, Arek, Arin, Aronek, Aronne, Aronos

Aban (Persian) Mythology: a figure associated with water and the arts.

Abasi (Swahili) stern.

Abbey (Hebrew) a familiar form of Abe.
Abey

Abbott (Hebrew) father; abbot.

Abbud (Arabic) devoted.

Abdirahman (Arabic) a form of Abdulrahman.

Abdul (Arabic) servant.
Abdal, Abdeel, Abdel, Abdoul, Abdual, Abul

Abdulaziz (Arabic) servant of the Mighty.

Abdullah (Arabic) servant of Allah.
Abdalah, Abdalla, Abdallah, Abdualla, Abdulah, Abdulahi

Abdulrahman (Arabic) servant of the Merciful.

Abe (Hebrew) a short form of Abel, Abraham.

Abel (Hebrew) breath. (Assyrian) meadow. (German) a short form of Abelard. Bible: Adam and Eve's second son.
Abele, Abell, Able, Adal

Abelard (German) noble; resolute.

Abi (Turkish) older brother.

Abiah (Hebrew) God is my father.

Abie (Hebrew) a familiar form of Abraham.

Abiel (Hebrew) a form of Abiah.

Abir (Hebrew) strong.

Abisha (Hebrew) gift of God.

Abner (Hebrew) father of light. Bible: the commander of Saul's army.

Abraham (Hebrew) father of many nations. Bible: the first Hebrew patriarch. See also Avram, Bram, Ibrahim.
Abarran, Aberham, Abey, Abhiram, Abrahamo, Abrahán, Abrahim, Abrahm, Abramo, Abrán, Abrao, Arraun

Abrahan (Spanish) a form of Abraham.

Abram (Hebrew) a short form of Abraham. See also Bram.
Abramo

Absalom (Hebrew) father of peace. Bible: the rebellious third son of King David. See also Avshalom, Axel.

Acar (Turkish) bright.

Ace (Latin) unity.

Achilles (Greek) Mythology: a hero of the Trojan War. Literature: the hero of Homer's epic poem *Iliad*.

Ackerley (English) meadow of oak trees.

Acton (English) oak-tree settlement.

Adahy (Cherokee) in the woods.

Adair (Scottish) oak-tree ford.

Adam ★ (Phoenician) man; mankind. (Hebrew) earth; man of the red earth. Bible: the first man created by God. See also Adamson, Addison, Damek, Keddy, Macadam.
Ad, Adama, Adamo, Adão, Adas, Addam, Addams, Addis, Adem, Adbamb, Adné, Adok, Adomas

Adamec (Czech) a form of Adam.

Adamson (Hebrew) son of Adam.

Adan (Irish) a form of Aidan.

Adar (Syrian) ruler; prince. (Hebrew) noble; exalted.

Adarius (American) a combination of Adam + Darius.

Addison (English) son of Adam.
Addis, Adison, Adisson

Addy (Hebrew) a familiar form of Adam, Adlai. (German) a familiar form of Adelard.

Ade (Yoruba) royal.

Adelard (German) noble; courageous.
Adal

Aden (Arabic) Geography: a region in southern Yemen. (Irish) a form of Aidan, Aiden.

Adham (Arabic) black.

Adil (Arabic) just; wise.

Adin (Hebrew) pleasant.

Adir (Hebrew) majestic; noble.

Adiv (Hebrew) pleasant; gentle.

Adlai (Hebrew) my ornament.
Ad

Adler (German) eagle.
Ad

Adli (Turkish) just; wise.

Admon (Hebrew) peony.

Adnan (Arabic) pleasant.

Adney (English) noble's island.

Adolf (German) noble wolf. History: Adolf Hitler's German army was defeated in World War II. See also Dolf.
Ad

Adolfo (Spanish) a form of Adolf.

Adolph (German) a form of Adolf.

Adom (Akan) help from God.

Adon (Hebrew) Lord. (Greek) a short form of Adonis.

Adonis (Greek) highly attractive. Mythology: the attractive youth loved by Aphrodite.

Adri (Indo-Pakistani) rock.

Adrian ★ (Greek) rich. (Latin) dark. (Swedish) a short form of Hadrian.
Adarian, Adorjan, Adrain, Adreian, Adreyan, Adriaan, Adriane, Adrion, Adron, Adryan, Adryon

Adriano (Italian) a form of Adrian.

Adriel (Hebrew) member of God's flock.
Adrial

Adrien (French) a form of Adrian.
Adriene

Adrik (Russian) a form of Adrian.

Aeneas (Greek) praised. (Scottish) a
form of Angus. Literature: the Trojan
hero of Vergil's epic poem *Aeneid*. See
also Eneas.

Afram (African) Geography: a river in
Ghana, Africa.

Afton (English) from Afton, England.

Agamemnon (Greek) resolute.
Mythology: the king of Mycenae who
led the Greeks in the Trojan War.

Agni (Hindi) Religion: the Hindu fire
god.

Agu (Ibo) leopard.

Agustin (Latin) a form of Augustine.

Ahab (Hebrew) father's brother.
Literature: the captain of the Pequod in
Herman Melville's novel *Moby-Dick*.

Ahanu (Native American) laughter.

Ahdik (Native American) caribou; rein-
deer.

Ahearn (Scottish) lord of the horses.
(English) heron.

Ahir (Turkish) last.

Ahmad (Arabic) most highly praised.
See also Muhammad.
*Achmad, Achmed, Ahamad,
Ahamada, Ahamed, Ahmaad,
Ahmaud, Amad, Amahd, Amed*

Ahmed (Swahili) praiseworthy.

Ahsan (Arabic) charitable.

Aidan ☽ (Irish) fiery.
Aydan

Aiden ☽ (Irish) a form of Aidan.

Aiken (English) made of oak.

Aimery (French) a form of Emery.

Aimon (French) house. (Irish) a form
of Eamon.

Aindrea (Irish) a form of Andrew.

Ainsley (Scottish) my own meadow.

Aizik (Russian) a form of Isaac.

Ajala (Yoruba) potter.

Ajay (Punjabi) victorious; undefeatable.
(American) a combination of the
initials A. + J.
Aj, Aja, Ajai, Ajaz

Ajit (Sanskrit) unconquerable.

Akar (Turkish) flowing stream.

Akash (Hindi) sky.

Akbar (Arabic) great.

Akecheta (Sioux) warrior.

Akeem, Akim (Hebrew) short forms of
Joachim.
*Achim, Ackeem, Ackim, Ahkieme,
Akeam, Akee, Akiem, Akima, Arkeem*

Akemi (Japanese) dawn.

Akil (Arabic) intelligent. (Greek) a form
of Achilles.

Akins (Yoruba) brave.

Akira (Japanese) intelligent.

Akiva (Hebrew) a form of Jacob.

Akmal (Arabic) perfect.

Aksel (Norwegian) father of peace.

Akshay (American) a form of Akash.

Akshat (Sanskrit) uninjurable.

Akule (Native American) he looks up.

Al (Irish) a short form of Alan, Albert, Alexander.

Aladdin (Arabic) height of faith. Literature: the hero of a story in the *Arabian Nights*.

Alain (French) a form of Alan.
Alaen, Alainn, Alayn, Allain

Alaire (French) joyful.

Alam (Arabic) universe.

Alan (Irish) handsome; peaceful.
Ailan, Ailin, Alair, Aland, Alani, Alano, Alanson, Alao, Alun

Alaric (German) ruler of all. See also Ulrich.

Alastair (Scottish) a form of Alexander.

Alban (Latin) from Alba, Italy.

Albern (German) noble; courageous.

Albert (German, French) noble and bright. See also Elbert, Ulbrecht.
Adelbert, Ailbert, Albertik, Alberts, Albrecht, Alvertos, Aubert

Alberto (Italian) a form of Albert.

Albie, Alby (German, French) familiar forms of Albert.

Albin (Latin) a form of Alvin.

Albion (Latin) white cliffs. Geography: a reference to the white cliffs in Dover, England.

Alcandor (Greek) manly; strong.

Alcott (English) old cottage.

Aldair (German, English) a form of Alder.

Alden (English) old; wise protector.
Aldin

Alder (German, English) alder tree.

Aldo (Italian) old; elder. (German) a short form of Aldous.

Aldous (German) a form of Alden.

Aldred (English) old; wise counselor.

Aldrich (English) wise.

Aldwin (English) old friend.

Alec, Alek (Greek) short forms of Alexander.
Aleck, Alekko

Alejandro ☙ (Spanish) a form of Alexander.
Aléjo, Alexjándro

Alejándro (Spanish) a form of Alexander.

Aleksandar, Aleksander (Greek) forms of Alexander.
Aleksandr, Aleksandras, Aleksandur

Aleksei (Russian) a short form of Alexander.
Alexei, Alexey

Alekzander, Alexzander (Greek) forms of Alexander.

Alem (Arabic) wise.

Aleric (German) a form of Alaric.

Aleron (Latin) winged.

Alessandro (Italian) a form of Alexander.
Alessand, Allessandro

Alex ✓ (Greek) a short form of Alexander.
Alax, Alix, Allax, Allex

Alexander ✓ (Greek) defender of mankind. History: Alexander the Great was the conqueror of the civilized world. See also Alastair, Alistair, Iskander, Jando, Leks, Lex, Lexus, Macallister, Oleksandr, Olés, Sander, Sándor, Sandro, Sandy, Sasha, Xan, Xander, Zander, Zindel.
Alecsandar, Alekos, Alexandar, Alexandor, Alexandr, Alexandros, Alexxander, Alick

Alexandre (French) a form of Alexander.

Alexandro (Greek) a form of Alexander.
Alexandros

Alexi (Russian) a form of Aleksei. (Greek) a short form of Alexander.
Alexey, Alexie, Alexio, Alexy

Alexis (Greek) a short form of Alexander.
Alexei, Alexes, Alexey, Alexios, Alexius, Alexiz

Alfie (English) a familiar form of Alfred.

Alfonso (Italian, Spanish) a form of Alphonse.
Affonso, Alfons, Alfonse, Alfonsus, Alfonza, Alfonzo, Alfonzus

Alford (English) old river ford.

Alfred (English) elf counselor; wise counselor. See also Fred.
Ailfrid, Ailfryd, Alf, Alfeo, Alured

Alfredo (Italian, Spanish) a form of Alfred.
Alfrido

Alger (German) noble spearman. (English) a short form of Algernon. See also Elger.

Algernon (English) bearded, wearing a moustache.

Algie (English) a familiar form of Algernon.

Algis (German) spear.

Ali (Arabic) greatest. (Swahili) exalted.
Aly

Alic (Greek) a short form of Alexander.
Alick

Alim (Arabic) scholar. (Arabic) a form of Alem.

Alisander (Greek) a form of Alexander.

Alistair (English) a form of Alexander.

Alixander (Greek) a form of Alexander.
Alixandre

Allan (Irish) a form of Alan.
Allayne

Allard (English) noble, brave.

Allen (Irish) a form of Alan.
Alen, Alley, Alleyn, Alleyne, Allie, Allin, Allon, Allyn

Almon (Hebrew) widower.

Alois (German) a short form of Aloysius.

Aloisio (Spanish) a form of Louis.

Alok (Sanskrit) victorious cry.

Alon (Hebrew) oak.

Alonso, Alonzo (Spanish) forms of Alphonse.
Alano, Alanzo, Alonza

Aloysius (German) a form of Louis.

Alphonse (German) noble and eager.
Alf, Alphons, Alphonsa, Alphonsus, Alphonza, Alphonzus

Alphonso (Italian) a form of Alphonse.
Alphanso, Alphonzo

Alpin (Irish) attractive.

Alroy (Spanish) king.

Alston (English) noble's settlement.

Altair (Greek) star. (Arabic) flying.

Altman (German) old man.

Alton (English) old town.
Alten

Alva (Hebrew) sublime.

Alvan (German) a form of Alvin.

Alvar (English) army of elves.

Alvaro (Spanish) just; wise.

Alvern (Latin) spring.

Alvin (Latin) white; light skinned. (German) friend to all; noble friend; friend of elves. See also Albin, Elvin.
Aloin, Aluin, Aluino, Alven, Alvie, Alvino, Alvy, Alvyn, Elwin

Alvis (Scandinavian) all-knowing.

Alwin (German) a form of Alvin.

Amadeo (Italian) a form of Amadeus.

Amadeus (Latin) loves God. Music: Wolfgang Amadeus Mozart was a famous eighteenth-century Austrian composer.
Amad

Amal (Hebrew) worker. (Arabic) hopeful.

Amandeep (Punjabi) light of peace.
Amandip, Amanjit, Amanjot, Amanpreet

Amando (French) a form of Amadeus.

Amani (Arabic) believer. (Yoruba) strength; builder.

Amar (Punjabi) immortal. (Arabic) builder.
Amari, Amario, Amaris, Amarjit, Amarpreet, Ammar, Ammer

Amato (French) loved.

Ambar (Sanskrit) sky.

Ambrose (Greek) immortal.

Ameer (Hebrew) a form of Amir.

Amerigo (Teutonic) industrious. History: Amerigo Vespucci was the Italian explorer for whom America is named.

Ames (French) friend.

Amicus (English, Latin) beloved friend.

Amiel (Hebrew) God of my people.

Amin (Hebrew, Arabic) trustworthy; honest. (Hindi) faithful.

Amir (Hebrew) proclaimed. (Punjabi) wealthy; king's minister. (Arabic) prince.

Amish (Sanskrit) honest.

Amit (Punjabi) unfriendly. (Arabic) highly praised.
Amitan, Amreet

Ammon (Egyptian) hidden. Mythology: the ancient god associated with reproduction.

Amol (Hindi) priceless, valuable.

Amon (Hebrew) trustworthy; faithful.

Amory (German) a form of Emory.

Amos (Hebrew) burdened, troubled. Bible: an Old Testament prophet.

Amram (Hebrew) mighty nation.

Amrit (Sanskrit) nectar. (Punjabi, Arabic) a form of Amit.

An (Chinese, Vietnamese) peaceful.

Anand (Hindi) blissful.

Anastasius (Greek) resurrection.

Anatole (Greek) east.

Anchali (Taos) painter.

Anders (Swedish) a form of Andrew.
Ander

Anderson (Swedish) son of Andrew.
Andersen

Andonios (Greek) a form of Anthony.
Andonis

Andor (Hungarian) a form of Andrew.

András (Hungarian) a form of Andrew.

Andre, André (French) forms of Andrew.
Andra, Andrae, Andrecito, Andree, Aundré

Andrea (Greek) a form of Andrew.

Andreas (Greek) a form of Andrew.
Andries

Andrei (Bulgarian, Romanian, Russian) a form of Andrew.

Andres (Spanish) a form of Andrew.
Andras, Andrés, Andrez

Andrew ☆ (Greek) strong; manly; courageous. Bible: one of the Twelve Apostles. See also Bandi, Drew, Endre, Evangelos, Kendrew, Ondro.
Andery, Andonis, Andrews, Andru, Andrue, Andrus, Anndra, Audrew

Andros (Polish) sea. Mythology: the god of the sea.
Andrus

Andy (Greek) a short form of Andrew.
Andino, Andis, Andje

Aneurin (Welsh) honorable; gold. See also Nye.

Anfernee (Greek) a form of Anthony.
Anferny

Angel ☆ (Greek) angel. (Latin) messenger. See also Gotzon.
Ange, Angell, Angie, Angy

Angelo (Italian) a form of Angel.
Angelito, Angelos, Anglo

Angus (Scottish) exceptional; outstanding. Mythology: Angus Og was the Celtic god of youth, love, and beauty. See also Ennis, Gus.
Aonghas

Anh (Vietnamese) peace; safety.

Anibal (Phoenician) a form of Hannibal.

Anil (Hindi) wind god.

Anka (Turkish) phoenix.

Anker (Danish) a form of Andrew.

Annan (Scottish) brook. (Swahili) fourth-born son.

Annas (Greek) gift from God.

Anno (German) a familiar form of Johann.

Anoki (Native American) actor.

Ansel (French) follower of a nobleman.

Anselm (German) divine protector. See also Elmo.

Ansis (Latvian) a form of Janis.

Ansley (Scottish) a form of Ainsley.

Anson (German) divine. (English) Anne's son.
Ansun

Antal (Hungarian) a form of Anthony.
Antos

Antares (Greek) giant, red star. Astronomy: the brightest star in the constellation Scorpio.

Antavas (Lithuanian) a form of Anthony.

Anthany (Latin, Greek) a form of Anthony.

Anthonie (Latin, Greek) a form of Anthony.
Anthoni

Anthony ✼ (Latin) praiseworthy. (Greek) flourishing. See also Tony.
Anathony, Anothony, Anthawn, Anthey, Anthian, Anthino, Anthoney, Anthonio, Anthonu, Anthoy, Anthyoine, Anthyonny

Antione (French) a form of Anthony.
Antionne

Antjuan (Spanish) a form of Anthony.

Antoan (Vietnamese) safe, secure.

Antoine (French) a form of Anthony.
Anntoin, Antoiné, Atoine

Anton (Slavic) a form of Anthony.
Antone, Antons, Antos

Antonio ✼ (Italian) a form of Anthony. See also Tino, Tonio.
Anthonio, Antinio, Antoino, Antonello, Antonin, Antonín, Antonino, Antonnio, Antonios, Antonius, Antonyia, Antonyio, Antonyo

Antony (Latin) a form of Anthony.
Antin, Antini, Antius, Antoney, Antoni, Antonie, Antonin, Antonios, Antonius, Antonyia, Antonyio, Antonyo, Anty

Antti (Finnish) manly.
Anthey

Antwan (Arabic) a form of Anthony.
Antaw, Antawan, Antawn, Anthawn, Antowine, Antowne, Antowyn, Antwain, Antwaina, Antwaine, Antwaion, Antwane, Antwann, Antwanne, Antwarn, Antwaun, Antwen, Antwian, Antwine, Antwuan

Antwon (Arabic) a form of Anthony.
Antwion, Antwoan, Antwoin,
Antwoine, Antwone, Antwonn,
Antwonne, Antwyon, Antyon,
Antywon

Anwar (Arabic) luminous.

Apiatan (Kiowa) wooden lance.

Apollo (Greek) manly. Mythology: the god
of prophecy, healing, music, poetry, and
light. See also Polo.

Aquila (Latin, Spanish) eagle.

Araldo (Spanish) a form of Harold.

Aram (Syrian) high, exalted.
Arram

Aramis (French) Literature: one of the
title characters in Alexandre Dumas's
novel *The Three Musketeers*.

Aran (Tai) forest. (Danish) a form of
Aren. (Hebrew, Scottish) a form of
Arran.

Archer (English) bowman.

Archibald (German) bold. See also
Arkady.

Archie (German, English) a familiar
form of Archer, Archibald.
Archy

Ardal (Irish) a form of Arnold.

Ardell (Latin) eager; industrious.

Arden (Latin) ardent; fiery.

Ardon (Hebrew) bronzed.

Aren (Danish) eagle; ruler. (Hebrew,
Arabic) a form of Aaron.

Aretino (Greek, Italian) victorious.

Argus (Danish) watchful, vigilant.

Ari (Hebrew) a short form of Ariel.
(Greek) a short form of Aristotle.
Aria, Arias, Arie, Arih, Arij, Ario, Arri

Arian (Greek) a form of Arion.

Aric (German) a form of Richard.
(Scandinavian) a form of Eric.
Aaric, Areck, Arick, Arik, Arric, Arrick,
Arrik

Ariel (Hebrew) lion of God. Bible:
another name for Jerusalem.
Literature: the name of a sprite in the
Shakespearean play *The Tempest*.
Airel, Arel, Areli, Ariya, Ariyel, Arrial,
Arriel

Aries (Latin) ram. Astrology: the first
sign of the zodiac.
Arie

Arif (Arabic) knowledgeable.

Arion (Greek) enchanted. (Hebrew)
melodious.
Ario

Aristides (Greek) son of the best.

Aristotle (Greek) best; wise. History: a
third-century B.C. philosopher who
tutored Alexander the Great.

Arjun (Hindi) white; milk colored.

Arkady (Russian) a form of Archibald.

Arkin (Norwegian) son of the eternal
king.

Arledge (English) lake with the hares.

Arlen (Irish) pledge.
Arlan, Arland, Arlend, Arlin, Arlyn,
Arlynn

Arley (English) a short form of Harley.

Arlo (Spanish) barberry. (English) fortified hill. A form of Harlow. (German) a form of Charles.

Arman (Persian) desire, goal.

Armand (Latin, German) a form of Herman. See also Mandek.
Armad, Armanda, Armands, Armanno, Armaude, Armenta, Armond

Armando (Spanish) a form of Armand.
Armondo

Armani (Hungarian) sly. (Hebrew) a form of Armon.

Armon (Hebrew) high fortress, stronghold.

Armstrong (English) strong arm. History: astronaut Neil Armstrong was the commander of Apollo 11 and the first person to walk on the moon.

Arnaud (French) a form of Arnold.

Arne (German) a form of Arnold.

Arnette (English) little eagle.

Arnie (German) a familiar form of Arnold.

Arno (German) a short form of Arnold. (Czech) a short form of Ernest.

Arnold (German) eagle ruler.
Arnald, Arnaldo

Arnon (Hebrew) rushing river.

Arnulfo (German) a form of Arnold.

Aron, Arron (Hebrew) forms of Aaron. (Danish) forms of Aren.

Aroon (Tai) dawn.

Arran (Scottish) island dweller. Geography: an island off the west coast of Scotland. (Hebrew) a form of Aaron.

Arrigo (Italian) a form of Harry.

Arrio (Spanish) warlike.
Ario

Arsenio (Greek) masculine; virile. History: Saint Arsenius was a teacher in the Roman Empire.

Arsha (Persian) venerable.

Art (English) a short form of Arthur.

Artemus (Greek) gift of Artemis. Mythology: Artemis was the goddess of the hunt and the moon.

Arthur (Irish) noble; lofty hill. (Scottish) bear. (English) rock. (Icelandic) follower of Thor. See also Turi.

Artie (English) a familiar form of Arthur.

Arturo (Italian) a form of Arthur.
Arthuro, Artur

Arun (Cambodian, Hindi) sun.

Arundel (English) eagle valley.

Arve (Norwegian) heir, inheritor.

Arvel (Welsh) wept over.

Arvid (Hebrew) wanderer. (Norwegian) eagle tree. See also Ravid.

Arvin (German) friend of the people; friend of the army.

Aryeh (Hebrew) lion.

Asa (Hebrew) physician, healer. (Yoruba) falcon.

Asád (Arabic) lion.

Asadel (Arabic) prosperous.

Ascot (English) eastern cottage; style of necktie. Geography: a village near London and the site of the Royal Ascot horseraces.

Asgard (Scandinavian) court of the gods.

Ash (Hebrew) ash tree.

Ashanti (Swahili) from a tribe in West Africa.

Ashby (Scandinavian) ash-tree farm. (Hebrew) a form of Ash.

Asher (Hebrew) happy; blessed.
Ashar, Ashor

Ashford (English) ash-tree ford.
Ashtin

Ashley (English) ash-tree meadow.
Asheley, Ashelie, Ashely, Ashlan, Ashleigh, Ashlen, Ashlie, Ashlin, Ashling, Ashlinn, Ashlone, Ashly, Ashlyn, Ashlynn, Aslan

Ashon (Swahili) seventh-born son.

Ashton (English) ash-tree settlement.
Ashtin

Ashur (Swahili) Mythology: the principal Assyrian deity.

Ashwani (Hindi) first. Religion: the first of the twenty-seven galaxies revolving around the moon.

Ashwin (Hindi) star.

Asiel (Hebrew) created by God.

Asker (Turkish) soldier.

Aspen (English) aspen tree.

Aston (English) eastern town.
Astin

Aswad (Arabic) dark skinned, black.

Ata (Fante) twin.

Atek (Polish) a form of Tanek.

Athan (Greek) immortal.

Atherton (English) town by a spring.

Atid (Tai) sun.

Atif (Arabic) caring.

Atlas (Greek) lifted; carried. Mythology: Atlas was forced by Zeus to carry the heavens on his shoulders as a punishment for his share of the war of the Titans.

Atley (English) meadow.

Attila (Gothic) little father. History: the Hun leader who invaded the Roman Empire.

Atwater (English) at the water's edge.

Atwell (English) at the well.

Atwood (English) at the forest.

Atworth (English) at the farmstead.

Auberon (German) a form of Oberon.

Aubrey (German) noble; bearlike. (French) a familiar form of Auberon. See also Avery.
Aubary, Aube, Aubery, Aubry, Aubury

Auburn (Latin) reddish brown.

Auden (English) old friend.

Audie (German) noble; strong. (English) a familiar form of Edward.

Audon (French) old; rich.

Audrey (English) noble strength.

Audric (English) wise ruler.

Audun (Scandinavian) deserted, desolate.

Augie (Latin) a familiar form of August.

August (Latin) a short form of Augustine, Augustus.
Agosto, Auguste, Augusto

Augustine (Latin) majestic. Religion: Saint Augustine was the first archbishop of Canterbury. See also Austin, Gus, Tino.

Augustus (Latin) majestic; venerable. History: an honorary title given to the first Roman emperor, Octavius Caesar.

Aukai (Hawaiian) seafarer.

Aundre (Greek) a form of Andre.

Aurek (Polish) golden haired.

Aurelio (Latin) a short form of Aurelius.

Aurelius (Latin) golden. History: Marcus Aurelius was a second-century a.d. philosopher and emperor of Rome.

Aurick (German) protecting ruler.

Austen, Auston, Austyn (Latin) short forms of Augustine.

Austin ✶ (Latin) a short form of Augustine.
Astin, Austine

Avel (Greek) breath.

Avent (French) born during Advent.

Averill (French) born in April.

Avery (English) a form of Aubrey.
Avary, Aveary, Averey, Averie, Avry

Avi (Hebrew) God is my father.

Aviv (Hebrew) youth; springtime.

Avner (Hebrew) a form of Abner.

Avram (Hebrew) a form of Abraham, Abram.
Arram

Avshalom (Hebrew) father of peace. See also Absalom.

Awan (Native American) somebody.

Axel (Latin) axe. (German) small oak tree; source of life. (Scandinavian) a form of Absalom.
Ax, Axe, Axell, Axil, Axill

Ayden (Irish) a form of Aidan.

Aydin (Turkish) intelligent.

Ayers (English) heir to a fortune.

Ayinde (Yoruba) we gave praise and he came.

Aylmer (English) a form of Elmer.

Aymil (Greek) a form of Emil.

Aymon (French) a form of Raymond.

Ayo (Yoruba) happiness.

Azad (Turkish) free.

Azeem (Arabic) a form of Azim.

Azi (Nigerian) youth.

Azim (Arabic) defender.

Aziz (Arabic) strong.

Azizi (Swahili) precious.

Azriel (Hebrew) God is my aid.

Azuriah (Hebrew) aided by God.

B

Baden (German) bather.

Bahir (Arabic) brilliant, dazzling.

Bahram (Persian) ancient king.

Bailey (French) bailiff, steward.

Bain (Irish) a short form of Bainbridge.

Bainbridge (Irish) fair bridge.

Baird (Irish) traveling minstrel, bard; poet.

Bakari (Swahili) noble promise.

Baker (English) baker. See also Baxter.

Bal (Sanskrit) child born with lots of hair.

Balasi (Basque) flat footed.

Balbo (Latin) stammerer.

Baldemar (German) bold; famous.

Balder (Scandinavian) bald. Mythology: the Norse god of light, summer, purity, and innocence.

Baldric (German) brave ruler.

Baldwin (German) bold friend.

Balfour (Scottish) pastureland.

Balin (Hindi) mighty soldier.

Ballard (German) brave; strong.

Balraj (Hindi) strongest.

Baltazar (Greek) a form of Balthasar.

Balthasar (Greek) God save the king. Bible: one of the three wise men who bore gifts for the infant Jesus.

Bancroft (English) bean field.

Bandi (Hungarian) a form of Andrew.

Bane (Hawaiian) a form of Bartholomew.

Banner (Scottish, English) flag bearer.

Banning (Irish) small and fair.

Barak (Hebrew) lightning bolt. Bible: the valiant warrior who helped Deborah.

Baran (Russian) ram.

Barasa (Kikuyu) meeting place.

Barclay (Scottish, English) birch-tree meadow.
Bar

Bard (Irish) a form of Baird.
Bar

Bardolf (German) bright wolf.

Bardrick (Teutonic) axe ruler.

Baris (Turkish) peaceful.

Barker (English) lumberjack; advertiser at a carnival.

Barlow (English) bare hillside.

Barnabas (Greek, Hebrew, Aramaic, Latin) son of the missionary. Bible:

Christian apostle and companion of Paul on his first missionary journey.

Barnaby (English) a form of Barnabas.
Bernabé

Barnard (French) a form of Bernard.

Barnes (English) bear; son of Barnett.

Barnett (English) nobleman; leader.
Barrie, Barron

Barney (English) a familiar form of Barnabas, Barnett.

Barnum (German) barn; storage place. (English) baron's home.

Baron (German, English) nobleman, baron.
Baaron, Baronie, Barrion, Barron, Baryn

Barrett (German) strong as a bear.
Bar, Baret, Barrat, Barret, Barrette

Barric (English) grain farm.

Barrington (English) fenced town. Geography: a town in England.

Barry (Welsh) son of Harry. (Irish) spear, marksman. (French) gate, fence.
Barri, Barrie, Barris, Bary

Bart (Hebrew) a short form of Bartholomew, Barton.
Barrt, Bartel, Bartie, Barty

Bartholomew (Hebrew) son of Talmaí. Bible: one of the Twelve Apostles. See also Jerney, Parlan, Parthalán.

Bartlet (English) a form of Bartholomew.

Barto (Spanish) a form of Bartholomew.

Barton (English) barley town; Bart's town.
Barrton

Bartram (English) a form of Bertram.

Baruch (Hebrew) blessed.

Basam (Arabic) smiling.

Basil (Greek, Latin) royal, kingly. Religion: a saint and founder of monasteries. Botany: an herb often used in cooking. See also Vasilis, Wasili.
Bas, Base, Baseal, Basel, Basle, Basile, Basilio, Basilios, Basilius, Bassel, Bazek, Bazel, Bazil, Bazyli

Basir (Turkish) intelligent, discerning.

Bassett (English) little person.

Bastien (German) a short form of Sebastian.
Bastian

Bat (English) a short form of Bartholomew.

Baul (Gypsy) snail.

Bavol (Gypsy) wind; air.

Baxter (English) a form of Baker.

Bay (Vietnamese) seventh son. (French) chestnut brown color; evergreen tree. (English) howler.

Bayard (English) reddish brown hair.

Bayley (French) a form of Bailey.

Beacan (Irish) small.

Beacher (English) beech trees.

Beagan (Irish) small.

Beale (French) a form of Beau.

Beaman (English) beekeeper.

Beamer (English) trumpet player.

Beasley (English) field of peas.

Beattie (Latin) blessed; happy; bringer of joy.

Beau (French) handsome.

Beaufort (French) beautiful fort.

Beaumont (French) beautiful mountain.

Beauregard (French) handsome; beautiful; well regarded.

Beaver (English) beaver.

Bebe (Spanish) baby.

Beck (English, Scandinavian) brook.

Bede (English) prayer. Religion: the patron saint of lectors.

Bela (Czech) white. (Hungarian) bright.

Belden (French, English) pretty valley.

Belen (Greek) arrow.

Bell (French) handsome. (English) bell ringer.

Bellamy (French) beautiful friend.

Bello (African) helper or promoter of Islam.

Belmiro (Portuguese) good-looking; attractive.

Bem (Tiv) peace.

Ben (Hebrew) a short form of Benjamin.
Behn, Benio, Benn, Benne, Benno

Ben-ami (Hebrew) son of my people.

Benedict (Latin) blessed. See also Venedictos, Venya.

Benedikt (German, Slavic) a form of Benedict.

Bengt (Scandinavian) a form of Benedict.
Bent

Beniam (Ethiopian) a form of Benjamin.

Benito (Italian) a form of Benedict. History: Benito Mussolini led Italy during World War II.
Benedo, Benino, Benno, Betto

Benjamen (Hebrew) a form of Benjamin.
Benejamen, Benjjmen

Benjamin ☀ (Hebrew) son of my right hand. See also Peniamina, Veniamin.
Behnjamin, Bejamin, Bemjiman, Benejaminas, Benja, Benjaim, Benjamaim, Benjaman, Benjamine, Benjamino, Benjamon, Benjamyn, Benjemin, Benjermain, Benji, Benjie, Benjy, Benkamin, Benyamin, Benyamino, Binyamin

Benjiman (Hebrew) a form of Benjamin.
Benjimen

Benjiro (Japanese) enjoys peace.

Bennett (Latin) little blessed one.
Benet, Benett, Bennet

Benny (Hebrew) a familiar form of Benjamin.
Bennie

Beno (Hebrew) son. (Mwera) band member.

Benoit (French) a form of Benedict.

Benoni (Hebrew) son of my sorrow.
Bible: Ben-oni was the son of Jacob and
Rachel.

Benson (Hebrew) son of Ben. A short
form of Ben Zion.
Bensen, Benssen, Bensson

Bentley (English) moor; coarse grass
meadow.
Bent

Benton (English) Ben's town; town on
the moors.
Bent

Benzi (Hebrew) a familiar form of Ben
Zion.

Ben Zion (Hebrew) son of Zion.

Beppe (Italian) a form of Joseph.

Ber (English) boundary. (Yiddish) bear.

Beredei (Russian) a form of Hubert.

Berg (German) mountain.

Bergen (German, Scandinavian) hill
dweller.

Berger (French) shepherd.

Bergren (Scandinavian) mountain
stream.

Berk (Turkish) solid, rugged.

Berkeley (English) a form of Barclay.

Berl (German) a form of Burl.

Berlyn (German) boundary line. See
also Burl.

Bern (German) a short form of Bernard.

Bernal (German) strong as a bear.
Bernel

Bernard (German) brave as a bear. See
also Bjorn.
*Bear, Bearnard, Benek, Berend,
Bernabé, Bernadas, Bernardel,
Bernardin, Bernardus, Bernardyn,
Bernarr, Bernat, Bernek, Bernel,
Bernerd, Berngards, Bernhard,
Bernhards, Bernhardt, Burnard*

Bernardo (Spanish) a form of Bernard.

Bernie (German) a familiar form of
Bernard.

Berry (English) berry; grape.

Bersh (Gypsy) one year.

Bert (German, English) bright, shining.
A short form of Berthold, Berton,
Bertram, Bertrand, Egbert, Filbert.
Bertus, Birt

Berthold (German) bright; illustrious;
brilliant ruler.

Bertie (English) a familiar form of Bert,
Egbert.
Birt

Bertín (Spanish) distinguished friend.

Berto (Spanish) a short form of Alberto.

Berton (English) bright settlement;
fortified town.

Bertram (German) bright; illustrious.
(English) bright raven. See also
Bartram.

Bertrand (German) bright shield.

Berwyn (Welsh) white head.

Bevan (Welsh) son of Evan.

Beverly (English) beaver meadow.

Bevis (French) from Beauvais, France; bull.

Bhagwandas (Hindi) servant of God.

Bickford (English) axe-man's ford.

Bienvenido (Filipino) welcome.

Bijan (Persian) ancient hero.

Bilal (Arabic) chosen.
Bila, Billal

Bill (German) a short form of William.
Bil, Billijo, Byll

Billy (German) a familiar form of Bill, William.
Bille, Billey, Billie, Bily

Binah (Hebrew) understanding; wise.

Bing (German) kettle-shaped hollow.

Binh (Vietnamese) peaceful.

Binkentios (Greek) a form of Vincent.

Binky (English) a familiar form of Bancroft, Vincent.

Birch (English) white; shining; birch tree.

Birger (Norwegian) rescued.

Birkey (English) island with birch trees.

Birkitt (English) birch-tree coast.

Birley (English) meadow with the cow barn.

Birney (English) island with a brook.

Birtle (English) hill with birds.

Bishop (Greek) overseer. (English) bishop.

Bjorn (Scandinavian) a form of Bernard.
Bjarne

Blackburn (Scottish) black brook.

Blade (English) knife, sword.

Bladimir (Russian) a form of Vladimir.

Blaine (Irish) thin, lean. (English) river source.
Blain

Blair (Irish) plain, field. (Welsh) place.
Blaire, Blayr, Blayre

Blaise, Blaize (French) forms of Blaze.
Ballas, Balyse, Blaisot, Blas, Blase, Blasi, Blasien, Blasius

Blake ✺ (English) attractive; dark.
Blakeman, Blakey

Blakely (English) dark meadow.

Blanco (Spanish) light skinned; white; blond.

Blane (Irish) a form of Blaine.
Blaney

Blayne (Irish) a form of Blaine.
Blayney

Blaze (Latin) stammerer. (English) flame; trail mark made on a tree.

Bliss (English) blissful; joyful.

Bly (Native American) high.

Blythe (English) carefree; merry, joyful.

Bo (English) a form of Beau, Beauregard. (German) a form of Bogart.

Boaz (Hebrew) swift; strong.

Bob (English) a short form of Robert.
Bobb

Bobby (English) a familiar form of Bob,
Robert.
Bobbey, Bobbi, Bobbie, Boby

Bobek (Czech) a form of Bob, Robert.

Boden (Scandinavian) sheltered.
(French) messenger, herald.

Bodie (Scandinavian) a familiar form
of Boden.

Bodil (Norwegian) mighty ruler.

Bodua (Akan) animal's tail.

Bogart (German) strong as a bow.
(Irish, Welsh) bog, marshland.

Bohdan (Ukrainian) a form of Donald.

Bonaro (Italian, Spanish) friend.

Bonaventure (Italian) good luck.

Bond (English) tiller of the soil.

Boniface (Latin) do-gooder.

Booker (English) bookmaker; book
lover; Bible lover.

Boone (Latin, French) good. History:
Daniel Boone was an American pio-
neer.

Booth (English) hut. (Scandinavian)
temporary dwelling.

Borak (Arabic) lightning. Mythology:
the horse that carried Muhammad to
seventh heaven.

Borden (French) cottage. (English)
valley of the boar; boar's den.

Borg (Scandinavian) castle.

Boris (Slavic) battler, warrior. Religion:
the patron saint of Moscow, princes,
and Russia.

Borka (Russian) fighter.

Boseda (Tiv) born on Saturday.

Bosley (English) grove of trees.

Botan (Japanese) blossom, bud.

Bourey (Cambodian) country.

Bourne (Latin, French) boundary.
(English) brook, stream.

Boutros (Arabic) a form of Peter.

Bowen (Welsh) son of Owen.

Bowie (Irish) yellow haired. History:
James Bowie was an American-born
Mexican colonist who died during the
defense of the Alamo.

Boyce (French) woods, forest.

Boyd (Scottish) yellow haired.
Boid, Boyde

Brad (English) a short form of Bradford,
Bradley.
Bradd, Brade

Bradburn (English) broad stream.

Braden (English) broad valley.
Bradan, Bradden, Bradin, Bradine

Bradford (English) broad river crossing.
Braddford

Bradlee (English) a form of Bradley.
Bradlea, Bradleigh, Bradlie

Bradley (English) broad meadow.
Bradlay, Bradney

Bradly (English) a form of Bradley.

Bradon (English) broad hill.
Braidon

Bradshaw (English) broad forest.

Brady (Irish) spirited. (English) broad
island.
Bradey

Bradyn (English) a form of Braden.

Braeden, Braiden (English) forms of
Braden.

Braedon (English) a form of Bradon.

Bragi (Scandinavian) poet. Mythology:
the god of poetry, eloquence, and song.

Braham (Hindi) creator.

Brainard (English) bold raven; prince.

Bram (Scottish) bramble, brushwood.
(Hebrew) a short form of Abraham,
Abram.

Bramwell (English) bramble spring.

Branch (Latin) paw; claw; tree branch.

Brand (English) firebrand; sword. A
short form of Brandon.

Brandeis (Czech) dweller on a burned
clearing.

Branden (English) beacon valley.
Brandin, Breandan

Brandon ❦ (English) beacon hill.
*Bran, Brandan, Branddon,
Brandone, Brandonn, Branndan*

Brandt (English) a form of Brant.

Brandy (Dutch) brandy. (English) a
familiar form of Brand.

Brandyn (English) a form of Branden,
Brandon.

Brannon (Irish) a form of Brandon.

Branson (English) son of Brandon,
Brant. A form of Bronson.
Bransen, Bransin

Brant (English) proud.
Brannt

Brantley (English) a form of Brant.
Brantlie

Braulio (Italian) a form of Brawley.

Brawley (English) meadow on the
hillside.

Braxton (English) Brock's town.

Brayan (Irish, Scottish) a form of Brian.

Brayden ❦ (English) a form of
Braden.

Braydon (English) a form of Bradon.

Breck (Irish) freckled.
Brec, Breckie, Brexton

Brede (Scandinavian) iceberg, glacier.

Brencis (Latvian) a form of Lawrence.

Brendan (Irish) little raven. (English)
sword.
*Breandan, Bren, Brendis, Brenn,
Brenndan, Bryn*

Brenden (Irish) a form of Brendan.
Bren, Brendene, Brendin, Brendine

Brendon (English) a form of Brandon.
(Irish, English) a form of Brendan.

Brennan, Brennen (English, Irish)
forms of Brendan.
Bren, Brenn, Brennin, Brennon

Brent (English) a short form of Brenton.
Brendt, Brentson

Brenton (English) steep hill.
Brentan, Brenten, Brentin, Brentton, Brentyn

Bret, Brett (Scottish) from Great Britain. See also Britton.
Bhrett, Braten, Braton, Brayton, Breton, Brette, Bretten, Bretton

Brewster (English) brewer.

Breyon (Irish, Scottish) a form of Brian.

Brian ✹ (Irish, Scottish) strong; virtuous; honorable. History: Brian Boru was an eleventh-century Irish king and national hero. See also Palaina.
Briano, Briant, Briante, Brien, Brience, Brient, Brin, Briny, Bryen

Briar (French) heather.

Brice (Welsh) alert; ambitious. (English) son of Rice.
Bricen, Briceton

Brick (English) bridge.

Bridger (English) bridge builder.

Brigham (English) covered bridge. (French) troops, brigade.

Brighton (English) bright town.

Brion (Irish, Scottish) a form of Brian.

Brit, Britt (Scottish) forms of Bret, Brett. See also Britton.
Brityce

Britton (Scottish) from Great Britain. See also Bret, Brett, Brit, Britt.
Britain, Briton, Brittain, Brittan, Britten

Brock (English) badger.
Broc, Brocke, Brockett, Brockie, Brockley, Brockton, Brocky, Brok, Broque

Brod (English) a short form of Broderick.
Broden

Broderick (Welsh) son of the famous ruler. (English) broad ridge. See also Roderick.
Broddie, Broddy, Broderic

Brodie (Irish) a form of Brody.
Brodi

Brodrick (Welsh, English) a form of Broderick.
Brodric, Brodryck

Brody (Irish) ditch; canal builder.
Brodee, Broden, Brodey, Broedy

Brogan (Irish) a heavy work shoe.

Bromley (English) brushwood meadow.

Bron (Afrikaans) source.

Bronislaw (Polish) weapon of glory.

Bronson (English) son of Brown.
Bransen, Bransin, Bronnie, Bronnson, Bronny, Bronsen, Bronsin, Bronsonn, Bronsson, Bronsun

Brook (English) brook, stream.
Brooke, Brooker, Brookin, Brooklyn

Brooks (English) son of Brook.
Brookes, Broox

Brown (English) brown; bear.

Bruce (French) brushwood thicket; woods.
Brucey, Brucy, Brue, Bruis

Bruno (German, Italian) brown haired; brown skinned.
Brunon, Bruns

Bryan ✼ (Irish) a form of Brian.
Bryen

Bryant (Irish) a form of Bryan.
Bryent

Bryce (Welsh) a form of Brice.
Brycen, Bryceton, Bryston

Bryon (German) cottage. (English) bear.
Bryn

Bryson (Welsh) son of Brice.

Bryton (English) a form of Brighton.
Brayton

Bubba (German) a boy.

Buck (German, English) male deer.

Buckley (English) deer meadow.

Buckminster (English) preacher.

Bud (English) herald, messenger.

Buddy (American) a familiar form of Bud.
Budde, Buddey, Buddie

Buell (German) hill dweller. (English) bull.

Buford (English) ford near the castle.

Burgess (English) town dweller; shopkeeper.

Burian (Ukrainian) lives near weeds.

Burke (German, French) fortress, castle.

Burl (English) cup bearer; wine servant; knot in a tree. (German) a short form of Berlyn.

Burleigh (English) meadow with knotted tree trunks.

Burne (English) brook.

Burney (English) island with a brook. A familiar form of Rayburn.

Burr (Swedish) youth. (English) prickly plant.

Burris (English) town dweller.

Burt (English) a form of Bert. A short form of Burton.

Burton (English) fortified town.

Busby (Scottish) village in the thicket; tall military hat made of fur.

Buster (American) hitter, puncher.

Butch (American) a short form of Butcher.

Butcher (English) butcher.

Buzz (Scottish) a short form of Busby.

Byford (English) by the ford.

Byram (English) cattle yard.

Byrd (English) birdlike.

Byrne (English) a form of Burne.

Byron (French) cottage. (English) barn.
Beyron, Biren, Biron, Buiron, Byran, Byrann, Byren, Byrom, Byrone

C

Cable (French, English) rope maker.

Cadao (Vietnamese) folksong.

Cadby (English) warrior's settlement.

Caddock (Welsh) eager for war.

Cade (Welsh) a short form of Cadell.

Cadell (Welsh) battler.

Caden ☼ (American) a form of Kadin.

Cadmus (Greek) from the east. Mythology: a Phoenician prince who founded Thebes and introduced writing to the Greeks.

Caelan (Scottish) a form of Nicholas.
Cailean

Caesar (Latin) long-haired. History: a title for Roman emperors. See also Kaiser, Kesar, Sarito.

Cahil (Turkish) young, naive.

Cai (Welsh) a form of Gaius.

Cain (Hebrew) spear; gatherer. Bible: Adam and Eve's oldest son. See also Kabil, Kane, Kayne.

Cairn (Welsh) landmark made of a mound of stones.

Cairo (Arabic) Geography: the capital of Egypt.

Cal (Latin) a short form of Calvert, Calvin.

Calder (Welsh, English) brook, stream.

Caldwell (English) cold well.

Cale (Hebrew) a short form of Caleb.

Caleb ☼ (Hebrew) dog; faithful. (Arabic) bold, brave. Bible: one of the twelve spies sent by Moses. See also Kaleb, Kayleb.
Caeleb, Calab

Calen, Calin (Scottish) forms of Caelan.

Caley (Irish) a familiar form of Caleb.

Calhoun (Irish) narrow woods. (Scottish) warrior.

Callahan (Irish) descendant of Ceallachen.

Callum (Irish) dove.

Calvert (English) calf herder.

Calvin (Latin) bald. See also Kalvin, Vinny.
Calv

Cam (Gypsy) beloved. (Scottish) a short form of Cameron. (Latin, French, Scottish) a short form of Campbell.

Camaron (Scottish) a form of Cameron.
Camar

Camden (Scottish) winding valley.

Cameron ☼ (Scottish) crooked nose. See also Kameron.
Cameran, Camerson, Camiren

Camille (French) young ceremonial attendant.

Camilo (Latin) child born to freedom; noble.

Campbell (Latin, French) beautiful field. (Scottish) crooked mouth.

Camron (Scottish) a short form of Cameron.

Canaan (French) a form of Cannon. History: an ancient region between the Jordan River and the Mediterranean.

Candide (Latin) pure; sincere.

Cannon (French) church official; large gun. See also Kannon.

Canute (Latin) white haired. (Scandinavian) knot. History: a Danish king who became king of England after 1016. See also Knute.

Cappi (Gypsy) good fortune.

Car (Irish) a short form of Carney.

Carey (Greek) pure. (Welsh) castle; rocky island. See also Karey.
Care

Carl (German, English) a short form of Carlton. A form of Charles. See also Carroll, Kale, Kalle, Karl, Karlen, Karol.
Carle, Carles, Carless, Carlis, Carll, Carlson, Carlston, Carlus, Carolos

Carlin (Irish) little champion.
Carlan, Carlen, Carley, Carlie, Carling, Carlino, Carly

Carlisle (English) Carl's island.

Carlito (Spanish) a familiar form of Carlos.

Carlo (Italian) a form of Carl, Charles.
Carolo

Carlos ✖ (Spanish) a form of Carl, Charles.

Carlton (English) Carl's town.
Carleton, Carllton, Carlston, Carltonn, Carltton

Carmel (Hebrew) vineyard, garden. See also Carmine.
Carmello, Carmelo

Carmichael (Scottish) follower of Michael.

Carmine (Latin) song; crimson. (Italian) a form of Carmel.
Carman, Carmen, Carmon

Carnelius (Greek, Latin) a form of Cornelius.

Carnell (English) defender of the castle. (French) a form of Cornell.

Carney (Irish) victorious. (Scottish) fighter. See also Kearney.

Carr (Scandinavian) marsh. See also Kerr.

Carrick (Irish) rock.

Carrington (Welsh) rocky town.

Carroll (Irish) champion. (German) a form of Carl.
Carolo

Carson ✖ (English) son of Carr.
Carrson

Carsten (Greek) a form of Karsten.

Carter (English) cart driver.
Cart

Cartwright (English) cart builder.

Carvell (French, English) village on the marsh.

Carver (English) wood-carver; sculptor.

Cary (Welsh) a form of Carey. (German, Irish) a form of Carroll.

Case (Irish) a short form of Casey.
(English) a short form of Casimir.

Casey (Irish) brave.
Casie, Casy, Cayse, Caysey

Cash (Latin) vain. (Slavic) a short form
of Casimir.

Casimir (Slavic) peacemaker.

Casper (Persian) treasurer. (German)
imperial. See also Gaspar, Jasper,
Kasper.

Cass (Irish, Persian) a short form of
Casper, Cassidy.

Cassidy (Irish) clever; curly haired. See
also Kazio.
Cassady

Cassie (Irish) a familiar form of
Cassidy.
Casie, Casy

Cassius (Latin, French) box; protective
cover.

Castle (Latin) castle.

Castor (Greek) beaver. Astrology: one of
the twins in the constellation Gemini.
Mythology: one of the patron saints of
mariners.

Cater (English) caterer.

Cato (Latin) knowledgeable, wise.

Cavan (Irish) handsome. See also
Kevin.

Cayden (American) a form of Caden.

Caylan (Scottish) a form of Caelan.

Cazzie (American) a familiar form of
Cassius.

Ceasar (Latin) a form of Caesar.

Cecil (Latin) blind.
*Cece, Cecile, Cecilio, Cecilius, Cecill,
Celio*

Cedric (English) battle chieftain. See
also Kedrick, Rick.
*Cad, Caddaric, Ced, Cedrec, Cédric,
Cedryche*

Cedrick (English) a form of Cedric.

Ceejay (American) a combination of
the initials C. + J.

Cemal (Arabic) attractive.

Cephas (Latin) small rock. Bible: the
term used by Jesus to describe Peter.

Cerdic (Welsh) beloved.

Cerek (Polish) lordly. (Greek) a form of
Cyril.

Cesar (Spanish) a form of Caesar.
*Casar, César, Cesare, Cesareo, Cesario,
Cesaro*

Cestmir (Czech) fortress.

Cezar (Slavic) a form of Caesar.

Chace (French) a form of Chase.

Chad (English) warrior. A short form of
Chadwick. Geography: a country in
north-central Africa.
*Ceadd, Chaad, Chadd, Chaddie,
Chaddy, Chade, Chadleigh, Chadler,
Chadley, Chadlin, Chadlyn,
Chadmen, Chado, Chadron, Chady*

Chadrick (German) mighty warrior.

Chadwick (English) warrior's town.
Chadvic, Chadwyck

Chago (Spanish) a form of Jacob.

Chaim (Hebrew) life. See also Hyman.

Chaise (French) a form of Chase.

Chal (Gypsy) boy; son.

Chalmers (Scottish) son of the lord.

Cham (Vietnamese) hard worker.

Chan (Sanskrit) shining. (English) a
form of Chauncey. (Spanish) a form of
Juan.
Chann

Chanan (Hebrew) cloud.

Chance (English) a short form of
Chancellor, Chauncey.
*Chanc, Chancey, Chancy, Chansy,
Chants, Chantz, Chanz*

Chancellor (English) record keeper.

Chander (Hindi) moon.
Chand

Chandler (English) candle maker.
Chandlan

Chane (Swahili) dependable.

Chaney (French) oak.

Chankrisna (Cambodian) sweet
smelling tree.

Channing (English) wise. (French)
canon; church official.
Chann

Chanse (English) a form of Chance.

Chante (French) singer.

Chapman (English) merchant.

Charles ☙ (German) farmer.
(English) strong and manly. See also
Carl, Searlas, Tearlach, Xarles.
*Charl, Charle, Charlen, Charlot,
Charlzell*

Charlie (German, English) a familiar
form of Charles.
Charle, Charley, Charly

Charlton (English) a form of Carlton.

Charro (Spanish) cowboy.

Chase ☙ (French) hunter.
*Chasen, Chason, Chass, Chasten,
Chaston, Chasyn*

Chaska (Sioux) first-born son.

Chauncey (English) chancellor; church
official.
*Chancey, Chaunce, Chauncei,
Chauncy*

Chavez (Hispanic) a surname used as a
first name.

Chayse (French) a form of Chase.

Chayton (Lakota) falcon.

Chaz (English) a familiar form of Charles.
Chas, Chazwick, Chazz

Ché (Spanish) a familiar form of José.
History: Ernesto "Che" Guevara was a
revolutionary who fought at Fidel
Castro's side in Cuba.

Checha (Spanish) a familiar form of
Jacob.

Cheche (Spanish) a familiar form of
Joseph.

Chen (Chinese) great, tremendous.

Chencho (Spanish) a familiar form of
Lawrence.

Chepe (Spanish) a familiar form of Joseph.

Cherokee (Cherokee) people of a different speech.

Chesmu (Native American) gritty.

Chester (English) a short form of Rochester.
Ches, Cheslav, Cheston

Chet (English) a short form of Chester.

Cheung (Chinese) good luck.

Chevalier (French) horseman, knight.

Chevy (French) a familiar form of Chevalier. Geography: Chevy Chase is a town in Maryland. Culture: a short form of Chevrolet, an American automobile company.

Cheyenne (Cheyenne) a tribal name.

Chi (Chinese) younger generation. (Nigerian) personal guardian angel.

Chick (English) a familiar form of Charles.

Chico (Spanish) boy.

Chik (Gypsy) earth.

Chike (Ibo) God's power.

Chiko (Japanese) arrow; pledge.

Chilo (Spanish) a familiar form of Francisco.

Chilton (English) farm by the spring.

Chim (Vietnamese) bird.

Chinua (Ibo) God's blessing.

Chioke (Ibo) gift of God.

Chip (English) a familiar form of Charles.

Chiram (Hebrew) exalted; noble.

Chris (Greek) a short form of Christian, Christopher. See also Kris.
Chriss, Christ, Chrys, Cris, Crist

Christain (Greek) a form of Christian.
Christai

Christian ★ (Greek) follower of Christ; anointed. See also Jaan, Kerstan, Khristian, Kit, Krister, Kristian, Krystian.
Chretien, Christa, Christé, Christen, Christensen, Christiaan, Christiana, Christiano, Christianos, Christin, Christino, Christion, Christon, Christyan, Chritian, Chrystian

Christien (Greek) a form of Christian.

Christofer (Greek) a form of Christopher.
Christafer, Christifer, Christoffer, Christofper

Christoff (Russian) a form of Christopher.

Christophe (French) a form of Christopher.
Christoph

Christopher ★ (Greek) Christ-bearer. Religion: the patron saint of travelers. See also Cristopher, Kester, Kit, Kristopher, Risto, Stoffel, Tobal, Topher.
Chrisopherson, Christepher, Christhoper, Christipher, Christobal, Christoher, Christopehr, Christoper, Christopherr, Christorpher, Christovao, Christpher, Christphere, Christpor, Christrpher

Christophoros (Greek) a form of Christopher.

Christos (Greek) a form of Christopher. See also Khristos.

Chucho (Hebrew) a familiar form of Jesus.

Chuck (American) a familiar form of Charles.

Chui (Swahili) leopard.

Chul (Korean) firm.

Chuma (Ibo) having many beads, wealthy. (Swahili) iron.

Chuminga (Spanish) a familiar form of Dominic.

Chumo (Spanish) a familiar form of Thomas.

Chun (Chinese) spring.

Chung (Chinese) intelligent.

Churchill (English) church on the hill. History: Sir Winston Churchill served as British prime minister and won a Nobel Prize for literature.

Cian (Irish) ancient.
Kian

Cicero (Latin) chickpea. History: a famous Roman orator, philosopher, and statesman.

Cid (Spanish) lord. History: title for Rodrigo Díaz de Vivar, an eleventh-century Spanish soldier and national hero.

Ciqala (Dakota) little.

Cirillo (Italian) a form of Cyril.
Cirillo, Ciro

Cisco (Spanish) a short form of Francisco.

Clancy (Irish) redheaded fighter.

Clare (Latin) a short form of Clarence.

Clarence (Latin) clear; victorious.
Clarance, Clarrance, Clarrence, Clearence

Clark (French) cleric; scholar.
Clarke, Clerc, Clerk

Claude (Latin, French) lame.
Claud, Claudan, Claudel, Claudell, Claudian, Claudianus, Claudien, Claudin, Claudius

Claudio (Italian) a form of Claude.

Claus (German) a short form of Nicholas. See also Klaus.

Clay (English) clay pit. A short form of Clayborne, Clayton.

Clayborne (English) brook near the clay pit.

Clayton (English) town built on clay.

Cleary (Irish) learned.

Cleavon (English) cliff.

Clem (Latin) a short form of Clement.

Clement (Latin) merciful. Bible: a coworker of Paul. See also Klement, Menz.

Clemente (Italian, Spanish) a form of Clement.

Cleon (Greek) famous.

Cletus (Greek) illustrious. History: a Roman pope and martyr.

Cleveland (English) land of cliffs.

Cliff (English) a short form of Clifford, Clifton.
Clif, Clift, Clyff, Clyph

Clifford (English) cliff at the river crossing.
Cliford, Clyfford

Clifton (English) cliff town.
Cliffton, Clift, Cliften, Clyfton

Clint (English) a short form of Clinton.

Clinton (English) hill town.
Clinten, Clintton, Clynton

Clive (English) a form of Cliff.

Clovis (German) famous soldier. See also Louis.

Cluny (Irish) meadow.

Clyde (Welsh) warm. (Scottish) Geography: a river in Scotland.
Cly, Clywd

Coby (Hebrew) a familiar form of Jacob.

Cochise (Apache) hardwood. History: a famous Chiricahua Apache leader.

Coco (French) a familiar form of Jacques.

Codey (English) a form of Cody.
Coday

Codi, Codie (English) forms of Cody.

Cody ❦ (English) cushion. History: William "Buffalo Bill" Cody was an American frontier scout who toured America and Europe with his Wild West show. See also Kody.
Code, Codee, Codell, Codiak, Coedy

Coffie (Ewe) born on Friday.

Cola (Italian) a familiar form of Nicholas, Nicola.

Colar (French) a form of Nicholas.

Colbert (English) famous seafarer.

Colby (English) dark; dark haired.
Colbey, Collby

Cole ❦ (Latin) cabbage farmer. (English) a short form of Coleman.
Colet, Coley, Colie

Coleman (Latin) cabbage farmer. (English) coal miner.
Colemann, Colm, Colman

Colin ❦ (Irish) young cub. (Greek) a short form of Nicholas.
Cailean, Colan, Colen, Colyn

Colley (English) black haired; swarthy.
Collis

Collier (English) miner.

Collin (Scottish) a form of Colin, Collins.
Collen, Collon, Collyn

Collins (Greek) son of Colin. (Irish) holly.
Collis

Colson (Greek, English) son of Nicholas.

Colt (English) young horse; frisky. A short form of Colter, Colton.

Colten (English) a form of Colton.

Colter (English) herd of colts.

Colton (English) coal town.
Coltin, Coltrane

Columba (Latin) dove.

Colwyn (Welsh) Geography: a river in Wales.

Coman (Arabic) noble. (Irish) bent.

Conall (Irish) high, mighty.

Conan (Irish) praised; exalted. (Scottish) wise.

Conary (Irish) a form of Conan.

Conlan (Irish) hero.

Conner (Irish) a form of Connor.

Connie (English, Irish) a familiar form of Conan, Conrad, Constantine, Conway.
Conny

Connor ☀ (Scottish) wise. (Irish) a form of Conan.

Conor (Irish) a form of Connor.

Conrad (German) brave counselor.
Conrade, Conrado

Conroy (Irish) wise.

Constant (Latin) a short form of Constantine.

Constantine (Latin) firm, constant. History: Constantine the Great was the Roman emperor who adopted the Christian faith. See also Dinos, Konstantin, Stancio.

Conway (Irish) hound of the plain.

Cook (English) cook.

Cooper (English) barrel maker. See also Keiffer.
Coop, Couper

Corbett (Latin) raven.

Corbin (Latin) raven.
Corban, Corben, Corbey, Corbie, Corby

Corcoran (Irish) ruddy.

Cordaro (Spanish) a form of Cordero.

Cordell (French) rope maker.
Cord, Cordae, Corday, Cordeal, Cordel, Cordelle, Cordie, Cordy

Cordero (Spanish) little lamb.
Cordeal, Cordeara, Cordearo, Cordeiro, Cordelro, Cordera, Corderall, Corderro, Corderun, Cordiaro, Cordy, Corrderio

Corey (Irish) hollow. See also Korey, Kory.
Core, Coreaa, Cori, Corian, Corie, Corio, Correy, Corria, Corrie, Corrye

Cormac (Irish) raven's son. History: a third-century king of Ireland who was a great lawmaker.

Cornelius (Greek) cornel tree. (Latin) horn colored. See also Kornel, Kornelius, Nelek.
Conny, Cornealous, Corneili, Corneilius, Corneliaus, Cornelious, Cornelis, Corneliu, Cornellis, Cornellius, Cornelus, Corney, Cornie, Corniellus, Corny, Cournelius

Cornell (French) a form of Cornelius.
Cornall, Corney, Cornie, Corny

Cornwallis (English) from Cornwall.

Corrado (Italian) a form of Conrad.

Corrigan (Irish) spearman.

Corrin (Irish) spear carrier.

Corry (Latin) a form of Corey.

Cort (German) bold. (Scandinavian) short. (English) a short form of Courtney.

Cortez (Spanish) conqueror. History: Hernando Cortés was a Spanish conquistador who conquered Aztec Mexico. *Cartez, Cortes, Courtez*

Corwin (English) heart's companion; heart's delight.

Cory (Latin) a form of Corey. (French) a familiar form of Cornell. (Greek) a short form of Corydon.

Corydon (Greek) helmet, crest.

Cosgrove (Irish) victor, champion.

Cosmo (Greek) orderly; harmonious; universe.

Costa (Greek) a short form of Constantine.

Coty (French) slope, hillside. *Cotee, Cotey, Cotie, Cotty*

Courtland (English) court's land. *Court, Courtlana, Courtlandt, Courtlin, Courtlyn*

Courtney (English) court. *Cortnay, Cortne, Cortney, Court, Courteney, Courtnay*

Cowan (Irish) hillside hollow.

Coy (English) woods. *Coyie, Coyt*

Coyle (Irish) leader in battle.

Coyne (French) modest.

Craddock (Welsh) love.

Craig (Irish, Scottish) crag; steep rock. *Crag, Craige, Craigen, Craigery, Craigon, Creag, Cregg, Creig, Criag*

Crandall (English) crane's valley.

Crawford (English) ford where crows fly.

Creed (Latin) belief.

Creighton (English) town near the rocks.

Crepin (French) a form of Crispin.

Crispin (Latin) curly haired. *Cris*

Cristian (Greek) a form of Christian. *Crétien, Cristhian, Cristiano, Cristino, Cristle, Criston, Cristos, Cristy*

Cristobal (Greek) a form of Christopher. *Cristóbal, Cristóbal, Cristoval, Cristovao*

Cristoforo (Italian) a form of Christopher.

Cristopher (Greek) a form of Christopher. *Cristaph, Cristofer, Cristoph, Cristophe*

Crofton (Irish) town with cottages.

Cromwell (English) crooked spring, winding spring.

Crosby (Scandinavian) shrine of the cross.

Crosley (English) meadow of the cross.

Crowther (English) fiddler.

Cruz (Portuguese, Spanish) cross.

Crystek (Polish) a form of Christian.

D

Cullen (Irish) handsome.
Cull, Cullan, Cullie, Cullin

Culley (Irish) woods.
Cullie

Culver (English) dove.
Cull, Cullie

Cunningham (Irish) village of the milk pail.

Curran (Irish) hero.

Currito (Spanish) a form of Curtis.

Curt (Latin) a short form of Courtney, Curtis. See also Kurt.

Curtis (Latin) enclosure. (French) courteous. See also Kurtis.
Curio, Curtice, Curtiss, Curtus

Cuthbert (English) brilliant.

Cutler (English) knife maker.

Cy (Persian) a short form of Cyrus.

Cyle (Irish) a form of Kyle.

Cyprian (Latin) from the island of Cyprus.

Cyrano (Greek) from Cyrene, an ancient city in North Africa. Literature: *Cyrano de Bergerac* is a play by Edmond Rostand about a great guardsman and poet whose large nose prevented him from pursuing the woman he loved.

Cyril (Greek) lordly. See also Kiril.
Cerel, Ceril, Ciril, Cirillo, Cyra, Cyrel, Cyrell, Cyrelle, Cyrill, Cyrille, Cyrillus

Cyrus (Persian) sun. Historical: Cyrus the Great was a king in ancient Persia. See also Kir.
Ciro, Cyris

Dabi (Basque) a form of David.

Dabir (Arabic) tutor.

Dacey (Latin) from Dacia, an area now in Romania. (Irish) southerner.

Dada (Yoruba) curly haired.

Daegel (English) from Daegel, England.

Daelen (English) a form of Dale.

Daemon (Greek) a form of Damian. (Greek, Latin) a form of Damon.
Daemean, Daemien, Daemyen

Daequan (American) a form of Daquan.

Daeshawn (American) a combination of the prefix Da + Shawn.

Daevon (American) a form of Davon.

Dafydd (Welsh) a form of David.

Dag (Scandinavian) day; bright.

Dagan (Hebrew) corn; grain.

Dagwood (English) shining forest.

Dai (Japanese) big.

Daimian (Greek) a form of Damian.
Daimean, Daimen, Daimien, Daimyan

Daimon (Greek, Latin) a form of Damon.

Daiquan (American) a form of Dajuan.

Daivon (American) a form of Davon.

Dajon (American) a form of Dajuan.

Dajuan (American) a combination of the prefix Da + Juan. See also Dejuan. *Dujuan, D'Juan*

Dakarai (Shona) happy.

Dakoda (Dakota) a form of Dakota. *Dacoda*

Dakota (Dakota) friend; partner; tribal name. *Dac, Dack, Dacota, Dak, Dakoata, Dakotha*

Dakotah (Dakota) a form of Dakota.

Daksh (Hindi) efficient.

Dalal (Sanskrit) broker.

Dalbert (English) bright, shining. See also Delbert.

Dale (English) dale, valley. *Dael, Dal, Dalibor, Daly, Dayl, Dayle*

Dalen (English) a form of Dale. *Dalibor*

Daley (Irish) assembly. (English) a familiar form of Dale. *Daly*

Dallan (English) a form of Dale.

Dallas (Scottish) valley of the water; resting place. Geography: a town in Scotland; a city in Texas. *Dal, Dalieass, Dall, Dalles, Dallis, Dalys, Dellis*

Dallin, Dallyn (English) pride's people.

Dalston (English) Daegel's place.

Dalton (English) town in the valley. *Dal, Dallton, Dalt, Dalten*

Dalvin (English) a form of Delvin.

Dalziel (Scottish) small field.

Damar (American) a short form of Damarcus, Damario.

Damarcus (American) a combination of the prefix Da + Marcus. *Damarco*

Damario (Greek) gentle. (American) a combination of the prefix Da + Mario.

Damek (Slavic) a form of Adam.

Dameon (Greek) a form of Damian. *Dameion, Dameone*

Dametrius (Greek) a form of Demetrius.

Damian (Greek) tamer; soother. *Damaiaon, Dame, Damean, Damián, Damiann, Damiano, Damianos, Damján, Damyan, Dema, Demyan*

Damien (Greek) a form of Damian. Religion: Father Damien ministered to the leper colony on the Hawaiian island Molokai. *Daemien, Daimien, Damie, Damyen*

Damion (Greek) a form of Damian. *Damin, Damyon*

Damon (Greek) constant, loyal. (Latin) spirit, demon. *Daemen, Daemond, Daman, Damen, Damonn, Damonta, Damontez, Damontis, Daymon, Daymond*

Dan (Vietnamese) yes. (Hebrew) a short form of Daniel. *Dahn, Danh, Danne*

Dana (Scandinavian) from Denmark.
Dain, Daina

Dandin (Hindi) holy man.

Dandré (French) a combination of the
prefix De + André.
D'andrea

Dane (English) from Denmark. See also
Halden.
Dain, Daine, Danie, Dhane

Danek (Polish) a form of Daniel.

Danforth (English) a form of Daniel.

Danial (Hebrew) a form of Daniel.
Danal, Daneal, Danieal

Danick, Dannick (Slavic) familiar
forms of Daniel.

Daniel ❀ (Hebrew) God is my judge.
Bible: a Hebrew prophet. See also
Danno, Kanaiela.
*Dacso, Daneel, Daneil, Danel,
Dániel, Daniël, Danielius, Daniell,
Daniels, Danielson, Daniyel, Dan'l,
Dannel, Danniel, Dannil, Danukas,
Dasco, Deniel, Doneal, Doniel,
Donois, Dusan*

Daniele (Hebrew) a form of Daniel.

Danilo (Slavic) a form of Daniel.
Danila, Danilka

Danior (Gypsy) born with teeth.

Danladi (Hausa) born on Sunday.

Danno (Hebrew) a familiar form of
Daniel. (Japanese) gathering in the
meadow. (Hebrew) a familiar form of
Daniel.

Dannon (American) a form of Danno.

Danny, Dany (Hebrew) familiar forms
of Daniel.
Dani, Dannee, Dannie, Dannye

Dano (Czech) a form of Daniel.

Dante, Danté (Latin) lasting, enduring.
*Danatay, Danaté, Dant, Dauntay,
Dauntaye, Daunté, Dauntrae*

Dantrell (American) a combination of
Dante + Darell.

Danyel (Hebrew) a form of Daniel.

Daoud (Arabic) a form of David.

Daquan (American) a combination of
the prefix Da + Quan.

Dar (Hebrew) pearl.

Dara (Cambodian) stars.

Daran (Irish) a form of Darren.
Darran

Darby (Irish) free. (English) deer park.

Darcy (Irish) dark. (French) from Arcy,
France.
*Daray, D'Aray, Darce, Darcee,
Darcel, Darcey, Darcio, D'Arcy,
Darsey, Darsy*

Dareh (Persian) wealthy.

Darell (English) a form of Darrell.
Daralle, Dareal, Darel, Darral

Daren (Hausa) born at night. (Irish,
English) a form of Darren.
Dare, Dayren, Dheren

Darian, Darrian (Irish) forms of
Darren.

Darick (German) a form of Derek.
Darek

Darien, Darrien (Irish) forms of Darren.

Darin (Irish) a form of Darren.
Daryn, Darynn, Dayrin, Dearin, Dharin

Dario (Spanish) affluent.

Darion, Darrion (Irish) forms of Darren.

Darius (Greek) wealthy.
Dairus, Dare, Darieus, Darioush

Darnell (English) hidden place.
Darn, Darnall, Darnel

Daron (Irish) a form of Darren.
Darone, Dayron, Dearon, Dharon, Diron

Darrell (French) darling, beloved; grove of oak trees.
Dare, Darel, Darral, Darrel, Darrill, Darrol

Darren (Irish) great. (English) small; rocky hill.
Dare, Darran, Darrience, Darryn, Darun, Daryn, Dearron, Deren, Dereon, Derron

Darrick (German) a form of Derek.
Darrec, Darrik, Darryk

Darrin (Irish) a form of Darren.

Darrion (Irish) a form of Darren.
Derrion

Darrius (Greek) a form of Darius.
Darrias, Darrious, Darris, Darrus, Derrious, Derris, Derrius

Darron (Irish) a form of Darren.

Darryl (French) darling, beloved; grove of oak trees. A form of Darrell.
Dahril, Darryle, Darryll, Daryle, Daryll

Darshan (Hindi) god; godlike. Religion: another name for the Hindu god Shiva.

Darton (English) deer town.

Darwin (English) dear friend. History: Charles Darwin was the British naturalist who established the theory of evolution.
Darwyn, Derwynn

Daryl (French) a form of Darryl.
Darel, Daril, Darl, Darly, Daryell, Daryle, Daryll, Darylle, Daroyl

Dasan (Pomo) leader of the bird clan.

Dashawn (American) a combination of the prefix Da + Shawn.
Dasean, Dashaun

Dauid (Swahili) a form of David.

Daulton (English) a form of Dalton.

Davante (American) a form of Davonte.
Davinte

Davaris (American) a combination of Dave + Darius.

Dave (Hebrew) a short form of David, Davis.

Davey (Hebrew) a familiar form of David.

David ☀ (Hebrew) beloved. Bible: the second king of Israel. See also Dov, Havika, Kawika, Taaveti, Taffy, Tevel.

Davin (Scandinavian) brilliant Finn.
Daevin, Dawin, Dawine, Deaven

Davion (American) a form of Davin.

Davis (Welsh) son of David.
Davidson, Davies, Davison

Davon (American) a form of Davin.
Davone, Davonn, Davonne, Deavon

Davonte (American) a combination of
Davon + the suffix Te.

Dawan (American) a form of Davin.
Dawayne, Dawyne

Dawit (Ethiopian) a form of David.

Dawson (English) son of David.

Dax (French, English) water.
(American) a form of Dillon.

Daymian (Greek) a form of Damian.

Dayne (Scandinavian) a form of Dane.

Dayquan (American) a form of Daquan.

Dayshawn (American) a form of
Dashawn.

Dayton (English) day town; bright,
sunny town.
Daeton, Daiton, Deyton

Dayvon (American) a form of Davin.

De (Chinese) virtuous.

Deacon (Greek) one who serves.

Dean (French) leader. (English) valley.
See also Dino.
Deane, Deen, Dene, Deyn

Deandre (French) a combination of the
prefix De + André.
*D'andre, D'andré, D'andrea,
Deandra, Deandrae, Déandre,
Deandré, De André, Deandrea, De
Andrea, Deaundera, Deaundra,
Deaundre, De Aundre, Deaundrey*

Deangelo (Italian) a combination of
the prefix De + Angelo.
Dang, Dangelo, D'Angelo, Danglo,

*Deaengelo, Déangelo, De Angelo,
Deangleo, Deanglo, Diangelo,
Di'angelo*

Deante (Latin) a form of Dante.
Deanté, De Anté, Deaunta

Deanthony (Italian) a combination of
the prefix De + Anthony.

Dearborn (English) deer brook.

Decarlos (Spanish) a combination of
the prefix De + Carlos.

Decha (Tai) strong.

Decimus (Latin) tenth.

Declan (Irish) man of prayer. Religion:
Saint Declan was a fifth-century Irish
bishop.

Dedrick (German) ruler of the people.
See also Derek, Theodoric.

Deems (English) judge's child.

Deion (Greek) a form of Dion.

Dejuan (American) a combination of
the prefix De + Juan. See also Dajuan.
*Dejan, Dejon, Dejun, Dewan,
Dewaun, Dewon, Dijaun, D'Juan,
Dujuan, D'Won*

Dekel (Hebrew, Arabic) palm tree, date
tree.

Dekota (Dakota) a form of Dakota.
Dekotes

Del (English) a short form of Delbert,
Delvin, Delwin.

Delaney (Irish) descendant of the challenger.

Delano (French) nut tree. (Irish) dark.

Delbert (English) bright as day. See also Dalbert.
Dilbert

Delfino (Latin) dolphin.

Délì (Chinese) virtuous.

Dell (English) small valley. A short form of Udell.

Delling (Scandinavian) scintillating.

Delmar (Latin) sea.

Delon (American) a form of Dillon.

Delroy (French) belonging to the king. See also Elroy, Leroy.

Delshawn (American) a combination of Del + Shawn.

Delsin (Native American) he is so.

Delton (English) a form of Dalton.

Delvin (English) proud friend; friend from the valley.
Delavan, Delvyn

Delwin (English) a form of Delvin.

Deman (Dutch) man.

Demarco (Italian) a combination of the prefix De + Marco.
Damarco, D'Marco

Demarcus (American) a combination of the prefix De + Marcus.
Damarcius, Demarkes, Demarkis, Demarkus, D'Marcus

Demario (Italian) a combination of the prefix De + Mario.
Demarreio, Demarrio, Demerrio

Demarius (American) a combination of the prefix De + Marius.

Demarquis (American) a combination of the prefix De + Marquis.

Dembe (Luganda) peaceful.

Demetri, Demitri (Greek) short forms of Demetrius.

Demetris (Greek) a short form of Demetrius.
Demeatric, Demeatrice, Demeatris, Demetres, Demetress, Demetric, Demetrice, Demetrick, Demetrics, Demetricus, Demetrik, Demitrez

Demetrius (Greek) lover of the earth. Mythology: a follower of Demeter, the goddess of the harvest. See also Dimitri, Mimis, Mitsos.
Damitriuz, Demeitrius, Demeterious, Demetreus, Demetrias, Demetrio, Demetrios, Demetrious, Demetriu, Demetrium, Demetrois, Demetruis, Demetrus, Demitirus, Demitrias, Demitriu, Demitrius, Demitrus, Demtriu, Demtrus, Dmetrius, Dymek

Demichael (American) a combination of the prefix De + Michael.

Demond (Irish) a short form of Desmond.

Demont (French) mountain.

Demorris (American) a combination of the prefix De + Morris.

Demos (Greek) people.

Demothi (Native American) talks while walking.

Dempsey (Irish) proud.

Dempster (English) one who judges.

Denby (Scandinavian) Geography: a Danish village.
Den, Denney, Dennie

Denham (English) village in the valley.

Denholm (Scottish) Geography: a town in Scotland.

Denis (Greek) a form of Dennis.
Deniz

Denley (English) meadow; valley.

Denman (English) man from the valley.

Dennis (Greek) Mythology: a follower of Dionysus, the god of wine. See also Dion, Nicho.
Den, Dénes, Denies, Deniz, Dennes, Dennet, Dennys, Denya, Denys, Dinis

Dennison (English) son of Dennis. See also Dyson, Tennyson.
Den

Denny (Greek) a familiar form of Dennis.
Den, Denney, Dennie, Deny

Denton (English) happy home.

Denver (English) green valley. Geography: the capital of Colorado.

Denzel (Cornish) a form of Denzil.

Denzell (Cornish) Geography: a location in Cornwall, England.

Deon (Greek) a form of Dennis. See also Dion.
Deone, Deonno

Deondre (French) a form of Deandre.
Deondray, Deondré

Deontae (American) a combination of the prefix De + Dontae.

Deonte, Deonté (American) forms of Deontae.

Deontre (American) a form of Deontae.

Dequan (American) a combination of the prefix De + Quan.

Dereck, Derick (German) forms of Derek.
Dericka, Derico, Deriek, Derique, Deryck, Deryk, Deryke, Detrek

Derek (German) a short form of Theodoric. See also Dedrick, Dirk.
Darek, Derak, Derecke, Derele, Derk, Derke, Deryek

Deric, Derik (German) forms of Derek.
Deriek, Derikk

Dermot (Irish) free from envy. (English) free. (Hebrew) a short form of Jeremiah. See also Kermit.

Deron (Hebrew) bird; freedom. (American) a combination of the prefix De + Ron.
Daaron, Da-Ron, Darone, Dayron, Dereon, Deronn, Deronne, Derrin, Derrion, Derron, Derronn, Derronne, Derryn, Diron, Duron, Durron, Dyron

Deror (Hebrew) lover of freedom.

Derrek (German) a form of Derek.
Derrec, Derreck

Derrell (French) a form of Darrell.
Derele, Derrel, Dérrell, Derriel, Derril, Derrill

Derren (Irish, English) a form of Darren.
Deren, Derrin, Derrion, Derron, Derryn

Derrick (German) ruler of the people. A form of Derek.
Derric, Derrik, Derryck, Derryk

Derry (Irish) redhead. Geography: a city in Northern Ireland.

Derryl (French) a form of Darryl.

Derward (English) deer keeper.

Derwin (English) a form of Darwin.

Desean (American) a combination of the prefix De + Sean.
Dasean, D'Sean, Dusean

Deshane (American) a combination of the prefix De + Shane.

Deshaun (American) a combination of the prefix De + Shaun.
Deshaune, D'shaun, Dushaun

Deshawn (American) a combination of the prefix De + Shawn.
Dashaun, Deshauwn, Deshawan, D'shawn, Dushan

Deshea (American) a combination of the prefix De + Shea.

Déshì (Chinese) virtuous.

Deshon (American) a form of Deshawn.

Desiderio (Spanish) desired.

Desmond (Irish) from south Munster.
Des, Desi, Desmon, Desmund

Destin (French) destiny, fate.

Destry (American) a form of Destin.

Detrick (German) a form of Dedrick.
Detrek

Devan (Irish) a form of Devin.

Devante (American) a combination of Devan + the suffix Te.

Devaughn (American) a form of Devin.

Devayne (American) a form of Dewayne.

Deven (Hindi) for God. (Irish) a form of Devin.
Deaven, Deiven

Deverell (English) riverbank.

Devin ☝ (Irish) poet.
Deavin, Deivin, Dev, Devlyn, Devy, Dyvon

Devine (Latin) divine. (Irish) ox.

Devlin (Irish) brave, fierce.
Dev, Devlyn

Devon (Irish) a form of Devin.
Deavon, Deivon, Deivone, Deivonne, Devoen, Devohn, Devone, Devonn, Devonne, Devontaine, Dewon

Devonta (American) a combination of Devon + the suffix Ta.
Devontae, Devontay

Devonte (American) a combination of Devon + the suffix Te.

Devyn (Irish) a form of Devin.

Dewayne (Irish) a form of Dwayne. (American) a combination of the prefix De + Wayne.
Dewwayne, Dewain, Dewaine, Dewan, Dewaun, Dewon, Dewune

Dewei (Chinese) highly virtuous.

Dewey (Welsh) prized.
Dew, Dewi, Dewie

DeWitt (Flemish) blond.

Dexter (Latin) dexterous, adroit.
(English) fabric dyer.
*Daxter, Decca, Deck, Decka, Dekka,
Dex, Dextar, Dextor, Dextrel, Dextron*

Dezmon, Dezmond (Irish) forms of
Desmond.

Diamond (English) brilliant gem;
bright guardian.

Dick (German) a short form of
Frederick, Richard.

Dickran (Armenian) History: an ancient
Armenian king.

Dickson (English) son of Dick.

Didi (Hebrew) a familiar form of
Jedidiah, Yedidyah.

Didier (French) desired, longed for.

Diedrich (German) a form of Dedrick,
Dietrich.

Diego ☼ (Spanish) a form of Jacob,
James.
Diaz

Dietbald (German) a form of Theobald.

Dieter (German) army of the people.

Dietrich (German) a form of Dedrick.

Digby (Irish) ditch town; dike town.

Dillan (Irish) a form of Dillon.
Dilan

Dillon (Irish) loyal, faithful. See also
Dylan.
*Dil, Dill, Dillen, Dillie, Dillin, Dillion,
Dilly, Dillyn, Dilon, Dilyn*

Dilwyn (Welsh) shady place.

Dima (Russian) a familiar form of
Vladimir.

Dimitri (Russian) a form of Demetrius.
*Dimetra, Dimetri, Dimetric,
Dimetrie, Dimitr, Dimitric, Dimitrie,
Dimitrik, Dimitris, Dimitry, Dimmy,
Dymitr, Dymitry*

Dimitrios (Greek) a form of Demetrius.
Dhimitrios, Dimos, Dmitrios

Dimitrius (Greek) a form of Demetrius.

Dingbang (Chinese) protector of the
country.

Dinh (Vietnamese) calm, peaceful.

Dino (German) little sword. (Italian) a
form of Dean.
Deano

Dinos (Greek) a familiar form of
Constantine, Konstantin.

Dinsmore (Irish) fortified hill.

Diogenes (Greek) honest. History: an
ancient philosopher who searched with
a lantern in daylight for an honest
man.

Dion (Greek) a short form of Dennis,
Dionysus.
*Dio, Dione, Dionigi, Dionis, Dionn,
Diontae, Diontray*

Dionte (American) a form of Deontae.
Diontae

Dionysus (Greek) celebration.
Mythology: the god of wine.

Diquan (American) a combination of
the prefix Di + Quan.

Dirk (German) a short form of Derek,
Theodoric.
Derk, Dirck, Dirke, Durc, Durk, Dyrk

Dixon (English) son of Dick.

Dmitri (Russian) a form of Dimitri.

Doane (English) low, rolling hills.

Dob (English) a familiar form of Robert.

Dobry (Polish) good.

Doherty (Irish) harmful.

Dolan (Irish) dark haired.

Dolf, Dolph (German) short forms of
Adolf, Adolph, Rudolf, Rudolph.

Dom (Latin) a short form of Dominic.

Domenic (Latin) a form of Dominic.
Domenick

Domenico (Italian) a form of Dominic.
Domicio, Dominico

Domingo (Spanish) born on Sunday.
See also Mingo.

Dominic ✦ (Latin) belonging to the
Lord. See also Chuminga.
*Deco, Demenico, Domanic, Domeka,
Domini, Dominie, Dominitric,
Dominy, Domnenique, Domonic*

Dominick (Latin) a form of Dominic.
*Domiku, Domineck, Dominicke,
Dominiek, Domminick, Domnick,
Domonick, Donek, Dumin*

Dominik (Latin) a form of Dominic.

Dominique (French) a form of
Dominic.
*Domeniqu, Domenque, Dominiqu,
Dominiqueia, Domnenique,
Domnique, Domoniqu, Domonique*

Domokos (Hungarian) a form of
Dominic.

Don (Scottish) a short form of Donald.
See also Kona.
Donn

Donahue (Irish) dark warrior.

Donal (Irish) a form of Donald.

Donald (Scottish) world leader; proud
ruler. See also Bohdan, Tauno.
*Dónal, Donaldo, Donall, Donalt,
Donát, Donaugh*

Donatien (French) gift.

Donato (Italian) gift.

Donavan (Irish) a form of Donovan.
Donavin, Donavon, Donavyn

Dondre (French) a form of Deandre.

Dong (Vietnamese) easterner.

Donkor (Akan) humble.

Donnell (Irish) brave; dark.
*Doneal, Donell, Donelle, Doniel,
Donielle, Donnel,, Donnelle, Donniel*

Donnelly (Irish) a form of Donnell.

Donnie, Donny (Irish) familiar forms
of Donald.

Donovan (Irish) dark warrior.
*Dohnovan, Donevon, Donoven,
Donovin, Donovon, Donvan*

Dontae, Donté (American) forms of
Dante.
*Donta, Dontai, Dontao, Dontate,
Dontay, Dontaye, Dontea, Dontee,
Dontez*

Dontrell (American) a form of Dantrell.

Donzell (Cornish) a form of Denzell.

Dooley (Irish) dark hero.

Dor (Hebrew) generation.

Doran (Greek, Hebrew) gift. (Irish) stranger; exile.

Dorian (Greek) from Doris, Greece. See also Isidore.

Dorrell (Scottish) king's doorkeeper. See also Durell.

Dotan (Hebrew) law.

Doug (Scottish) a short form of Dougal, Douglas.

Dougal (Scottish) dark stranger. See also Doyle.

Douglas (Scottish) dark river, dark stream. See also Koukalaka.
Douglass, Dougles, Dugaid, Dughlas

Dov (Yiddish) bear. (Hebrew) a familiar form of David.

Dovev (Hebrew) whisper.

Dow (Irish) dark haired.

Doyle (Irish) a form of Dougal.
Doy, Doyal, Doyel

Drago (Italian) a form of Drake.

Drake (English) dragon; owner of the inn with the dragon trademark.

Draper (English) fabric maker.

Draven (American) a combination of the letter D + Raven.

Dreng (Norwegian) hired hand; brave.

Dreshawn (American) a combination of Drew + Shawn.

Drevon (American) a form of Draven.

Drew (Welsh) wise. (English) a short form of Andrew.
Drewe

Dru (English) a form of Drew.

Drummond (Scottish) druid's mountain.

Drury (French) loving. Geography: Drury Lane is a street in London's theater district.

Dryden (English) dry valley.

Duane (Irish) a form of Dwayne.
Deune, Duain, Duaine, Duana

Duarte (Portuguese) rich guard. See also Edward.

Duc (Vietnamese) moral.

Dudd (English) a short form of Dudley.

Dudley (English) common field.

Duer (Scottish) heroic.

Duff (Scottish) dark.

Dugan (Irish) dark.

Duke (French) leader; duke.

Dukker (Gypsy) fortuneteller.

Dulani (Nguni) cutting.

Dumaka (Ibo) helping hand.

Duman (Turkish) misty, smoky.

Duncan (Scottish) brown warrior. Literature: King Duncan was Macbeth's victim in Shakespeare's play *Hamlet.*
Dunc

Dunham (Scottish) brown.

Dunixi (Basque) a form of Dionysus.

Dunley (English) hilly meadow.

Dunlop (Scottish) muddy hill.

Dunmore (Scottish) fortress on the hill.

Dunn (Scottish) a short form of Duncan.

Dunstan (English) brownstone fortress.

Dunton (English) hill town.

Dur (Hebrew) stacked up. (English) a short form of Durwin.

Durand (Latin) a form of Durant.

Durant (Latin) enduring.

Durell (Scottish, English) king's door-keeper. See also Dorrell.
Durel, Durial, Durreil, Durrell, Durrelle

Durko (Czech) a form of George.

Durriken (Gypsy) fortuneteller.

Durril (Gypsy) gooseberry.
Durrell

Durward (English) gatekeeper.

Durwin (English) a form of Darwin.

Dushawn (American) a combination of the prefix Du + Shawn.
Dusan, Dusean, Dushan, Dushaun

Dustin (German) valiant fighter. (English) brown rock quarry.
Dust, Dustan, Dusten, Dustie, Dustine, Duston, Dustyn

Dusty (English) a familiar form of Dustin.

Dustyn (English) a form of Dustin.

Dutch (Dutch) from the Netherlands; from Germany.

Duval (French) a combination of the prefix Du + Val.

Dwaun (American) a form of Dajuan.
Dwan

Dwayne (Irish) dark. See also Dewayne.
Dawayne, Dawyne, Duwain, Duwan, Duwane, Duwayn, Duwayne, Dwain, Dwaine, Dwan, Dwane, Dwyane, Dywane

Dwight (English) a form of DeWitt.

Dyami (Native American) soaring eagle.

Dyer (English) fabric dyer.

Dyke (English) dike; ditch.

Dylan ★ (Welsh) sea. See also Dillon.
Dyllan

Dylon (Welsh) a form of Dylan.
Dyllon

Dyre (Norwegian) dear heart.

Dyson (English) a short form of Dennison.

E

Ea (Irish) a form of Hugh.

Eachan (Irish) horseman.

Eagan (Irish) very mighty.

Eamon (Irish) a form of Edmond, Edmund.

Ean (English) a form of Ian.

Earl (Irish) pledge. (English) nobleman.
*Airle, Earld, Earle, Earlie, Earlson,
Early, Eorl, Erl, Erle*

Earnest (English) a form of Ernest.
Earn, Earnesto, Earnie, Eranest

Easton (English) eastern town.

Eaton (English) estate on the river.

Eb (Hebrew) a short form of Ebenezer.

Eben (Hebrew) rock.

Ebenezer (Hebrew) foundation stone.
Literature: Ebenezer Scrooge is a
miserly character in Charles Dickens's
A Christmas Carol.

Eberhard (German) courageous as a
boar. See also Everett.

Ebner (English) a form of Abner.

Ebo (Fante) born on Tuesday.

Ed (English) a short form of Edgar,
Edsel, Edward.

Edan (Scottish) fire.

Edbert (English) wealthy; bright.

Eddie (English) a familiar form of
Edgar, Edsel, Edward.
Eddee

Eddy (English) a form of Eddie.
Eddye, Edy

Edel (German) noble.

Eden (Hebrew) delightful. Bible: the
garden that was first home to Adam
and Eve.

Eder (Hebrew) flock.

Edgar (English) successful spearman.
See also Garek, Gerik, Medgar.
Edek, Edgard, Edgars

Edgardo (Spanish) a form of Edgar.

Edison (English) son of Edward.

Edmond (English) a form of Edmund.
*Edmon, Edmonde, Edmondo,
Edmondson*

Edmund (English) prosperous protector.
Eadmund, Edmunds

Edmundo (Spanish) a form of Edmund.

Edo (Czech) a form of Edward.

Edoardo (Italian) a form of Edward.

Edorta (Basque) a form of Edward.

Edouard (French) a form of Edward.
Édouard

Edric (English) prosperous ruler.

Edsel (English) rich man's house.

Edson (English) a short form of Edison.

Eduardo (Spanish) a form of Edward.

Edur (Basque) snow.

Edward (English) prosperous guardian.
See also Audie, Duarte, Ekewaka, Ned,
Ted, Teddy.
*Edik, Edko, Édouard, Eduard, Edus,
Edvard, Edvardo, Edwardo,
Edwards, Edwy, Edzio, Etzio, Ewart*

Edwin (English) prosperous friend. See
also Ned, Ted.
*Eadwinn, Edik, Edlin, Eduino,
Edwyn*

Efrain (Hebrew) fruitful.
Efrane

Efrat (Hebrew) honored.

Efrem (Hebrew) a short form of Ephraim.

Efren (Hebrew) a form of Efrain, Ephraim.

Egan (Irish) ardent, fiery.

Egbert (English) bright sword. See also Bert, Bertie.

Egerton (English) Edgar's town.

Egil (Norwegian) awe inspiring.

Eginhard (German) power of the sword.

Egon (German) formidable.

Egor (Russian) a form of George. See also Igor, Yegor.

Ehren (German) honorable.

Eikki (Finnish) ever powerful.

Einar (Scandinavian) individualist.

Eion (Irish) a form of Ean, Ian.

Eitan (Hebrew) a form of Ethan.

Ejau (Ateso) we have received.

Ekewaka (Hawaiian) a form of Edward.

Ekon (Nigerian) strong.

Elam (Hebrew) highlands.

Elan (Hebrew) tree. (Native American) friendly.

Elbert (English) a form of Albert.

Elchanan (Hebrew) a form of John.

Elden (English) a form of Alden, Aldous.

Elder (English) dweller near the elder trees.

Eldon (English) holy hill.

Eldred (English) a form of Aldred.

Eldridge (English) a form of Aldrich.
El

Eldwin (English) a form of Aldwin.

Eleazar (Hebrew) God has helped. See also Lazarus.

Elek (Hungarian) a form of Alec, Alex.

Elger (German) a form of Alger.

Elgin (English) noble; white.

Eli (Hebrew) uplifted. A short form of Elijah, Elisha. Bible: the high priest who trained the prophet Samuel. See also Elliot.
Elier, Eloi

Elia (Zuni) a short form of Elijah.
Elio, Eliya

Elian (English) a form of Elijah. See also Trevelyan.

Elias (Greek) a form of Elijah.
Eliasz, Elice, Ellice, Elyas

Eliazar (Hebrew) a form of Eleazar.

Elie (Hebrew) a form of Eli.

Eliezer (Hebrew) a form of Eleazar.

Elihu (Hebrew) a short form of Eliyahu.

Elijah ☙ (Hebrew) a form of Eliyahu. Bible: a Hebrew prophet. See also Eli, Elisha, Elliot, Ilias, Ilya.
El, Elija, Elijuo, Elisjsha, Eliya

Elika (Hawaiian) a form of Eric.

Eliseo (Hebrew) a form of Elisha.
Elisee, Elisée

Elisha (Hebrew) God is my salvation.
Bible: a Hebrew prophet, successor to
Elijah. See also Eli, Elijah.
*Elijsha, Elish, Elisher, Elishia, Elishua,
Lisha*

Eliyahu (Hebrew) the Lord is my God.

Elkan (Hebrew) God is jealous.

Elki (Moquelumnan) hanging over the
top.

Ellard (German) sacred; brave.

Ellery (English) from a surname
derived from the name Hilary.

Elliot, Elliott (English) forms of Eli,
Elijah.
*Elio, Eliot, Eliott, Eliud, Eliut, Elyot,
Elyott*

Ellis (English) a form of Elias.

Ellison (English) son of Ellis.

Ellsworth (English) nobleman's estate.

Elman (German) like an elm tree.

Elmer (English) noble; famous.
Elemér, Ellmer, Elmir

Elmo (Greek) lovable, friendly. (Italian)
guardian. (Latin) a familiar form of
Anselm. (English) a form of Elmer.

Elmore (English) moor where the elm
trees grow.

Elonzo (Spanish) a form of Alonzo.

Eloy (Latin) chosen.
Eloi

Elrad (Hebrew) God rules.

Elroy (French) a form of Delroy, Leroy.

Elsdon (English) nobleman's hill.

Elston (English) noble's town.

Elsu (Native American) swooping, soaring falcon.

Elsworth (English) noble's estate.

Elton (English) old town.
Ellton

Elvern (Latin) a form of Alvern.

Elvin (English) a form of Alvin.
El, Elvyn, Elwin, Elwyn, Elwynn

Elvio (Spanish) light skinned; blond.

Elvis (Scandinavian) wise.
El, Elvys

Elvy (English) elfin warrior.

Elwell (English) old well.

Elwood (English) old forest. See also
Wood, Woody.

Ely (Hebrew) a form of Eli. Geography: a
region of England with extensive
drained fens.

Eman (Czech) a form of Emmanuel.

Emanuel (Hebrew) a form of
Emmanuel.
*Emaniel, Emanual, Emanuele,
Emanuell*

Emerson (German, English) son of
Emery.
Emmerson, Emreson

Emery (German) industrious leader.
*Emari, Emeri, Emerich, Emerio,
Emmerich, Emmerie, Emmery,
Emmo*

Emil (Latin) flatterer. (German) industrious. See also Milko, Milo.
Emilek, Emill, Emils, Emilyan

Émile (French) a form of Emil.

Emiliano (Italian) a form of Emil.

Emilien (Latin) friendly; industrious.

Emilio (Italian, Spanish) a form of Emil.
Emilios, Emilo

Emlyn (Welsh) waterfall.

Emmanuel (Hebrew) God is with us. See also Immanuel, Maco, Mango, Manuel.
Emanuell, Emek, Emmaneuol, Emmanle, Emmanueal, Emmanuele, Emmanuil

Emmett (German) industrious; strong. (English) ant. History: Robert Emmett was an Irish patriot.
Em, Emitt, Emmet, Emmot, Emmott, Emmy

Emmitt (German, English) a form of Emmett.
Emmit

Emory (German) a form of Emery.
Emmory

Emre (Turkish) brother.
Emreson

Emrick (German) a form of Emery.

Enapay (Sioux) brave appearance; he appears.

Endre (Hungarian) a form of Andrew.

Eneas (Greek) a form of Aeneas.

Engelbert (German) bright as an angel. See also Ingelbert.

Enli (Dene) that dog over there.

Ennis (Greek) mine. (Scottish) a form of Angus.

Enoch (Hebrew) dedicated, consecrated. Bible: the father of Methuselah.

Enos (Hebrew) man.

Enric (Romanian) a form of Henry.

Enrick (Spanish) a form of Henry.

Enrico (Italian) a form of Henry.

Enrikos (Greek) a form of Henry.

Enrique (Spanish) a form of Henry. See also Quiqui.
Enrigué, Enriqué, Enriquez, Enrrique

Enver (Turkish) bright; handsome.

Enyeto (Native American) walks like a bear.

Enzi (Swahili) powerful.

Eoin (Welsh) a form of Evan.

Ephraim (Hebrew) fruitful. Bible: the second son of Joseph.

Erasmus (Greek) lovable.

Erastus (Greek) beloved.

Erbert (German) a short form of Herbert.

Ercole (Italian) splendid gift.

Erek (Scandinavian) a form of Eric.

Erhard (German) strong; resolute.

Eriberto (Italian) a form of Herbert.

Eric ☙ (Scandinavian) ruler of all. (English) brave ruler. (German) a short form of Frederick. History: Eric the Red was a Norwegian explorer who founded Greenland's first colony.
Ehrich, Éric, Erica, Erico, Erric, Eryc

Erich (Czech, German) a form of Eric.

Erick (English) a form of Eric.
Errick

Erickson (English) son of Eric.
Ericson, Erikson

Erik (Scandinavian) a form of Eric.
Eriks, Errick, Eryk

Erikur (Icelandic) a form of Eric, Erik.

Erin (Irish) peaceful. History: an ancient name for Ireland.
Erine, Erinn, Erino, Eryn, Erynn

Erland (English) nobleman's land.

Erling (English) nobleman's son.

Ermanno (Italian) a form of Herman.

Ermano (Spanish) a form of Herman.

Ernest (English) earnest, sincere. See also Arno.
Ernestino, Ernestus

Ernesto (Spanish) a form of Ernest.
Ernester

Ernie (English) a familiar form of Ernest.
Earnie

Erno (Hungarian) a form of Ernest.

Ernst (German) a form of Ernest.

Erol (Turkish) strong, courageous.

Eron (Irish) a form of Erin.

Errando (Basque) bold.

Errol (Latin) wanderer. (English) a form of Earl.
Erold, Erroll, Erryl

Erroman (Basque) from Rome.

Erskine (Scottish) high cliff. (English) from Ireland.

Ervin, Erwin (English) sea friend. Forms of Irving, Irwin.

Ervine (English) a form of Irving.

Esau (Hebrew) rough; hairy. Bible: Jacob's twin brother.

Esequiel (Hebrew) a form of Ezekiel.

Eshkol (Hebrew) grape clusters.

Eskil (Norwegian) god vessel.

Esmond (English) rich protector.

Espen (Danish) bear of the gods.

Essien (Ochi) sixth-born son.

Este (Italian) east.

Estéban (Spanish) a form of Stephen.
Estabon, Esteban, Estefan, Estephan

Estebe (Basque) a form of Stephen.

Estevan (Spanish) a form of Stephen.

Estevao (Spanish) a form of Stephen.

Ethan ☙ (Hebrew) strong; firm.
Eathan, Etan, Ethe

Étienne (French) a form of Stephen.

Ettore (Italian) steadfast.

Etu (Native American) sunny.

Euclid (Greek) intelligent. History: the founder of Euclidean geometry.

Eugen (German) a form of Eugene.

Eugene (Greek) born to nobility. See also Ewan, Gene, Gino, Iukini, Jenö, Yevgenyi, Zenda.
Eoghan, Eugéne, Eugeni, Eugenius

Eugenio (Spanish) a form of Eugene.

Eulises (Latin) a form of Ulysses.

Eustace (Greek) productive. (Latin) stable, calm. See also Stacey.

Evan ✻ (Irish) young warrior. (English) a form of John. See also Bevan, Owen.
Ev, Evann, Evans, Even, Evens, Evyn, Ewen

Evangelos (Greek) a form of Andrew.

Evelyn (English) hazelnut.

Everardo (German) strong as a boar.

Everett (English) a form of Eberhard.
Ev, Evered, Everet, Everette, Everitt, Evert, Evrett

Everley (English) boar meadow.

Everton (English) boar town.

Evgeny (Russian) a form of Eugene. See also Zhek.

Evin (Irish) a form of Evan.

Ewald (German) always powerful. (English) powerful lawman.

Ewan (Scottish) a form of Eugene, Evan. See also Keon.
Ewen

Ewert (English) ewe herder, shepherd.
Ewart

Ewing (English) friend of the law.

Exavier (Basque) a form of Xavier.

Eyota (Native American) great.

Ezekiel (Hebrew) strength of God. Bible: a Hebrew prophet. See also Haskel, Zeke.
Ezéchiel, Ezeck, Ezeeckel, Ezekeial, Ezekial, Ezell, Eziakah, Eziechiele

Ezequiel (Hebrew) a form of Ezekiel.
Eziequel

Ezer (Hebrew) a form of Ezra.

Ezra (Hebrew) helper; strong. Bible: a Jewish priest who led the Jews back to Jerusalem.
Esdras, Esra, Ezera, Ezri

Ezven (Czech) a form of Eugene.

Faber (German) a form of Fabian.

Fabian (Latin) bean grower.
Fabayan, Fabe, Fabek, Fabeon, Fabert, Fabi, Fabien, Fabius, Fabiyan, Fabiyus, Fabyan, Fabyen, Faybian, Faybien

Fabiano (Italian) a form of Fabian.

Fabio (Latin) a form of Fabian. (Italian) a short form of Fabiano.

Fabrizio (Italian) craftsman.

Fabron (French) little blacksmith; apprentice.

Fadey (Ukrainian) a form of Thaddeus.

Fadi (Arabic) redeemer.

Fadil (Arabic) generous.

Fagan (Irish) little fiery one.

Fahd (Arabic) lynx.

Fai (Chinese) beginning.

Fairfax (English) blond.

Faisal (Arabic) decisive.

Fakhir (Arabic) excellent.

Fakih (Arabic) thinker; reader of the Koran.

Falco (Latin) falconer.

Falito (Italian) a familiar form of Rafael, Raphael.

Falkner (English) trainer of falcons. See also Falco.

Fane (English) joyful, glad.

Faraji (Swahili) consolation.

Farid (Arabic) unique.

Faris (Arabic) horseman.

Farley (English) bull meadow; sheep meadow. See also Lee.

Farnell (English) fern-covered hill.

Farnham (English) field of ferns.

Farnley (English) fern meadow.

Faroh (Latin) a form of Pharaoh.

Farold (English) mighty traveler.

Farquhar (Scottish) dear.

Farr (English) traveler.

Farrell (Irish) heroic; courageous.

Farrow (English) piglet.

Farruco (Spanish) a form of Francis, Francisco.

Faruq (Arabic) honest.

Faste (Norwegian) firm.

Fath (Arabic) victor.

Fatin (Arabic) clever.

Faust (Latin) lucky, fortunate. History: the sixteenth-century German necromancer who inspired many legends.

Faustino (Italian) a form of Faust.

Fausto (Italian) a form of Faust.

Favian (Latin) understanding.

Faxon (German) long-haired.

Federico (Italian, Spanish) a form of Frederick.

Feivel (Yiddish) God aids.

Feliks (Russian) a form of Felix.

Felipe (Spanish) a form of Philip. *Feeleep, Felipino, Felo, Filippo, Filips, Fillip*

Felippo (Italian) a form of Philip. *Filippo, Pippo*

Felix (Latin) fortunate; happy. See also Pitin. *Felo*

Felton (English) field town.

Fenton (English) marshland farm.

Feodor (Slavic) a form of Theodore.

Feoras (Greek) smooth rock.

Ferdinand (German) daring, adventurous. See also Hernando.
Ferdie, Ferdynand

Ferenc (Hungarian) a form of Francis.

Fergus (Irish) strong; manly.

Fermin (French, Spanish) firm, strong.

Fernando (Spanish) a form of Ferdinand.
Ferdinando, Ferdnando, Ferdo, Fernand, Fernandez

Feroz (Persian) fortunate.

Ferran (Arabic) baker.

Ferrand (French) iron gray hair.

Ferrell (Irish) a form of Farrell.

Ferris (Irish) a form of Peter.

Fico (Spanish) a familiar form of Frederick.

Fidel (Latin) faithful. History: Fidel Castro was the Cuban revolutionary who overthrew a dictatorship in 1959 and established a communist regime in Cuba.

Field (English) a short form of Fielding.

Fielding (English) field; field worker.

Fife (Scottish) from Fife, Scotland.

Fifi (Fante) born on Friday.

Fil (Polish) a form of Phil.

Filbert (English) brilliant. See also Bert.

Filiberto (Spanish) a form of Filbert.

Filip (Greek) a form of Philip.
Filippo

Fillipp (Russian) a form of Philip.
Filips, Fillip

Filmore (English) famous.

Filya (Russian) a form of Philip.

Fineas (Irish) a form of Phineas.

Finian (Irish) light skinned; white.

Finlay (Irish) blond-haired soldier.

Finn (German) from Finland. (Irish) blond haired; light skinned. A short form of Finlay. (Norwegian) from the Lapland.

Finnegan (Irish) light skinned; white.

Fiorello (Italian) little flower.

Firas (Arabic) persistent.

Firman (French) firm; strong.

Firth (English) woodland.

Fischel (Yiddish) a form of Phillip.

Fiske (English) fisherman.

Fitch (English) weasel, ermine.

Fitz (English) son.

Fitzgerald (English) son of Gerald.

Fitzhugh (English) son of Hugh.

Fitzpatrick (English) son of Patrick.

Fitzroy (Irish) son of Roy.

Flaminio (Spanish) Religion: Marcantonio Flaminio coauthored one of the most important texts of the Italian Reformation.

Flann (Irish) redhead.

Flavian (Latin) blond, yellow haired.

Flavio (Italian) a form of Flavian.

Fleming (English) from Denmark; from Flanders.

Fletcher (English) arrow featherer, arrow maker.
Flecher, Fletch

Flint (English) stream; flint stone.

Flip (Spanish) a short form of Felipe. (American) a short form of Philip.

Florencio (Italian) a form of Florent.

Florent (French) flowering.

Florian (Latin) flowering, blooming.

Floyd (English) a form of Lloyd.

Flurry (English) flourishing, blooming.

Flynn (Irish) son of the red-haired man.

Folke (German) a form of Volker.

Foluke (Yoruba) given to God.

Foma (Bulgarian, Russian) a form of Thomas.

Fonso (German, Italian) a short form of Alphonso.

Fontaine (French) fountain.

Fonzie (German) a familiar form of Alphonse.

Forbes (Irish) prosperous.

Ford (English) a short form of names ending in "ford."

Fordel (Gypsy) forgiving.

Forest (French) a form of Forrest.

Forester (English) forest guardian.
Forrie

Forrest (French) forest; woodsman.
Forrie

Fortino (Italian) fortunate, lucky.

Fortune (French) fortunate, lucky.

Foster (Latin) a short form of Forester.

Fowler (English) trapper of wildfowl.

Fran (Latin) a short form of Francis.

Francesco (Italian) a form of Francis.

Franchot (French) a form of Francis.

Francis (Latin) free; from France. Religion: Saint Francis of Assisi was the founder of the Franciscan order. See also Farruco, Ferenc.
France, Francessco, Franciskus, Frang, Frannie, Franny, Franscis, Fransis, Franta, Frants, Franus, Frencis

Francisco (Portuguese, Spanish) a form of Francis. See also Chilo, Cisco, Farruco, Paco, Pancho.

Franco (Latin) a short form of Francis.
Franko

François (French) a form of Francis.

Frank (English) a short form of Francis, Franklin. See also Palani, Pancho.
Franc, Franck, Franek, Frang, Franio, Franke, Franko

Frankie (English) a familiar form of Frank.
Franke, Franky

Franklin (English) free landowner.
Francklin, Francklyn, Frankin,
Franklinn, Franquelin

Franklyn (English) a form of Franklin.
Franklynn

Frans (Swedish) a form of Francis.
Frants

Frantisek (Czech) a form of Francis.
Franta

Franz (German) a form of Francis.

Fraser (French) strawberry. (English)
curly haired.
Fraizer, Frasier, Fraze, Frazer,
Frazier

Frayne (French) dweller at the ash tree.
(English) stranger.

Fred (German) a short form of Alfred,
Frederick, Manfred.
Fredd, Fredson

Freddie (German) a familiar form of
Frederick.
Freddi, Fredi

Freddy, Fredy (German) familiar forms
of Frederick.

Frederic (German) a form of Frederick.
Frédéric, Frederich, Frederric,
Fredric, Fredrich

Frederick (German) peaceful ruler. See
also Dick, Eric, Fico, Peleke, Rick.
Fredderick, Freddrick, Fredek,
Fréderick, Frédérick, Frederrick,
Fredwick, Fredwyck

Frederico (Spanish) a form of
Frederick.

Frederik (German) a form of Frederick.
Frédérik, Fredrik

Frederique (French) a form of
Frederick.

Fredo (Spanish) a form of Fred.

Fredrick (German) a form of Frederick.
Fredric

Freeborn (English) child of freedom.

Freeman (English) free.

Fremont (German) free; noble protector.

Frewin (English) free; noble friend.

Frey (English) lord. (Scandinavian)
Mythology: the Norse god who dis-
penses peace and prosperity.

Frick (English) bold.

Fridolf (English) peaceful wolf.

Friedrich (German) a form of
Frederick.

Frisco (Spanish) a short form of
Francisco.

Fritz (German) a familiar form of
Frederick.
Fritson, Fritts, Fritzchen, Fritzl

Frode (Norwegian) wise.

Fulbright (German) very bright.

Fuller (English) cloth thickener.

Fulton (English) field near town.

Funsoni (Nguni) requested.

Fyfe (Scottish) a form of Fife.

Fynn (Ghanaian) Geography: another
name for the Offin River in Ghana.

Fyodor (Russian) a form of Theodore.

G

Gabby (American) a familiar form of Gabriel.

Gabe (Hebrew) a short form of Gabriel.

Gabino (American) a form of Gabriel. *Gabin*

Gábor (Hungarian) God is my strength.

Gabrial (Hebrew) a form of Gabriel. *Gaberial, Gabrail*

Gabriel ✻ (Hebrew) devoted to God. Bible: the angel of the Annunciation. *Gab, Gabis, Gabreil, Gabriël, Gabriele, Gabriell, Gabris, Gabys, Gebereal, Ghabriel*

Gabrielli (Italian) a form of Gabriel.

Gadi (Arabic) God is my fortune.

Gaetan (Italian) from Gaeta, a region in southern Italy.

Gage (French) pledge.

Gaige (French) a form of Gage.

Gair (Irish) small.

Gaius (Latin) rejoicer. See also Cai.

Galbraith (Irish) Scotsman in Ireland.

Gale (Greek) a short form of Galen.

Galen (Greek) healer; calm. (Irish) little and lively. *Gaelan, Gaelen, Galan, Galin*

Galeno (Spanish) illuminated child. (Greek, Irish) a form of Galen.

Gallagher (Irish) eager helper.

Galloway (Irish) Scotsman in Ireland.

Galt (Norwegian) high ground.

Galton (English) owner of a rented estate.

Galvin (Irish) sparrow.

Gamal (Arabic) camel. See also Jamal.

Gamble (Scandinavian) old.

Gan (Chinese) daring, adventurous. (Vietnamese) near.

Gannon (Irish) light skinned, white.

Ganya (Zulu) clever.

Gar (English) a short form of Gareth, Garnett, Garrett, Garvin.

Garcia (Spanish) mighty with a spear.

Gardner (English) gardener.

Garek (Polish) a form of Edgar.

Garen (English) a form of Garry.

Gareth (Welsh) gentle. *Garith, Garreth, Garyth*

Garett (Irish) a form of Garrett. *Gared, Garet*

Garfield (English) field of spears; battlefield.

Garland (French) wreath of flowers; prize. (English) land of spears; battleground.

Garman (English) spearman.

Garner (French) army guard, sentry.

Garnett (Latin) pomegranate seed; garnet stone. (English) armed with a spear.

Garnock (Welsh) dweller by the alder river.

Garrad (English) a form of Garrett.
Gared, Garrard

Garret (Irish) a form of Garrett.

Garrett (Irish) brave spearman. See also Jarrett.

Garrick (English) oak spear.

Garren, Garrin (English) forms of Garry.

Garrison (French) troops stationed at a fort; garrison.
Garris

Garroway (English) spear fighter.

Garry (English) a form of Gary.
Garrey, Garri, Garrie

Garson (English) son of Gar.

Garth (Scandinavian) garden, gardener. (Welsh) a short form of Gareth.

Garvey (Irish) rough peace.

Garvin (English) comrade in battle.

Garwood (English) evergreen forest. See also Wood, Woody.

Gary (German) mighty spearman. (English) a familiar form of Gerald. See also Kali.
Gare, Garey, Gari

Gaspar (French) a form of Casper.

Gaston (French) from Gascony, France.

Gaute (Norwegian) great.

Gautier (French) a form of Walter.

Gavin ☀ (Welsh) white hawk.
Gav, Gavan, Gaven, Gavinn, Gavino, Gavyn, Gavynn

Gavriel (Hebrew) man of God.
Gav

Gavril (Russian) a form of Gavriel.

Gawain (Welsh) a form of Gavin.

Gaylen (Greek) a form of Galen.

Gaylord (French) merry lord; jailer.

Gaynor (Irish) son of the fair-skinned man.

Geary (English) variable, changeable.

Gedeon (Bulgarian, French) a form of Gideon.

Geffrey (English) a form of Geoffrey. See also Jeffrey.

Gellert (Hungarian) a form of Gerald.

Gena (Russian) a short form of Yevgenyi.

Genaro (Latin) consecrated to God.

Gene (Greek) a short form of Eugene.

Genek (Polish) a form of Gene.

Geno (Italian) a form of John. A short form of Genovese.

Genovese (Italian) from Genoa, Italy.

Gent (English) gentleman.

Genty (Irish, English) snow.

Geoff (English) a short form of Geoffrey.

Geoffery (English) a form of Geoffrey.

Geoffrey (English) a form of Jeffrey. See also Giotto, Godfrey, Gottfried, Jeff.
Geoffre, Geoffroi, Geoffroy, Geoffry, Geofrey, Geofri, Gofery

Geordan (Scottish) a form of Gordon.

Geordie (Scottish) a form of George.

Georg (Scandinavian) a form of George.

George (Greek) farmer. See also Durko, Egor, Iorgos, Jerzy, Jiri, Joji, Jörg, Jorge, Jorgen, Joris, Jorrín, Jur, Jurgis, Keoki, Mahiái, Serner, Yegor, Yorgos, Yoyi, Yrjo, Yuri, Zhora.
Georgas, Georget, Georgi, Georgii, Georgiy, Gevork, Gheorghe, Goerge, Goran, Gordios, Gorge, Gorje, Gorya, Grzegorz

Georges (French) a form of George.

Georgio (Italian) a form of George.

Georgios (Greek) a form of George.

Georgy (Greek) a familiar form of George.

Geovanni, Geovanny (Italian) forms of Giovanni.

Geraint (English) old.

Gerald (German) mighty spearman. See also Fitzgerald, Jarell, Jarrell, Jerald, Jerry, Kharald.
Garald, Garold, Garolds, Gearalt, Gérald, Geralde, Gerale, Geraud, Gerick, Gerold, Gerrald, Gerrell, Gérrick, Gerrild, Gerrin, Gerrold, Geryld, Giraldo, Giraud, Girauld

Geraldo (Italian, Spanish) a form of Gerald.

Gerard (English) brave spearman. See also Jerard, Jerry.
Garrard, Garrat, Garratt, Gearard, Gerad, Gerar, Gérard, Geraro, Gerd, Gerrard, Girard

Gerardo (Spanish) a form of Gerard.
Gherardo

Géraud (French) a form of Gerard.

Gerek (Polish) a form of Gerard.

Geremia (Hebrew) exalted by God.
(Italian) a form of Jeremiah.

Geremiah (Italian) a form of Jeremiah.

Gerhard (German) a form of Gerard.

Gerik (Polish) a form of Edgar.
Gerick

Germain (French) from Germany.
(English) sprout, bud. See also Jermaine.

Gerome (English) a form of Jerome.

Geronimo (Greek, Italian) a form of Jerome. History: a famous Apache chief.

Gerrit (Dutch) a form of Gerald.

Gerry (English) a familiar form of Gerald, Gerard. See also Jerry.
Geri, Gerre, Gerri, Gerrie, Gerryson

Gershom (Hebrew) exiled. (Yiddish) stranger in exile.

Gerson (English) son of Gar.

Gert (German, Danish) fighter.

Gervaise (French) honorable. See also Jervis.

Gerwin (Welsh) fair love.

Gethin (Welsh) dusky.

Ghazi (Arabic) conqueror.

Ghilchrist (Irish) servant of Christ. See also Gil.

Ghislain (French) pledge.

Gi (Korean) brave.

Gia (Vietnamese) family.

Giacinto (Portuguese, Spanish) a form of Jacinto.

Giacomo (Italian) a form of Jacob.

Gian (Italian) a form of Giovanni, John.

Giancarlo (Italian) a combination of John + Charles.
Giancarlos

Gianluca (Italian) a combination of John + Lucas.

Gianni (Italian) a form of Johnny.

Gianpaolo (Italian) a combination of John + Paul.

Gib (English) a short form of Gilbert.

Gibor (Hebrew) powerful.

Gibson (English) son of Gilbert.

Gideon (Hebrew) tree cutter. Bible: the judge who defeated the Midianites.
Gideone, Hedeon

Gidon (Hebrew) a form of Gideon.

Gifford (English) bold giver.

Gig (English) horse-drawn carriage.

Gil (Greek) shield bearer. (Hebrew) happy. (English) a short form of Ghilchrist, Gilbert.

Gilad (Arabic) camel hump; from Giladi, Saudi Arabia.

Gilamu (Basque) a form of William.

Gilbert (English) brilliant pledge; trustworthy. See also Gil, Gillett.
Gilburt, Giselbert, Giselberto, Giselbertus, Guilbert

Gilberto (Spanish) a form of Gilbert.

Gilby (Scandinavian) hostage's estate. (Irish) blond boy.

Gilchrist (Irish) a form of Ghilchrist.

Gilen (Basque, German) illustrious pledge.

Giles (French) goatskin shield.
Gide, Gilles, Gyles

Gillean (Irish) Bible: Saint John's servant.

Gillespie (Irish) son of the bishop's servant.

Gillett (French) young Gilbert.

Gilmer (English) famous hostage.

Gilmore (Irish) devoted to the Virgin Mary.

Gilon (Hebrew) circle.

Gilroy (Irish) devoted to the king.

Gino (Greek) a familiar form of Eugene. (Italian) a short form of names ending in "gene," "gino."
Ghino

Giona (Italian) a form of Jonah.

Giordano (Italian) a form of Jordan.

Giorgio (Italian) a form of George.

Giorgos (Greek) a form of George.

Giosia (Italian) a form of Joshua.

Giotto (Italian) a form of Geoffrey.

Giovani (Italian) a form of Giovanni.
Giavani

Giovanni (Italian) a form of John. See
also Jeovanni, Jiovanni.
*Giannino, Giovannie, Giovanno,
Giovonathon, Giovonni*

Giovanny (Italian) a form of Giovanni.
Giovany

Gipsy (English) wanderer.

Girvin (Irish) small; tough.

Gitano (Spanish) gypsy.

Giuliano (Italian) a form of Julius.

Giulio (Italian) a form of Julius.

Giuseppe (Italian) a form of Joseph.
Giuseppino

Giustino (Italian) a form of Justin.

Givon (Hebrew) hill; heights.

Gladwin (English) cheerful. See also
Win.

Glanville (English) village with oak
trees.

Glen (Irish) a form of Glenn.

Glendon (Scottish) fortress in the glen.

Glendower (Welsh) from Glyndwr,
Wales.

Glenn (Irish) a short form of Glendon.
*Gleann, Glennie, Glennis, Glennon,
Glenny, Glynn*

Glentworth (English) from Glenton,
England.

Glenville (Irish) village in the glen.

Glyn (Welsh) a form of Glen.
Glynn

Goddard (German) divinely firm.

Godfrey (Irish) God's peace. (German)
a form of Jeffrey. See also Geoffrey,
Gottfried.

Godwin (English) friend of God. See
also Win.

Goel (Hebrew) redeemer.

Goldwin (English) golden friend. See
also Win.

Goliath (Hebrew) exiled. Bible: the giant
Philistine whom David slew with a
slingshot.

Gomda (Kiowa) wind.

Gomer (Hebrew) completed, finished.
(English) famous battle.

Gonza (Rutooro) love.

Gonzalo (Spanish) wolf.

Gordon (English) triangular-shaped
hill.
Gord, Gordain, Gordan, Gorden

Gordy (English) a familiar form of
Gordon.

Gore (English) triangular-shaped land;
wedge-shaped land.

Gorman (Irish) small; blue eyed.

Goro (Japanese) fifth.

Gosheven (Native American) great leaper.

Gottfried (German) a form of Geoffrey, Godfrey.

Gotzon (German) a form of Angel.

Govert (Dutch) heavenly peace.

Gower (Welsh) pure.

Gowon (Tiv) rainmaker.

Gozol (Hebrew) soaring bird.

Grady (Irish) noble; illustrious.
Gradea, Gradee, Gradey, Gradleigh, Graidey, Graidy

Graeme (Scottish) a form of Graham.
Graem

Graham (English) grand home.
Graeham, Graehame, Graehme, Grahame, Grahme, Gram

Granger (French) farmer.

Grant (English) a short form of Grantland.
Grantham, Granthem, Grantley

Grantland (English) great plains.

Granville (French) large village.

Gray (English) gray haired.

Grayden (English) gray haired.

Graydon (English) gray hill.
Greydon

Grayson (English) bailiff's son. See also Sonny.

Greeley (English) gray meadow.

Greenwood (English) green forest.

Greg, Gregg (Latin) short forms of Gregory.
Graig, Greig, Gregson

Greggory (Latin) a form of Gregory.
Greggery

Gregor (Scottish) a form of Gregory.

Gregorio (Italian, Portuguese) a form of Gregory.

Gregory (Latin) vigilant watchman. See also Jörn, Krikor.
Gergely, Gergo, Greagoir, Greagory, Greer, Gregary, Greger, Gregery, Grégoire, Gregori, Grégorie, Gregorius, Gregors, Gregos, Gregrey, Gregroy, Gregry, Greogry, Gries, Grzegorz

Gresham (English) village in the pasture.

Greyson (English) a form of Grayson.

Griffin (Latin) hooked nose.
Griff, Griffen, Griffie, Griffon, Griffy, Gryphon

Griffith (Welsh) fierce chief; ruddy.
Griff, Griffie, Griffy, Gryphon

Grigori (Bulgarian) a form of Gregory.

Grimshaw (English) dark woods.

Grisha (Russian) a form of Gregory.

Griswold (German, French) gray forest.

Grosvener (French) big hunter.

Grover (English) grove.

Guadalupe (Arabic) river of black stones.

Gualberto (Spanish) a form of Walter.

Gualtiero (Italian) a form of Walter.

Guglielmo (Italian) a form of William.

Guido (Italian) a form of Guy.

Guilford (English) ford with yellow flowers.

Guilherme (Portuguese) a form of William.

Guillaume (French) a form of William.
Guillaums

Guillermo (Spanish) a form of William.

Gunnar (Scandinavian) a form of Gunther.

Gunther (Scandinavian) battle army; warrior.

Guotin (Chinese) polite; strong leader.

Gurion (Hebrew) young lion.

Gurpreet (Sikh) devoted to the guru; devoted to the Prophet.
Gurjeet, Gurmeet, Guruprit

Gurvir (Sikh) guru's warrior.

Gus (Scandinavian) a short form of Angus, Augustine, Gustave.

Gustaf (Swedish) a form of Gustave.
Gustaff

Gustave (Scandinavian) staff of the Goths. History: Gustavus Adolphus was a king of Sweden. See also Kosti, Tabo, Tavo.
Gustaff, Gustav, Gustus

Gustavo (Italian, Spanish) a form of Gustave.

Guthrie (German) war hero. (Irish) windy place.

Gutierre (Spanish) a form of Walter.

Guy (Hebrew) valley. (German) warrior. (French) guide. See also Guido.
Guyon

Guyapi (Native American) candid.

Gwayne (Welsh) a form of Gawain.

Gwidon (Polish) life.

Gwilym (Welsh) a form of William.

Gwyn (Welsh) fair; blessed.

Gyasi (Akan) marvelous baby.

Gyorgy (Russian) a form of George.

Gyula (Hungarian) youth.

H

Habib (Arabic) beloved.

Hackett (German, French) little wood cutter.

Hackman (German, French) wood cutter.

Hadar (Hebrew) glory.

Haddad (Arabic) blacksmith.

Hadden (English) heather-covered hill.

Haden (English) a form of Hadden.

Hadi (Arabic) guiding to the right.

Hadley (English) heather-covered meadow.

Hadrian (Latin, Swedish) dark.

Hadwin (English) friend in a time of war.

Hagan (German) strong defense.

Hagen (Irish) young, youthful.

Hagley (English) enclosed meadow.

Hagos (Ethiopian) happy.

Hahnee (Native American) beggar.

Hai (Vietnamese) sea.

Haidar (Arabic) lion.

Haiden (English) a form of Hayden. *Haidyn*

Haig (English) enclosed with hedges.

Hailey (Irish) a form of Haley.

Haji (Swahili) born during the pilgrimage to Mecca.

Hakan (Native American) fiery.

Hakeem (Arabic) a form of Hakim.

Hakim (Arabic) wise. (Ethiopian) doctor. *Hakiem*

Hakon (Scandinavian) of Nordic ancestry.

Hal (English) a short form of Halden, Hall, Harold.

Halbert (English) shining hero.

Halden (Scandinavian) half-Danish. See also Dane.

Hale (English) a short form of Haley. (Hawaiian) a form of Harry.

Halen (Swedish) hall.

Haley (Irish) ingenious.

Halford (English) valley ford.

Hali (Greek) sea.

Halian (Zuni) young.

Halil (Turkish) dear friend.

Halim (Arabic) mild, gentle.

Hall (English) manor, hall.

Hallam (English) valley.

Hallan (English) dweller at the hall; dweller at the manor.

Halley (English) meadow near the hall; holy.

Halliwell (English) holy well.

Hallward (English) hall guard.

Halsey (English) Hal's island.

Halstead (English) manor grounds.

Halton (English) estate on the hill.

Halvor (Norwegian) rock; protector.

Ham (Hebrew) hot. Bible: one of Noah's sons.

Hamal (Arabic) lamb. Astronomy: a bright star in the constellation of Aries.

Hamar (Scandinavian) hammer.

Hamid (Arabic) praised. See also Muhammad.

Hamill (English) scarred.

Hamilton (English) proud estate.

Hamish (Scottish) a form of Jacob, James.

Hamisi (Swahili) born on Thursday.

Hamlet (German, French) little village; home. Literature: one of Shakespeare's tragic heroes.

Hamlin (German, French) loves his home.

Hammet (English, Scandinavian) village.

Hammond (English) village.

Hampton (English) Geography: a town in England.

Hamza (Arabic) powerful.

Hanale (Hawaiian) a form of Henry.

Hanan (Hebrew) grace.

Hanbal (Arabic) pure. History: Ahmad Ibn Hanbal founded an Islamic school of thought.

Handel (German, English) a form of John. Music: George Frideric Handel was a German composer whose works include *Messiah* and *Water Music*.

Hanford (English) high ford.

Hanif (Arabic) true believer.

Hank (American) a familiar form of Henry.

Hanley (English) high meadow.

Hannes (Finnish) a form of John.

Hannibal (Phoenician) grace of God. History: a famous Carthaginian general who fought the Romans.

Hanno (German) a short form of Johan.

Hans (Scandinavian) a form of John. *Hanschen, Hants, Hanz*

Hansel (Scandinavian) a form of Hans.

Hansen (Scandinavian) son of Hans.

Hansh (Hindi) god; godlike.

Hanson (Scandinavian) a form of Hansen.

Hanus (Czech) a form of John.

Haoa (Hawaiian) a form of Howard.

Hara (Hindi) seizer. Religion: another name for the Hindu god Shiva.

Harald (Scandinavian) a form of Harold. *Haraldo, Haralds*

Harb (Arabic) warrior.

Harbin (German, French) little bright warrior.

Harcourt (French) fortified dwelling. *Court*

Hardeep (Punjabi) a form of Harpreet.

Harden (English) valley of the hares.

Harding (English) brave; hardy.

Hardwin (English) brave friend.

Hardy (German) bold, daring.

Harel (Hebrew) mountain of God.

Harford (English) ford of the hares.

Hargrove (English) grove of the hares.

Hari (Hindi) tawny.

Harith (Arabic) cultivator.

Harjot (Sikh) light of God.

Harkin (Irish) dark red.

Harlan (English) hare's land; army land.
Harlen, Harlenn, Harlin, Harlon, Harlyn, Harlynn

Harland (English) a form of Harlan.

Harley (English) hare's meadow; army meadow.
Harlea, Harlee, Harleigh, Harly

Harlow (English) hare's hill; army hill. See also Arlo.

Harman, Harmon (English) forms of Herman.
Harm

Harold (Scandinavian) army ruler. See also Jindra.
Garald, Garold, Haraldas, Haraldo, Haralds, Herold, Heronim, Herryck

Haroun (Arabic) lofty; exalted.

Harper (English) harp player.

Harpreet (Punjabi) loves God, devoted to God.

Harris (English) a short form of Harrison.
Haris, Hariss

Harrison (English) son of Harry.
Harrisen

Harrod (Hebrew) hero; conqueror.

Harry (English) a familiar form of Harold. See also Arrigo, Hale, Parry.
Harm, Harray, Harrey, Harri, Harrie

Hart (English) a short form of Hartley.

Hartley (English) deer meadow.

Hartman (German) hard; strong.

Hartwell (English) deer well.

Hartwig (German) strong advisor.

Hartwood (English) deer forest.

Harvey (German) army warrior.
Harv, Hervey, Hervy

Harvir (Sikh) God's warrior.

Hasad (Turkish) reaper, harvester.

Hasan (Arabic) a form of Hassan.

Hasani (Swahili) handsome.

Hashim (Arabic) destroyer of evil.

Hasin (Hindi) laughing.

Haskel (Hebrew) a form of Ezekiel.

Haslett (English) hazel-tree land.

Hassan (Arabic) handsome.

Hassel (German, English) witches' corner.

Hastin (Hindi) elephant.

Hastings (Latin) spear. (English) house council.

Hatim (Arabic) judge.

Hauk (Norwegian) hawk.

Havelock (Norwegian) sea battler.

Haven (Dutch, English) harbor, port; safe place.

Havika (Hawaiian) a form of David.

Hawk (English) hawk.

Hawley (English) hedged meadow.

Hawthorne (English) hawthorn tree.

Hayden ❦ (English) hedged valley.
Haydn, Haydon

Hayes (English) hedged valley.

Hayward (English) guardian of the
hedged area.

Haywood (English) hedged forest.

Hearn (Scottish, English) a short form
of Ahearn.

Heath (English) heath.
Heathe, Heith

Heathcliff (English) cliff near the
heath. Literature: the hero of Emily
Brontë's novel *Wuthering Heights*.

Heaton (English) high place.

Heber (Hebrew) ally, partner.

Hector (Greek) steadfast. Mythology: the
greatest hero of the Trojan War in
Homer's epic poem *Iliad*.

Hedley (English) heather-filled
meadow.

Heinrich (German) a form of Henry.

Heinz (German) a familiar form of
Henry.

Helaku (Native American) sunny day.

Helge (Russian) holy.

Helki (Moquelumnan) touching.

Helmer (German) warrior's wrath.

Helmut (German) courageous.

Heman (Hebrew) faithful.

Henderson (Scottish, English) son of
Henry.

Hendrick (Dutch) a form of Henry.

Heniek (Polish) a form of Henry.

Henley (English) high meadow.

Henning (German) a form of Hendrick,
Henry.

Henoch (Yiddish) initiator.

Henri (French) a form of Henry.

Henrick (Dutch) a form of Henry.

Henrique (Portuguese) a form of Henry.

Henry (German) ruler of the household.
See also Arrigo, Enric, Enrick, Enrico,
Enrikos, Enrique, Hanale, Honok, Kiki.
*Harro, Heike, Henery, Henraoi,
Henrim, Henrry, Heromin, Hersz*

Heraldo (Spanish) a form of Harold.

Herb (German) a short form of Herbert.

Herbert (German) glorious soldier.
*Harbert, Hebert, Hébert, Heberto,
Hurbert*

Hercules (Latin) glorious gift.
Mythology: a Greek hero of fabulous
strength, renowned for his twelve
labors.

Heriberto (Spanish) a form of Herbert.
Heribert

Herman (Latin) noble. (German) sol-
dier. See also Armand, Ermanno,
Ermano, Mandek.
*Hermann, Hermie, Herminio,
Hermino, Hermon, Hermy, Heromin*

Hermes (Greek) messenger. Mythology:
the divine herald of Greek mythology.

Hernan (German) peacemaker.

Hernando (Spanish) a form of Ferdinand.

Herrick (German) war ruler.
Herryck

Herschel (Hebrew) a form of Hershel.

Hersh (Hebrew) a short form of Hershel.

Hershel (Hebrew) deer.

Hertz (Yiddish) my strife.

Hervé (French) a form of Harvey.

Hesperos (Greek) evening star.

Hesutu (Moquelumnan) picking up a yellow jacket's nest.

Hew (Welsh) a form of Hugh.

Hewitt (German, French) little smart one.

Hewson (English) son of Hugh.

Hezekiah (Hebrew) God gives strength.

Hiamovi (Cheyenne) high chief.

Hibah (Arabic) gift.

Hideaki (Japanese) smart, clever.

Hieremias (Greek) God will uplift.

Hieronymos (Greek) a form of Jerome. Art: Hieronymus Bosch was a fifteenth-century Dutch painter.

Hieu (Vietnamese) respectful.

Hilario (Spanish) a form of Hilary.

Hilary (Latin) cheerful. See also Ilari.
Hi

Hildebrand (German) battle sword.

Hilel (Arabic) new moon.

Hillel (Hebrew) greatly praised. Religion: Rabbi Hillel originated the Talmud.

Hilliard (German) brave warrior.

Hilmar (Swedish) famous noble.

Hilton (English) town on a hill.

Hinto (Dakota) blue.

Hinun (Native American) spirit of the storm.

Hippolyte (Greek) horseman.

Hiram (Hebrew) noblest; exalted.
Hi, Hirom, Huram, Hyrum

Hiromasa (Japanese) fair, just.

Hiroshi (Japanese) generous.

Hisoka (Japanese) secretive, reserved.

Hiu (Hawaiian) a form of Hugh.

Ho (Chinese) good.

Hoang (Vietnamese) finished.

Hobart (German) Bart's hill.

Hobert (German) Bert's hill.

Hobson (English) son of Robert.

Hoc (Vietnamese) studious.

Hod (Hebrew) a short form of Hodgson.

Hodgson (English) son of Roger.

Hogan (Irish) youth.

Holbrook (English) brook in the hollow.

Holden (English) hollow in the valley.

Holic (Czech) barber.

Holland (French) Geography: a former province of the Netherlands.

Holleb (Polish) dove.

Hollis (English) grove of holly trees.

Holmes (English) river islands.

Holt (English) forest.

Homer (Greek) hostage; pledge; security. Literature: a renowned Greek epic poet. *Homere, Homère, Homero, Homeros, Homerus*

Hondo (Shona) warrior.

Honesto (Filipino) honest.

Honi (Hebrew) gracious.

Honok (Polish) a form of Henry.

Honon (Moquelumnan) bear.

Honorato (Spanish) honorable.

Honoré (Latin) honored.

Honovi (Native American) strong.

Honza (Czech) a form of John.

Hop (Chinese) agreeable.

Horace (Latin) keeper of the hours. Literature: a famous Roman lyric poet and satirist. *Horaz*

Horacio (Latin) a form of Horace.

Horatio (Latin) clan name. See also Orris.

Horst (German) dense grove; thicket.

Horton (English) garden estate.

Hosa (Arapaho) young crow.

Hosea (Hebrew) salvation. Bible: a Hebrew prophet.

Hotah (Lakota) white.

Hototo (Native American) whistler.

Houghton (English) settlement on the headland.

Houston (English) hill town. Geography: a city in Texas. *Huston*

Howard (English) watchman. See also Haoa.

Howe (German) high.

Howell (Welsh) remarkable.

Howi (Moquelumnan) turtledove.

Howie (English) a familiar form of Howard, Howland.

Howin (Chinese) loyal swallow.

Howland (English) hilly land.

Hoyt (Irish) mind; spirit.

Hu (Chinese) tiger.

Hubbard (German) a form of Hubert.

Hubert (German) bright mind; bright spirit. See also Beredei, Uberto. *Hubbert, Huber*

Huberto (Spanish) a form of Hubert.

Hubie (English) a familiar form of Hubert.

Hud (Arabic) Religion: a Muslim prophet.

Hudson (English) son of Hud.

Huey (English) a familiar form of Hugh.

Hugh (English) a short form of Hubert. See also Ea, Hewitt, Huxley, Maccoy, Ugo.
Hughes, Hugues

Hugo (Latin) a form of Hugh.

Hulbert (German) brilliant grace.

Humbert (German) brilliant strength. See also Umberto.

Humberto (Portuguese) a form of Humbert.

Humphrey (German) peaceful strength. See also Onofrio, Onufry.

Hung (Vietnamese) brave.

Hunt (English) a short form of names beginning with "Hunt."

Hunter ☙ (English) hunter.

Huntington (English) hunting estate.

Huntley (English) hunter's meadow.

Hurley (Irish) sea tide.

Hurst (English) a form of Horst.

Husam (Arabic) sword.

Husamettin (Turkish) sharp sword.

Huslu (Native American) hairy bear.

Hussain (Arabic) a form of Hussein.

Hussein (Arabic) little; handsome.

Hussien (Arabic) a form of Hussein.

Hutchinson (English) son of the hutch dweller.

Hute (Native American) star.

Hutton (English) house on the jutting ledge.

Huxley (English) Hugh's meadow.

Huy (Vietnamese) glorious.

Hy (Vietnamese) hopeful. (English) a short form of Hyman.

Hyacinthe (French) hyacinth.

Hyatt (English) high gate.

Hyde (English) cache; measure of land equal to 120 acres; animal hide.

Hyder (English) tanner, preparer of animal hides for tanning.

Hyman (English) a form of Chaim.

Hyun-Ki (Korean) wise.

Hyun-Shik (Korean) clever.

Iago (Spanish, Welsh) a form of Jacob, James. Literature: the villain in Shakespeare's *Othello*.

Iain (Scottish) a form of Ian.

Iakobos (Greek) a form of Jacob.

Ian ☙ (Scottish) a form of John. See also Ean, Eion.

Ianos (Czech) a form of John.

Ib (Phoenician, Danish) oath of Baal.

Iban (Basque) a form of John.

Ibon (Basque) a form of Ivor.

Ibrahim (Hausa) my father is exalted.
Ibraham, Ibrahem

Ichabod (Hebrew) glory is gone.
Literature: Ichabod Crane is the main
character of Washington Irving's story
"The Legend of Sleepy Hollow."

Idi (Swahili) born during the Idd festival.

Idris (Welsh) eager lord. (Arabic)
Religion: a Muslim prophet.

Iestyn (Welsh) a form of Justin.

Igashu (Native American) wanderer;
seeker.

Iggy (Latin) a familiar form of Ignatius.

Ignacio (Italian) a form of Ignatius.

Ignatius (Latin) fiery, ardent. Religion:
Saint Ignatius of Loyola founded the
Jesuit order. See also Inigo, Neci.

Igor (Russian) a form of Inger, Ingvar.
See also Egor, Yegor.

Ihsan (Turkish) compassionate.

Ike (Hebrew) a familiar form of Isaac.
History: the nickname of the thirty-
fourth U.S. president Dwight D.
Eisenhower.
Ikey

Iker (Basque) visitation.

Ilan (Hebrew) tree. (Basque) youth.

Ilari (Basque) a form of Hilary.

Ilias (Greek) a form of Elijah.

Illan (Basque, Latin) youth.

Ilom (Ibo) my enemies are many.

Ilya (Russian) a form of Elijah.

Imad (Arabic) supportive; mainstay.

Iman (Hebrew) a short form of
Immanuel.

Immanuel (Hebrew) a form of
Emmanuel.

Imran (Arabic) host.

Imre (Hungarian) a form of Emery.

Imrich (Czech) a form of Emery.

Inay (Hindi) god; godlike.

Ince (Hungarian) innocent.

Inder (Hindi) god; godlike.

Indiana (Hindi) from India.

Inek (Welsh) a form of Irvin.

Ing (Scandinavian) a short form of
Ingmar.

Ingelbert (German) a form of
Engelbert.

Inger (Scandinavian) son's army.

Ingmar (Scandinavian) famous son.

Ingram (English) angel.

Ingvar (Scandinavian) Ing's soldier.

Inigo (Basque) a form of Ignatius.

Iniko (Ibo) born during bad times.

Innis (Irish) island.

Innocenzio (Italian) innocent.

Inteus (Native American) proud;
unashamed.

Ioakim (Russian) a form of Joachim.

Ioan (Greek, Bulgarian, Romanian) a form of John.

Iokepa (Hawaiian) a form of Joseph.

Iolo (Welsh) the Lord is worthy.

Ionakana (Hawaiian) a form of Jonathan.

Iorgos (Greek) a form of George.

Iosif (Greek, Russian) a form of Joseph.

Iosua (Romanian) a form of Joshua.

Ipyana (Nyakyusa) graceful.

Ira (Hebrew) watchful.

Iram (English) bright.

Irumba (Rutooro) born after twins.

Irv (Irish, Welsh, English) a short form of Irvin, Irving.

Irvin (Irish, Welsh, English) a short form of Irving. See also Ervine.
Irvine

Irving (Irish) handsome. (Welsh) white river. (English) sea friend. See also Ervin, Ervine.
Irvington

Irwin (English) a form of Irving. See also Ervin.

Isa (Arabic) a form of Jesus.

Isaac ☝ (Hebrew) he will laugh. Bible: the son of Abraham and Sarah. See also Itzak, Izak, Yitzchak.
Icek, Ikey, Ikie, Isaakios, Isac, Isacco, Isack, Isiac, Isiacc, Issca

Isaak (Hebrew) a form of Isaac.
Isack, Isak

Isaiah ☝ (Hebrew) God is my salvation. Bible: a Hebrew prophet.
Isai, Isaia, Isaid, Isaih, Isaish, Isia, Isiah, Isiash, Issia, Izaiah, Izaiha

Isaias (Hebrew) a form of Isaiah.
Isais

Isam (Arabic) safeguard.

Isas (Japanese) meritorious.

Isekemu (Native American) slow-moving creek.

Isham (English) home of the iron one.

Ishan (Hindi) direction.

Ishaq (Arabic) a form of Isaac.

Ishmael (Hebrew) God will hear. Literature: the narrator of Herman Melville's novel *Moby-Dick*.
Isamail, Ishma, Ishmel

Isidore (Greek) gift of Isis. See also Dorian, Ysidro.

Isidro (Greek) a form of Isidore.

Iskander (Afghan) a form of Alexander.

Ismael (Arabic) a form of Ishmael.

Ismail (Arabic) a form of Ishmael.

Israel (Hebrew) prince of God; wrestled with God. History: the nation of Israel took its name from the name given Jacob after he wrestled with the angel of the Lord. See also Yisrael.
Iser, Isser, Izrael

Isreal (Hebrew) a form of Israel.

Issa (Swahili) God is our salvation.

Issac (Hebrew) a form of Isaac.
Issiac

Issiah (Hebrew) a form of Isaiah.
Issia

Istu (Native American) sugar pine.

István (Hungarian) a form of Stephen.

Ithel (Welsh) generous lord.

Ittamar (Hebrew) island of palms.

Itzak (Hebrew) a form of Isaac, Yitzchak.

Iukini (Hawaiian) a form of Eugene.

Iustin (Bulgarian, Russian) a form of Justin.

Ivan (Russian) a form of John.
Iván, Ivanchik, Ivanichek, Ivano, Ivas

Ivar (Scandinavian) a form of Ivor. See also Yves, Yvon.

Ives (English) young archer.

Ivo (German) yew wood; bow wood.

Ivor (Scandinavian) a form of Ivo.

Iwan (Polish) a form of John.

Iyapo (Yoruba) many trials; many obstacles.

Iye (Native American) smoke.

Izak (Czech) a form of Isaac.

Izzy (Hebrew) a familiar form of Isaac, Isidore, Israel.

J

J (American) an initial used as a first name.
J.

Ja (Korean) attractive, magnetic.

Jaali (Swahili) powerful.

Jaan (Estonian) a form of Christian.

Jaap (Dutch) a form of Jim.

Jabari (Swahili) fearless, brave.
Jabier

Jabez (Hebrew) born in pain.

Jabin (Hebrew) God has created.

Jabir (Arabic) consoler, comforter.

Jabril (Arabic) a form of Jibril.

Jabulani (Shona) happy.

Jacan (Hebrew) trouble.

Jacari (American) a form of Jacorey.

Jace (American) a combination of the initials J. + C.
JC, J.C., Jacey, Jaice

Jacen (Greek) a form of Jason.

Jacinto (Portuguese, Spanish) hyacinth. See also Giacinto.

Jack ❦ (American) a familiar form of Jacob, John. See also Keaka.
Jacko, Jackub, Jak, Jax, Jocko

Jackie, Jacky (American) familiar forms of Jack.

Jackson ❦ (English) son of Jack.
Jacson, Jakson

Jaco (Portuguese) a form of Jacob.

Jacob ☙ (Hebrew) supplanter, substitute. Bible: son of Isaac, brother of Esau. See also Akiva, Chago, Checha, Coby, Diego, Giacomo, Hamish, Iago, Iakobos, James, Kiva, Koby, Kuba, Tiago, Yakov, Yasha, Yoakim. *Jacbob, Jackub, Jacobb, Jacobe, Jacolby, Jalu, Jecis, Jeks, Jeska, Jocek, Jocoby, Jocolby, Jokubas*

Jacobi, Jacoby (Hebrew) forms of Jacob. *Jacobis*

Jacobo (Hebrew) a form of Jacob.

Jacobson (English) son of Jacob. *Jacobs, Jacobus*

Jacorey (American) a combination of Jacob + Corey.

Jacque (French) a form of Jacob.

Jacques (French) a form of Jacob, James. See also Coco. *Jacot, Jacquan, Jacquees, Jacquet, Jarques, Jarquis*

Jacquez, Jaquez (French) forms of Jacques. *Jaques*

Jacy (Tupi-Guarani) moon. *Jaycee*

Jade (Spanish) jade, precious stone.

Jaden ☙ (Hebrew) a form of Jadon.

Jadon (Hebrew) God has heard.

Jadrien (American) a combination of Jay + Adrien.

Jadyn (Hebrew) a form of Jadon.

Jaegar (German) hunter.

Jae-Hwa (Korean) rich, prosperous.

Jael (Hebrew) mountain goat.

Jaelen (American) a form of Jalen.

Ja'far (Sanskrit) little stream.

Jagger (English) carter.

Jago (English) a form of James.

Jaguar (Spanish) jaguar.

Jahi (Swahili) dignified.

Jahlil (Hindi) a form of Jalil.

Jahmar (American) a form of Jamar.

Jahvon (Hebrew) a form of Javan. *Jahvine*

Jai (Tai) heart.

Jaiden (Hebrew) a form of Jadon.

Jailen (American) a form of Jalen.

Jaime (Spanish) a form of Jacob, James. *Jaimey, Jaimie, Jaimito, Jaymie*

Jairo (Spanish) God enlightens.

Jaison (Greek) a form of Jason. *Jaisen*

Jaivon (Hebrew) a form of Javan.

Jaja (Ibo) honored.

Jajuan (American) a combination of the prefix Ja + Juan.

Jakari (American) a form of Jacorey.

Jake (Hebrew) a short form of Jacob. *Jakie, Jayk, Jayke*

Jakeem (Arabic) uplifted.

Jakob (Hebrew) a form of Jacob.
*Jakab, Jakiv, Jakov, Jakovian, Jakub,
Jakubek, Jekebs*

Jakome (Basque) a form of James.

Jal (Gypsy) wanderer.

Jalan (American) a form of Jalen.

Jaleel (Hindi) a form of Jalil.

Jalen (American) a combination of the
prefix Ja + Len.

Jalil (Hindi) revered.

Jalin, Jalyn (American) forms of Jalen.

Jalon (American) a form of Jalen.

Jam (American) a short form of Jamal,
Jamar.

Jamaal (Arabic) a form of Jamal.

Jamaine (Arabic) a form of Germain.

Jamal (Arabic) handsome. See also
Gamal.
*Jahmal, Jahmalle, Jahmel, Jahmil,
Jahmile, Jamael, Jamahl, Jamail,
Jamala, Jamale, Jamall, Jammal,
Jarmal, Jaumal*

Jamar (American) a form of Jamal.

Jamarcus (American) a combination
of the prefix Ja + Marcus.

Jamari (American) a form of Jamario.

Jamario (American) a combination of
the prefix Ja + Mario.

Jamarquis (American) a combination
of the prefix Ja + Marquis.

Jamel (Arabic) a form of Jamal.
*Jameel, Jamele, Jamell, Jamelle,
Jammel, Jarmel, Jaumal, Jaumell, Je-
Mell*

James ♓ (Hebrew) supplanter, substi-
tute. (English) a form of Jacob. Bible:
James the Great and James the Less
were two of the Twelve Apostles. See
also Diego, Hamish, Iago, Kimo,
Santiago, Seamus, Seumas, Yago,
Yasha.
Jaimes, Jamesie, Jamesy, Jemes

Jameson (English) son of James.
Jamerson, Jamesian, Jaymeson

Jamie (English) a familiar form of
James.
*Jaimey, Jaimie, Jame, Jamee, Jamey,
Jameyel, Jami, Jamian, Jammie,
Jammy, Jaymee, Jaymie*

Jamil (Arabic) a form of Jamal.
*Jamiel, Jamiell, Jamielle, Jamile,
Jamill, Jamille, Jamyl, Jarmil*

Jamin (Hebrew) favored.
Jamian

Jamison (English) son of James.
Jamiesen, Jamieson, Jamisen

Jamon (Hebrew) a form of Jamin.

Jamond (American) a combination of
James + Raymond.

Jamor (American) a form of Jamal.

Jamsheed (Persian) from Persia.

Jan (Dutch, Slavic) a form of John.
Jano, Jenda

Janco (Czech) a form of John.

Jando (Spanish) a form of Alexander.

Janeil (American) a combination of the
prefix Ja + Neil.

Janek (Polish) a form of John.
Janak

Janis (Latvian) a form of John.

Janne (Finnish) a form of John.

János (Hungarian) a form of John.
Jano

Janson (Scandinavian) son of Jan.
Jansen

Jantzen (Scandinavian) a form of Janson.

Janus (Latin) gate, passageway; born in January. Mythology: the Roman god of beginnings and endings.

Japheth (Hebrew) handsome. (Arabic) abundant. Bible: a son of Noah. See also Yaphet.

Jaquan (American) a combination of the prefix Ja + Quan.

Jaquarius (American) a combination of Jaquan + Darius.

Jaquavius (American) a form of Jaquan.

Jaquon (American) a form of Jaquan.

Jarad (Hebrew) a form of Jared.

Jarah (Hebrew) sweet as honey.

Jardan (Hebrew) a form of Jordan.

Jareb (Hebrew) contending.

Jared (Hebrew) a form of Jordan.
Jahred, Jaired, Jareid, Jarid, Jerryd

Jarek (Slavic) born in January.

Jarell (Scandinavian) a form of Gerald.
Jairell, Jareil, Jarel, Jarelle, Jarryl, Jayryl, Jharell

Jaren (Hebrew) a form of Jaron.

Jareth (American) a combination of Jared + Gareth.

Jarett (English) a form of Jarrett.
Jaret

Jarl (Scandinavian) earl, nobleman.

Jarlath (Latin) in control.

Jarman (German) from Germany.

Jarod (Hebrew) a form of Jared.

Jaron (Hebrew) he will sing; he will cry out.
Jaaron, Jairon, Jarone, Jayron, Jayronn, Je Ronn, J'ron

Jaroslav (Czech) glory of spring.

Jarred (Hebrew) a form of Jared.
Ja'red, Jarrad, Jarrayd, Jarrid, Jerrid

Jarrell (English) a form of Gerald.
Jarel, Jarrel

Jarren (Hebrew) a form of Jaron.

Jarrett (English) a form of Garrett, Jared.
Jairett, Jaretté, Jarhett, Jarratt, Jarret, Jarrette, Jarrot, Jarrott

Jarrod (Hebrew) a form of Jared.

Jarryd (Hebrew) a form of Jared.
Jarrayd, Jaryd

Jarvis (German) skilled with a spear.
Jaravis, Jarv, Jarvaris, Jarvas, Jarvaska, Jarvey, Jarvie, Jarvorice, Jarvoris, Jarvous, Jervey

Jaryn (Hebrew) a form of Jaron.

Jas (Polish) a form of John. (English) a familiar form of James.

Jasha (Russian) a familiar form of Jacob, James.

Jashawn (American) a combination of the prefix Ja + Shawn.

Jaskaran (Sikh) sings praises to the Lord.

Jasmin (Persian) jasmine flower.

Jason ☼ (Greek) healer. Mythology: the hero who led the Argonauts in search of the Golden Fleece.
Jaeson, Jahson, Jasan, Jase, Jasen, Jasin, Jasten, Jasun

Jaspal (Punjabi) living a virtuous lifestyle.

Jasper (French) brown, red, or yellow ornamental stone. (English) a form of Casper. See also Kasper.
Jaspar, Jazper, Jespar, Jesper

Jasson (Greek) a form of Jason.

Jatinra (Hindi) great Brahmin sage.

Javan (Hebrew) Bible: son of Japheth.
Jahvaughan, JaVaughn, Javen, Javin, Javine, Javoanta, Javona, Javone, Jayvin, Jayvion

Javante (American) a form of Javan.

Javaris (English) a form of Jarvis.
Javaor, Javar, Javares, Javario, Javarius, Javaro, Javaron, Javarous, Javarre, Javarrious, Javarro, Javarte, Javarus, Javoris, Javouris

Javas (Sanskrit) quick, swift.

Javier (Spanish) owner of a new house. See also Xavier.
Jabier

Javon (Hebrew) a form of Javan.
Jaavon, Javion, Javona, Javone, Javoney, Javoni, Javonn

Javonte (American) a form of Javan.
Javona

Jawaun (American) a form of Jajuan.

Jawhar (Arabic) jewel; essence.

Jaxon (English) a form of Jackson.

Jay (French) blue jay. (English) a short form of James, Jason.
Jae, Jave, Jaye, Jeays, Jeyes

Jayce (American) a combination of the initials J. + C.
JC, J.C., Jaycee, Jay Cee

Jaycob (Hebrew) a form of Jacob.

Jayde (American) a combination of the initials J. + D.

Jayden ☼ (American) a form of Jayde.

Jaylee (American) a combination of Jay + Lee.

Jaylen (American) a combination of Jay + Len.

Jaylin (American) a form of Jaylen.

Jaylon (American) a form of Jaylen.

Jaylyn (American) a form of Jaylen.

Jayme (English) a form of Jamie.
Jaymie

Jaymes (English) a form of James.
Jayms

Jayquan (American) a combination of Jay + Quan.

Jayson (Greek) a form of Jason.
Jaycent, Jaysen, Jaysin, Jayssen, Jaysson

Jayvon (American) a form of Javon.
Jayvion

Jazz (American) jazz.

Jean (French) a form of John.
Jean-Francois, Jean-Michel, Jean-Philippe, Jéan, Jeannah, Jeannie, Jeannot, Jeanot, Jeanty, Jene

Jeb (Hebrew) a short form of Jebediah.

Jebediah (Hebrew) a form of Jedidiah.

Jed (Hebrew) a short form of Jedidiah.
(Arabic) hand.
Jedd, Jeddy, Jedi

Jediah (Hebrew) hand of God.
Jedi

Jedidiah (Hebrew) friend of God, beloved of God. See also Didi.
Jedediah, Jedediha, Jedidia

Jedrek (Polish) strong; manly.

Jeff (English) a short form of Jefferson, Jeffrey. A familiar form of Geoffrey.
Jefe, Jeffe, Jeffey, Jeffie, Jeffy, Jhef

Jefferson (English) son of Jeff. History: Thomas Jefferson was the third U.S. president.
Jeferson, Jeffers

Jeffery (English) a form of Jeffrey.
Jefery, Jeffeory, Jefferay, Jeffereoy, Jefferey, Jefferie, Jeffory

Jefford (English) Jeff's ford.

Jeffrey (English) divinely peaceful. See also Geffrey, Geoffrey, Godfrey.
Jefferies, Jeffree, Jeffrie, Jeffrery, Jeffries, Jefre, Jefry, Jeoffroi, Joffre, Joffrey

Jeffry (English) a form of Jeffrey.

Jehan (French) a form of John.

Jehu (Hebrew) God lives. Bible: a military commander and king of Israel.

Jelani (Swahili) mighty.

Jem (English) a short form of James, Jeremiah.
Jemmy

Jemal (Arabic) a form of Jamal.

Jemel (Arabic) a form of Jemal.
Jemmy

Jemond (French) worldly.

Jenkin (Flemish) little John.
Jenkyn

Jenö (Hungarian) a form of Eugene.

Jens (Danish) a form of John.

Jeovanni (Italian) a form of Giovanni.

Jequan (American) a combination of the prefix Je + Quan.

Jerad, Jerrad (Hebrew) forms of Jared.
Jeread, Jeredd

Jerahmy (Hebrew) a form of Jeremy.

Jerald (English) a form of Gerald.
Jeraldo, Jerold, Jerral, Jerrald, Jerrold

Jerall (English) a form of Jarrell.
Jerrail, Jerral, Jerrel

Jeramie, Jeramy (Hebrew) forms of Jeremy.
Jerame, Jeramee, Jeramey, Jerami, Jerammie

Jerard (French) a form of Gerard.
Jarard, Jarrard, Jerardo, Jeraude, Jerrard

Jere (Hebrew) a short form of Jeremiah, Jeremy.
Jeree

Jered, Jerred (Hebrew) forms of Jared.
Jerryd

Jerel, Jerell, Jerrell (English) forms of Jarell.
Jerelle, Jeril, Jerrail, Jerral, Jerrall, Jerrel, Jerrill, Jerrol, Jerroll, Jerryll, Jeryl

Jereme, Jeremey (Hebrew) forms of Jeremy.
Jarame

Jeremiah ✼ (Hebrew) God will uplift. Bible: a Hebrew prophet. See also Dermot, Yeremey, Yirmaya.
Jaramia, Jemeriah, Jemiah, Jeramiah, Jeramiha, Jereias, Jeremaya, Jeremi, Jeremia, Jeremial, Jeremias, Jeremija, Jerimiah, Jerimiha, Jerimya, Jermija

Jeremie, Jérémie (Hebrew) forms of Jeremy.
Jeremi, Jérémie, Jeremii

Jeremy (English) a form of Jeremiah.
Jaremay, Jaremi, Jaremy, Jemmy, Jereamy, Jeremee, Jeremry, Jérémy, Jeremye, Jereomy, Jeriemy, Jerime, Jerimy, Jerremy

Jeriah (Hebrew) Jehovah has seen.

Jericho (Arabic) city of the moon. Bible: a city conquered by Joshua.

Jermaine (French) a form of Germain. (English) sprout, bud.
Jeremaine, Jeremane, Jerimane, Jermain, Jermane, Jermanie, Jermayn, Jermayne, Jermiane, Jermine, Jer-Mon, Jhirmaine

Jermal (Arabic) a form of Jamal.

Jermey (English) a form of Jeremy.
Jerme, Jermee, Jermere, Jermery, Jermie, Jhermie

Jermiah (Hebrew) a form of Jeremiah.

Jerney (Slavic) a form of Bartholomew.

Jerod, Jerrod (Hebrew) forms of Jarrod.

Jerolin (Basque, Latin) holy.

Jerome (Latin) holy. See also Geronimo, Hieronymos.
Jeroen, Jerom, Jérome, Jérôme, Jeromo, Jerónimo, Jerrome, Jerromy

Jeromy (Latin) a form of Jerome.
Jeromey, Jeromie

Jeron (English) a form of Jerome.
Jéron, Jerone, Jeronimo, Jerron, J'ron

Jerrett (Hebrew) a form of Jarrett.

Jerrick (American) a combination of Jerry + Derrick.

Jerry (German) mighty spearman. (English) a familiar form of Gerald, Gerard. See also Gerry, Kele.
Jebri, Jeree, Jeris, Jerison, Jerri, Jerrie

Jervis (English) a form of Gervaise, Jarvis.

Jerzy (Polish) a form of George.

Jeshua (Hebrew) a form of Joshua.

Jess (Hebrew) a short form of Jesse.

Jesse ☝ (Hebrew) wealthy. Bible: the father of David. See also Yishai.
Jesee, Jesi, Jessé, Jessee

Jessie (Hebrew) a form of Jesse.
Jesie, Jessi

Jessy (Hebrew) a form of Jesse.
Jescey, Jessey

Jestin (Welsh) a form of Justin.

Jesus ☝ (Hebrew) a form of Joshua. Bible: son of Mary and Joseph, believed by Christians to be the Son of God. See also Chucho, Isa, Yosu.
Jecho, Josu

Jesús (Hispanic) a form of Jesus.

Jethro (Hebrew) abundant. Bible: the father-in-law of Moses. See also Yitro.

Jett (English) hard, black mineral. (Hebrew) a short form of Jethro.

Jevan (Hebrew) a form of Javan.

Jevon (Hebrew) a form of Javan.

Jevonte (American) a form of Jevon.

Jibade (Yoruba) born close to royalty.

Jibben (Gypsy) life.

Jibril (Arabic) archangel of Allah.

Jilt (Dutch) money.

Jim (Hebrew, English) a short form of James. See also Jaap.

Jimbo (American) a familiar form of Jim.

Jimell (Arabic) a form of Jamel.

Jimiyu (Abaluhya) born in the dry season.

Jimmie (English) a form of Jimmy.
Jimi, Jimmee

Jimmy (English) a familiar form of Jim.
Jimmey, Jimmyjo, Jimy

Jimoh (Swahili) born on Friday.

Jin (Chinese) gold.

Jindra (Czech) a form of Harold.

Jing-Quo (Chinese) ruler of the country.

Jiovanni (Italian) a form of Giovanni.

Jirair (Armenian) strong; hard working.

Jiri (Czech) a form of George.

Jiro (Japanese) second son.

Jivin (Hindi) life giver.

Jo (Hebrew, Japanese) a form of Joe.

Joab (Hebrew) God is father. See also Yoav.

Joachim (Hebrew) God will establish. See also Akeem, Ioakim, Yehoyakem.
Joakim, Jov

João (Portuguese) a form of John.

Joaquim (Portuguese) a form of Joachim.

Joaquín (Spanish) a form of Joachim, Yehoyakem.
Jehoichin, Joaquin, Jocquin, Jocquinn

Job (Hebrew) afflicted. Bible: a righteous man whose faith in God survived the test of many afflictions.

Joben (Japanese) enjoys cleanliness.

Jobo (Spanish) a familiar form of Joseph.

Joby (Hebrew) a familiar form of Job.

Jock (American) a familiar form of Jacob.
Jocko, Jocoby, Jocolby

Jocquez (French) a form of Jacquez.

Jodan (Hebrew) a combination of Jo + Dan.

Jody (Hebrew) a familiar form of Joseph.
Jodey, Jodi, Jodie, Jodiha, Joedy

Joe (Hebrew) a short form of Joseph.
Joely

Joel (Hebrew) God is willing. Bible: an Old Testament Hebrew prophet.
Jôel, Joël, Joell, Joelle, Joely, Jole

Joeseph (Hebrew) a form of Joseph.

Joey (Hebrew) a familiar form of Joe, Joseph.

Johan, Johann (German) forms of John. See also Anno, Hanno, Yoan, Yohan.

Johannes (German) a form of Johan, Johann.

John ✡ (Hebrew) God is gracious. Bible: the name honoring John the Baptist and John the Evangelist. See also Elchanan, Evan, Geno, Gian, Giovanni, Handel, Hannes, Hans, Hanus, Honza, Ian, Ianos, Iban, Ioan, Ivan, Iwan, Keoni, Kwam, Ohannes, Sean, Ugutz, Yan, Yanka, Yanni, Yochanan, Yohance, Zane.
Jacsi, Jaenda, Jahn, Janak, Jansen, Jantje, Jen, Jenkyn, Jhan, Jhanick,
Jhon, Jian, Joáo, Joen, Johne, Johnl, Johnlee, Jonam, Jone, Jonté

Johnathan (Hebrew) a form of Jonathan.
Jhonathan, Johathe, Johnatan, Johnathaon, Johnathen, Johnatten, Johniathin, Johnothan, Johnthan

Johnathon (Hebrew) a form of Jonathon. See also Yanton.

Johnnie (Hebrew) a familiar form of John.
Johnie, Johnier, Johnni, Johnsie, Jonni, Jonnie

Johnny (Hebrew) a familiar form of John. See also Gianni.
Jantje, Jhonny, Johney, Johmney, Johny

Johnson (English) son of John.
Johnston, Jonson

Joji (Japanese) a form of George.

Jojo (Fante) born on Monday.

Jokim (Basque) a form of Joachim.

Jolon (Native American) valley of the dead oaks.
Jolyon

Jomar (American) a form of Jamar.

Jomei (Japanese) spreads light.

Jon (Hebrew) a form of John. A short form of Jonathan.
J'on, Joni, Jonn, Jonnie, Jony

Jonah (Hebrew) dove. Bible: an Old Testament prophet who was swallowed by a large fish.
Jona

Jonas (Hebrew) he accomplishes. (Lithuanian) a form of John.

*Jonelis, Jonukas, Jonus, Jonutis,
Joonas*

Jonatan (Hebrew) a form of Jonathan.
*Jonatane, Jonate, Jonattan,
Jonnattan*

Jonathan ☀ (Hebrew) gift of God.
Bible: the son of King Saul who
became a loyal friend of David. See also
Ionakana, Yanton, Yonatan.
*Janathan, Jonatha, Jonathen,
Jonethen, Jonnatha, Jonnathan,
Jonothan*

Jonathon (Hebrew) a form of Jonathan.
*Joanathon, Jonothon, Jounathon,
Yanaton*

Jones (Welsh) son of John.

Jonny (Hebrew) a familiar form of
John.
Joni, Jony

Jontae (French) a combination of Jon
+ the suffix Tae.

Jontay (American) a form of Jontae.
Jonté

Joop (Dutch) a familiar form of Joseph.
Jopie

Joost (Dutch) just.

Joquin (Spanish) a form of Joaquín.

Jora (Hebrew) teacher.

Joram (Hebrew) Jehovah is exalted.

Jordan ☀ (Hebrew) descending. See
also Giordano, Yarden.
*Jordaan, Jordae, Jordain, Jordaine,
Jordany, Jordão, Jordin, Jorrdan*

Jorden (Hebrew) a form of Jordan.
Jordenn

Jordon (Hebrew) a form of Jordan.
Jeordon, Johordan

Jordy (Hebrew) a familiar form of
Jordan.
Jordi, Jordie

Jordyn (Hebrew) a form of Jordan.

Jorell (American) he saves. Literature: a
name inspired by the fictional character Jor-El, Superman's father.

Jörg (German) a form of George.

Jorge (Spanish) a form of George.

Jorgen (Danish) a form of George.

Joris (Dutch) a form of George.

Jörn (German) a familiar form of
Gregory.

Jorrín (Spanish) a form of George.

Jory (Hebrew) a familiar form of
Jordan.
Joar, Joary, Jori, Jorie

José ☀ (Spanish) a form of Joseph.
See also Ché, Pepe.
*Josean, Josecito, Josee, Joseito, Joselito,
Josey*

Josef (German, Portuguese, Czech,
Scandinavian) a form of Joseph.
Joosef, Joseff, Josif, Jozef, József, Juzef

Joseluis (Spanish) a combination of
Jose + Luis.

Joseph ☼ (Hebrew) God will add, God
will increase. Bible: in the Old
Testament, the son of Jacob who came
to rule Egypt; in the New Testament,
the husband of Mary. See also Beppe,
Cheche, Chepe, Giuseppe, Iokepa, Iosif,
Osip, Pepa, Peppe, Pino, Sepp, Yeska,
Yosef, Yousef, Youssel, Yusif, Yusuf,
Zeusef.
*Jazeps, Joos, Jooseppi, Jopie, Joseba,
Josep, Josephat, Josephe, Josephie,
Josephus, Josheph, Josip, Jóska, Joza,
Joze, Jozef, Jozhe, Jozio, Jozka, Jozsi,
Jozzepi, Juziu*

Josh (Hebrew) a short form of Joshua.
Joshe

Josha (Hindi) satisfied.

Joshi (Swahili) galloping.

Joshua ☼ (Hebrew) God is my salva-
tion. Bible: led the Israelites into the
Promised Land. See also Giosia, Iosua,
Jesus, Yehoshua.
*Johsua, Johusa, Joshau, Joshaua,
Joshauh, Joshawa, Joshawah, Joshia,
Joshu, Joshuaa, Joshuah, Joshuea,
Joshula, Joshus, Joshusa, Joshuwa,
Joshwa, Jousha, Jozshua, Jozsua,
Jozua, Jushua*

Josiah (Hebrew) fire of the Lord. See
also Yoshiyahu.
*Joshiah, Josia, Josiahs, Josian, Josias,
Josie*

Joss (Chinese) luck; fate.

Josue (Hebrew) a form of Joshua.
Joshue, Josu, Josua, Josuha, Jozus

Jotham (Hebrew) may God complete.
Bible: a king of Judah.

Jourdan (Hebrew) a form of Jordan.
Jourdain

Jovan (Latin) Jove-like, majestic.
(Slavic) a form of John. Mythology:
Jove, also known as Jupiter, was the
supreme Roman deity.
*Jovaan, Jovanic, Jovann, Jovannis,
Jovenal, Jovenel, Jovi, Jovian, Jovin,
Jovito, Jovoan, Jovon, Jovonn,
Jovonne, Yovan*

Jovani, Jovanni (Latin) forms of
Jovan.
Jovannie

Jovanny, Jovany (Latin) forms of
Jovan.

Jr (Latin) a short form of Junior.
Jr.

Juan ☼ (Spanish) a form of John. See
also Chan.
*Juanch, Juanchito, Juanito, Juann,
Juaun*

Juancarlos (Spanish) a combination
of Juan + Carlos.

Juaquin (Spanish) a form of Joaquín.

Jubal (Hebrew) ram's horn. Bible: a
musician and a descendant of Cain.

Judah (Hebrew) praised. Bible: the
fourth of Jacob's sons. See also Yehudi.

Judas (Latin) a form of Judah. Bible:
Judas Iscariot was the disciple who
betrayed Jesus.

Judd (Hebrew) a short form of Judah.
Jud

Jude (Latin) a short form of Judah,
Judas. Bible: one of the Twelve Apostles,
author of "The Epistle of Jude."

Judson (English) son of Judd.

Juhana (Finnish) a form of John.

Juku (Estonian) a form of Richard.

Jules (French) a form of Julius.
Jule

Julian ♀ (Greek, Latin) a form of
Julius.
*Jolyon, Juliaan, Juliano, Jullian,
Julyan*

Julien (Latin) a form of Julian.

Julio (Hispanic) a form of Julius.

Julius (Greek, Latin) youthful, downy
bearded. History: Julius Caesar was a
great Roman dictator. See also
Giuliano.
*Jolyon, Julas, Jule, Julen, Julias, Julie,
Juliusz*

Jumaane (Swahili) born on Tuesday.

Jumah (Arabic, Swahili) born on Friday,
a holy day in the Islamic religion.

Jumoke (Yoruba) loved by everyone.

Jun (Chinese) truthful. (Japanese) obedient; pure.

Junior (Latin) young.
Junious, Junius

Jupp (German) a form of Joseph.

Jur (Czech) a form of George.

Jurgis (Lithuanian) a form of George.

Juro (Japanese) best wishes; long life.

Jurrien (Dutch) God will uplift.

Justen (Latin) a form of Justin.
Jasten

Justice (Latin) a form of Justis.

Justin ♀ (Latin) just, righteous. See
also Giustino, Iestyn, Iustin, Tutu,
Ustin, Yustyn.
*Jobst, Jost, Jusa, Just, Justain, Justan,
Justas, Justek, Justinas, Justine,
Justinian, Justinius, Justinn, Justino,
Justins, Justinus, Justo, Juston,
Justton, Justun*

Justis (French) just.

Justyn (Latin) a form of Justin.
Justn

Juvenal (Latin) young. Literature: a
Roman satirist.

Juwan (American) a form of Jajuan.

K

Kabiito (Rutooro) born while foreigners
are visiting.

Kabil (Turkish) a form of Cain.

Kabir (Hindi) History: an Indian mystic
poet.

Kabonero (Runyankore) sign.

Kabonesa (Rutooro) difficult birth.

Kacey (Irish) a form of Casey.
(American) a combination of the
initials K. + C. See also KC.
*Kace, Kacee, Kacy, Kaesy, Kase, Kasie,
Kasy, Kaycee*

Kadar (Arabic) powerful.

Kadarius (American) a combination of
Kade + Darius.

Kade (Scottish) wetlands. (American) a combination of the initials K. + D. *Kadee, Kaydee*

Kadeem (Arabic) servant.

Kaden (Arabic) a form of Kadin.

Kadin (Arabic) friend, companion.

Kadir (Arabic) spring greening.

Kado (Japanese) gateway.

Kaeden (Arabic) a form of Kadin.

Kaelan, Kaelin (Irish) forms of Kellen.

Kaeleb (Hebrew) a form of Kaleb.

Kaemon (Japanese) joyful; right-handed.

Kaenan (Irish) a form of Keenan.

Ka'eo (Hawaiian) victorious.

Kafele (Nguni) worth dying for.

Kaga (Native American) writer.

Kagan (Irish) a form of Keegan.

Kahale (Hawaiian) home.

Kahil (Turkish) young; inexperienced; naive.

Kahlil (Arabic) a form of Khalíl.

Kaholo (Hawaiian) runner.

Kahraman (Turkish) hero.

Kai (Welsh) keeper of the keys. (German) a form of Kay. (Hawaiian) sea.

Kaikara (Runyoro) Religion: a Banyoro deity.

Kailen (Irish) a form of Kellen.

Kaili (Hawaiian) Religion: a Hawaiian god.

Kain (Welsh, Irish) a form of Kane. *Kainan, Kaine, Kainen*

Kainoa (Hawaiian) name.

Kaipo (Hawaiian) sweetheart.

Kairo (Arabic) a form of Cairo.

Kaiser (German) a form of Caesar.

Kaiven (American) a form of Kevin.

Kaj (Danish) earth.

Kakar (Hindi) grass.

Kala (Hindi) black; phase. (Hawaiian) sun.

Kalama (Hawaiian) torch.

Kalan (Irish) a form of Kalen.

Kalani (Hawaiian) sky; chief.

Kale (Arabic) a short form of Kahlil. (Hawaiian) a familiar form of Carl. *Kalee, Kaleu, Kaley*

Kaleb (Hebrew) a form of Caleb. *Kal, Kalab, Kalb, Kalev, Kalib, Kïlab*

Kalen, Kalin (Arabic, Hawaiian) forms of Kale. (Irish) forms of Kellen.

Kalevi (Finnish) hero.

Kali (Arabic) a short form of Kalil. (Hawaiian) a form of Gary.

Kalil (Arabic) a form of Khalíl. *Kaleel*

Kaliq (Arabic) a form of Khaliq.

Kalkin (Hindi) tenth. Religion: Kalki is the final incarnation of the Hindu god Vishnu.

Kalle (Scandinavian) a form of Carl. (Arabic, Hawaiian) a form of Kale.

Kallen (Irish) a form of Kellen.

Kalon, Kalyn (Irish) forms of Kellen.

Kaloosh (Armenian) blessed event.

Kalvin (Latin) a form of Calvin.
Kal, Kalv

Kamaka (Hawaiian) face.

Kamakani (Hawaiian) wind.

Kamal (Hindi) lotus. (Arabic) perfect, perfection.

Kamau (Kikuyu) quiet warrior.

Kamden (Scottish) a form of Camden.

Kameron (Scottish) a form of Cameron.
Kam, Kamey, Kammy

Kami (Hindi) loving.

Kamil (Arabic) a form of Kamal.

Kamran, Kamron (Scottish) forms of Kameron.
Kamren

Kamuela (Hawaiian) a form of Samuel.

Kamuhanda (Runyankore) born on the way to the hospital.

Kamukama (Runyankore) protected by God.

Kamuzu (Nguni) medicine.

Kamya (Luganda) born after twin brothers.

Kana (Japanese) powerful; capable. (Hawaiian) Mythology: a demigod.

Kanaiela (Hawaiian) a form of Daniel.

Kane (Welsh) beautiful. (Irish) tribute. (Japanese) golden. (Hawaiian) eastern sky. (English) a form of Keene. See Kahan, Kain, Kaney, Kayne.

Kange (Lakota) raven.

Kaniel (Hebrew) stalk, reed.

Kannan (Hindi) Religion: another name for the Hindu god Krishna.

Kannon (Polynesian) free. (French) a form of Cannon.

Kanoa (Hawaiian) free.

Kantu (Hindi) happy.

Kanu (Swahili) wildcat.

Kaori (Japanese) strong.

Kapila (Hindi) ancient prophet.

Kapono (Hawaiian) righteous.

Kardal (Arabic) mustard seed.

Kare (Norwegian) enormous.
Karee

Kareem (Arabic) noble; distinguished.
Karee, Karem, Kareme, Karriem

Karel (Czech) a form of Carl.

Karey (Greek) a form of Carey.
Karee, Kari

Karif (Arabic) born in autumn.

Kariisa (Runyankore) herdsman.

Karim (Arabic) a form of Kareem.

Karl (German) a form of Carl.
Kaarle, Kaarlo, Kalman, Kálmán, Karcsi, Kari, Karlitis, Karlo, Karlos, Karlton, Karlus

Karlen (Latvian, Russian) a form of Carl.

Karmel (Hebrew) a form of Carmel.

Karney (Irish) a form of Carney.

Karol (Czech, Polish) a form of Carl.

Karr (Scandinavian) a form of Carr.

Karson (English) a form of Carson.

Karsten (Greek) anointed.

Karu (Hindi) cousin.

Karutunda (Runyankore) little.

Karwana (Rutooro) born during wartime.

Kaseem (Arabic) divided.

Kaseko (Rhodesian) mocked, ridiculed.

Kasem (Tai) happiness.

Kasen (Basque) protected with a helmet.

Kasey (Irish) a form of Casey.
Kaesy

Kashawn (American) a combination of the prefix Ka + Shawn.

Kasib (Arabic) fertile.

Kasim (Arabic) a form of Kaseem.

Kasimir (Arabic) peace. (Slavic) a form of Casimir.

Kasiya (Nguni) separate.

Kasper (Persian) treasurer. (German) a form of Casper.

Kass (German) blackbird.
Kase

Kassidy (Irish) a form of Cassidy.

Kateb (Arabic) writer.

Kato (Runyankore) second of twins.

Katungi (Runyankore) rich.

Kavan (Irish) handsome.

Kaveh (Persian) ancient hero.

Kavi (Hindi) poet.

Kavin, Kavon (Irish) forms of Kavan.

Kawika (Hawaiian) a form of David.

Kay (Greek) rejoicing. (German) fortified place. Literature: one of King Arthur's knights of the Round Table.
Kaycee

Kayden (Arabic) a form of Kadin.
Kaydee

Kayin (Nigerian) celebrated. (Yoruba) long-hoped-for child.

Kayle (Hebrew) faithful dog. (Arabic) a short form of Kahlil.

Kayleb (Hebrew) a form of Caleb.

Kaylen (Irish) a form of Kellen.

Kayne (Hebrew) a form of Cain.

Kayode (Yoruba) he brought joy.

Kayonga (Runyankore) ash.

Kazio (Polish) a form of Casimir, Kasimir. See also Cassidy.

Kazuo (Japanese) man of peace.

KC (American) a combination of the initials K. + C. See also Kacey.

Keagan (Irish) a form of Keegan.
Keagen

Keahi (Hawaiian) flames.

Keaka (Hawaiian) a form of Jack.

Kealoha (Hawaiian) fragrant.

Keanan (Irish) a form of Keenan.
Keanen, Keannan

Keandre (American) a combination of the prefix Ke + Andre.
Keondre

Keane (German) bold; sharp. (Irish) handsome. (English) a form of Keene.

Keanu (Irish) a form of Keenan.

Kearn (Irish) a short form of Kearney.

Kearney (Irish) a form of Carney.

Keary (Irish) a form of Kerry.

Keaton (English) where hawks fly.
Keaten, Keeton, Keetun

Keaven (Irish) a form of Kevin.

Keawe (Hawaiian) strand.

Keb (Egyptian) earth. Mythology: an ancient earth god, also known as Geb.

Kedar (Hindi) mountain lord. (Arabic) powerful. Religion: another name for the Hindu god Shiva.

Keddy (Scottish) a form of Adam.

Kedem (Hebrew) ancient.

Kedrick (English) a form of Cedric.

Keefe (Irish) handsome; loved.

Keegan (Irish) little; fiery.
Kaegan, Keagen

Keelan (Irish) little; slender.

Keeley (Irish) handsome.

Keenan (Irish) little Keene.
Keenon, Keynan, Kienan, Kienon

Keene (German) bold; sharp. (English) smart. See also Kane.

Keenen (Irish) a form of Keenan.
Kienen

Kees (Dutch) a form of Kornelius.

Keevon (Irish) a form of Kevin.
Keevin

Kegan (Irish) a form of Keegan.
Keghan, Kegun

Kehind (Yoruba) second-born twin.

Keiffer (German) a form of Cooper.

Keigan (Irish) a form of Keegan.

Keiji (Japanese) cautious ruler.

Keilan (Irish) a form of Keelan.

Keir (Irish) a short form of Kieran.

Keitaro (Japanese) blessed.

Keith (Welsh) forest. (Scottish) battle place. See also Kika.
Keath, Keeth

Keithen (Welsh, Scottish) a form of Keith.
Keithon

Keivan (Irish) a form of Kevin.

Kekapa (Hawaiian) tapa cloth.

Kekipi (Hawaiian) rebel.

Kekoa (Hawaiian) bold, courageous.

Kelby (German) farm by the spring.

Kele (Hopi) sparrow hawk. (Hawaiian) a form of Jerry.
Kelle

Kelemen (Hungarian) gentle; kind.

Kelevi (Finnish) hero.

Keli (Hawaiian) a form of Terry.

Keli'i (Hawaiian) chief.

Kelile (Ethiopian) protected.

Kell (Scandinavian) spring.

Kellan (Irish) a form of Kellen.
Keillan

Kellen (Irish) mighty warrior.
Kelden, Kelle, Kellin, Kelynn

Keller (Irish) little companion.

Kelly (Irish) warrior.
Kelle, Kelley, Kelli, Kely

Kelmen (Basque) merciful.

Kelsey (Scandinavian) island of ships.
Kelcy, Kelse, Kelsie, Kelsy, Kesley, Kesly

Kelton (English) keel town; port.
Kelden

Kelvin (Irish, English) narrow river. Geography: a river in Scotland.
Kelvan, Kelven, Kelvyn, Kelwin, Kelwyn

Kemal (Turkish) highest honor.

Kemen (Basque) strong.

Kemp (English) fighter; champion.

Kempton (English) military town.

Ken (Japanese) one's own kind. (Scottish) a short form of Kendall, Kendrick, Kenneth.
Kena, Keno

Kenan (Irish) a form of Keenan.

Kenaz (Hebrew) bright.

Kendal (English) a form of Kendall.
Kendale, Kendali, Kendel

Kendall (English) valley of the river Kent.
Kendrall, Kendryll

Kendarius (American) a combination of Ken + Darius.

Kendell (English) a form of Kendall.
Kendrell

Kendrew (Scottish) a form of Andrew.

Kendrick (Irish) son of Henry. (Scottish) royal chieftain.
Kendric, Kendricks, Kendrik, Kendrix, Kendryck, Keondric, Keondrick

Kenley (English) royal meadow.

Kenn (Scottish) a form of Ken.

Kennan (Scottish) little Ken.

Kennard (Irish) brave chieftain.

Kennedy (Irish) helmeted chief. History: John F. Kennedy was the thirty-fifth U.S. president.

Kenneth (Irish) handsome. (English) royal oath.
Keneth, Kennet, Kennethen, Kennett, Kennieth, Kennith, Kennth, Kennyth

Kenny (Scottish) a familiar form of
Kenneth.
Keni, Kenney, Kennie, Kinnie

Kenrick (English) bold ruler; royal
ruler.

Kent (Welsh) white; bright. (English) a
short form of Kenton. Geography: a
region in England.

Kentaro (Japanese) big boy.

Kenton (English) from Kent, England.
Kenten, Kentin, Kentonn

Kentrell (English) king's estate.

Kenward (English) brave; royal
guardian.

Kenya (Hebrew) animal horn.
(Russian) a form of Kenneth.
Geography: a country in east-central
Africa.

Kenyatta (American) a form of Kenya.

Kenyon (Irish) white haired, blond.

Kenzie (Scottish) wise leader. See also
Mackenzie.

Keoki (Hawaiian) a form of George.

Keola (Hawaiian) life.

Keon (Irish) a form of Ewan.
*Keeon, Keion, Keionne, Keondre,
Keone, Keony, Kian*

Keoni (Hawaiian) a form of John.

Keonte (American) a form of Keon.
Keontae, Keontrye

Kerbasi (Basque) warrior.

Kerel (Afrikaans) young.

Kerem (Turkish) noble; kind.

Kerey (Gypsy) homeward bound.

Kerman (Basque) from Germany.

Kermit (Irish) a form of Dermot.

Kern (Irish) a short form of Kieran.

Kerr (Scandinavian) a form of Carr.

Kerrick (English) king's rule.

Kerry (Irish) dark; dark haired.
Keri, Kerrey, Kerri, Kerrie

Kers (Todas) Botany: an Indian plant.

Kersen (Indonesian) cherry.

Kerstan (Dutch) a form of Christian.

Kerwin (Irish) little; dark. (English)
friend of the marshlands.

Kesar (Russian) a form of Caesar.

Keshawn (American) a combination of
the prefix Ke + Shawn.

Kesin (Hindi) long-haired beggar.

Kesse (Ashanti, Fante) chubby baby.

Kester (English) a form of Christopher.

Kestrel (English) falcon.

Keung (Chinese) universe.

Kevan (Irish) a form of Kevin.

Keven (Irish) a form of Kevin.
Keve

Kevin ☙ (Irish) handsome. See also
Cavan.
*Kev, Keverne, Kévin, Kevinn, Kevins,
Kevis, Kevn, Kevvy*

Kevon (Irish) a form of Kevin.
Keveon, Kevion, Kevron

Kevyn (Irish) a form of Kevin.

Key (English) key; protected.

Keyon (Irish) a form of Keon.

Keyshawn (American) a combination
of Key + Shawn.

Khachig (Armenian) small cross.

Khaim (Russian) a form of Chaim.

Khaldun (Arabic) forever.

Khalfani (Swahili) born to lead.

Khälid (Arabic) eternal.
Khaled, Khalid

Khalíl (Arabic) friend.
*Kaleel, Khalee, Khali, Khalial, Khalil,
Khaliyl*

Khaliq (Arabic) creative.

Khamisi (Swahili) born on Thursday.

Khan (Turkish) prince.

Kharald (Russian) a form of Gerald.

Khayru (Arabic) benevolent.

Khoury (Arabic) priest.

Khristian (Greek) a form of Christian,
Kristian.

Khristopher (Greek) a form of
Kristopher.

Khristos (Greek) a form of Christos.
Kristos

Kibo (Uset) worldly; wise.

Kibuuka (Luganda) brave warrior.
History: a Ganda warrior deity.

Kidd (English) child; young goat.

Kiefer (German) a form of Keifer.

Kiel (Irish) a form of Kyle.

Kiele (Hawaiian) gardenia.

Kieran (Irish) little and dark; little Keir.
Keiran, Keiren, Keiron, Kieron

Kiernan (Irish) a form of Kieran.
Kernan

Kiet (Tai) honor.

Kifeda (Luo) only boy among girls.

Kiho (Rutooro) born on a foggy day.

Kijika (Native American) quiet walker.

Kika (Hawaiian) a form of Keith.

Kiki (Spanish) a form of Henry.

Kile (Irish) a form of Kyle.
Kilen, Kiley

Killian (Irish) little Kelly.

Kim (English) a short form of Kimball.
Kimie, Kimmy

Kimball (Greek) hollow vessel.
(English) warrior chief.

Kimo (Hawaiian) a form of James.

Kimokeo (Hawaiian) a form of
Timothy.

Kin (Japanese) golden.

Kincaid (Scottish) battle chief.

Kindin (Basque) fifth.

King (English) king. A short form of names beginning with "King."

Kingsley (English) king's meadow.

Kingston (English) king's estate.

Kingswell (English) king's well.

Kini (Hawaiian) a short form of Iukini.

Kinnard (Irish) tall slope.

Kinsey (English) victorious royalty.

Kinton (Hindi) crowned.

Kion (Irish) a form of Keon.

Kioshi (Japanese) quiet.

Kipp (English) pointed hill.

Kir (Bulgarian) a familiar form of Cyrus.

Kiral (Turkish) king; supreme leader.

Kiran (Sanskrit) beam of light.

Kirby (Scandinavian) church village. (English) cottage by the water.
Kerbey, Kerbie, Kerby, Kirbey, Kirbie, Kirkby

Kiri (Cambodian) mountain.

Kiril (Slavic) a form of Cyril.

Kiritan (Hindi) wearing a crown.

Kirk (Scandinavian) church.
Kerk

Kirkland (English) church land.

Kirkley (English) church meadow.

Kirklin (English) a form of Kirkland.

Kirkwell (English) church well; church spring.

Kirkwood (English) church forest.

Kirton (English) church town.

Kishan (American) a form of Keshawn.

Kistna (Hindi) sacred, holy. Geography: a sacred river in India.

Kistur (Gypsy) skillful rider.

Kit (Greek) a familiar form of Christian, Christopher, Kristopher.

Kito (Swahili) jewel; precious child.

Kitwana (Swahili) pledged to live.

Kiva (Hebrew) a short form of Akiva, Jacob.

Kiyoshi (Japanese) quiet; peaceful.

Kizza (Luganda) born after twins.

Kjell (Swedish) a form of Karl.

Klaus (German) a short form of Nicholas. A form of Claus.

Klay (English) a form of Clay.

Klayton (English) a form of Clayton.

Kleef (Dutch) cliff.

Klement (Czech) a form of Clement.

Kleng (Norwegian) claw.

Knight (English) armored knight.

Knoton (Native American) a form of Nodin.

Knowles (English) grassy slope.

Knox (English) hill.

Knute (Scandinavian) a form of Canute.

Koby (Polish) a familiar form of Jacob.

Kodi (English) a form of Kody.
Kodie

Kody (English) a form of Cody.
Kodey, Koty

Kofi (Twi) born on Friday.

Kohana (Lakota) swift.

Koi (Choctaw) panther. (Hawaiian) a
form of Troy.

Kojo (Akan) born on Monday.

Koka (Hawaiian) Scotsman.

Kokayi (Shona) gathered together.

Kolby (English) a form of Colby.
Kollby

Kole (English) a form of Cole.

Koleman (English) a form of Coleman.

Kolin (English) a form of Colin.

Kolton (English) a form of Colton.

Kolya (Russian) a familiar form of
Nikolai, Nikolos.

Kona (Hawaiian) a form of Don.

Konane (Hawaiian) bright moonlight.

Kondo (Swahili) war.

Kong (Chinese) glorious; sky.

Konner (Irish) a form of Conner, Connor.

Konnor (Irish) a form of Connor.

Kono (Moquelumnan) squirrel eating a
pine nut.

Konrad (German) a form of Conrad.
*Khonrad, Koen, Koenraad, Kon,
Konn, Konney, Konni, Konnie,*

*Konny, Konrád, Konrade, Konrado,
Kord, Kunz*

Konstantin (German, Russian) a form
of Constantine. See also Dinos.

Kontar (Akan) only child.

Korb (German) basket.

Korbin (English) a form of Corbin.

Kordell (English) a form of Cordell.

Korey (Irish) a form of Corey, Kory.
Kore, Korio, Korria, Korrye

Kornel (Latin) a form of Cornelius,
Kornelius.

Kornelius (Latin) a form of Cornelius.
See also Kees, Kornel.

Korrigan (Irish) a form of Corrigan.

Kort (German, Dutch) a form of Cort,
Kurt.

Kortney (English) a form of Courtney.

Korudon (Greek) helmeted one.

Kory (Irish) a form of Corey.
Kori, Korie, Korrey, Korrie, Korry

Kosey (African) lion.

Kosmo (Greek) a form of Cosmo.

Kostas (Greek) a short form of
Konstantin.

Kosti (Finnish) a form of Gustave.

Kosumi (Moquelumnan) spear fisher.

Koukalaka (Hawaiian) a form of
Douglas.

Kourtland (English) a form of
Courtland.

Kovit (Tai) expert.

Kraig (Irish, Scottish) a form of Craig.
Kraggie, Kraggy

Krikor (Armenian) a form of Gregory.

Kris (Greek) a form of Chris. A short
form of Kristian, Kristofer, Kristopher.
Kriss, Krys

Krischan (German) a form of
Christian.

Krishna (Hindi) delightful, pleasurable.
Religion: the eighth and principal
avatar of the Hindu god Vishnu.

Krispin (Latin) a form of Crispin.

Krister (Swedish) a form of Christian.
Krist, Kristar

Kristian (Greek) a form of Christian,
Khristian.
*Krist, Kristar, Kristek, Kristjan, Kristos,
Krists, Krystek, Khrystiyan*

Kristo (Greek) a short form of Khristos.

Kristofer (Swedish) a form of
Kristopher.
Kristef, Kristoffer, Kristofor, Kristus

Kristoff (Greek) a short form of
Kristofer, Kristopher.
Kristóf

Kristophe (French) a form of
Kristopher.

Kristopher (Greek) a form of
Christopher. See also Topher.
*Kristfer, Kristfor, Kristoforo, Kristoph,
Kristophor, Kristos, Krists, Krzysztof*

Kruz (Spanish) a form of Cruz.

Krystian (Polish) a form of Christian.
Krys, Krystek

Kuba (Czech) a form of Jacob.

Kueng (Chinese) universe.

Kugonza (Rutooro) love.

Kuiril (Basque) lord.

Kumar (Sanskrit) prince.

Kunle (Yoruba) home filled with hon-
ors.

Kuper (Yiddish) copper.

Kurt (Latin, German, French) a short
form of Kurtis. A form of Curt.
Kuno

Kurtis (Latin, French) a form of Curtis.
Kurtice, Kurtiss

Kuruk (Pawnee) bear.

Kuzih (Carrier) good speaker.

Kwabena (Akan) born on Tuesday.

Kwacha (Nguni) morning.

Kwako (Akan) born on Wednesday.

Kwam (Zuni) a form of John.

Kwame (Akan) born on Saturday.

Kwan (Korean) strong.

Kwasi (Akan) born on Sunday.
(Swahili) wealthy.

Kwayera (Nguni) dawn.

Kwende (Nguni) let's go.

Kyele (Irish) a form of Kyle.

Kylan (Irish) a form of Kyle.
Kylen

Kyle ☀ (Irish) narrow piece of land; place where cattle graze. (Yiddish) crowned with laurels.
Kílan, Kílen, Kíley, Ky, Kye, Kylie, Kyrell

Kyler (English) a form of Kyle.

Kynan (Welsh) chief.

Kyndall (English) a form of Kendall.

Kyne (English) royal.

Kyran (Sanskrit) a form of Kiran.

Kyros (Greek) master.

Kyven (American) a form of Kevin.

Laban (Hawaiian) white.

Labaron (American) a combination of the prefix La + Baron.

Labib (Arabic) sensible; intelligent.

Labrentsis (Russian) a form of Lawrence.

Lachlan (Scottish) land of lakes.

Ladarian (American) a combination of the prefix La + Darian.

Ladarius (American) a combination of the prefix La + Darius.

Ladarrius (American) a form of Ladarius.

Ladd (English) attendant.

Laderrick (American) a combination of the prefix La + Derrick.

Ladislav (Czech) a form of Walter.

Lado (Fante) second-born son.

Lafayette (French) History: Marquis de Lafayette was a French soldier and politician who aided the American Revolution.

Laine (English) a form of Lane.

Laird (Scottish) wealthy landowner.

Lais (Arabic) lion.

Lajos (Hungarian) famous; holy.

Lake (English) lake.

Lakota (Dakota) a tribal name.

Lal (Hindi) beloved.

Lamar (German) famous throughout the land. (French) sea, ocean.
Lamair, Lamario, Lamaris, Lamarr, Lamarre, Larmar

Lambert (German) bright land.

Lamond (French) world.

Lamont (Scandinavian) lawyer.
Lamaunt, Lamonte, Lamontie, Lemont

Lance (German) a short form of Lancelot.
Lancy, Lantz, Launce

Lancelot (French) attendant. Literature: the knight who loved King Arthur's wife, Queen Guinevere.

Landen (English) a form of Landon.

Lander (Basque) lion man. (English) landowner.

Lando (Portuguese, Spanish) a short
form of Orlando, Rolando.

Landon ☝ (English) open, grassy
meadow.
Landan, Landin

Landry (French, English) ruler.

Lane (English) narrow road.
Laney, Lanie

Lang (Scandinavian) tall man.

Langdon (English) long hill.

Langford (English) long ford.

Langley (English) long meadow.

Langston (English) long, narrow town.

Langundo (Native American) peaceful.

Lani (Hawaiian) heaven.

Lanny (American) a familiar form of
Lawrence, Laurence.
Lannie, Lennie

Lanu (Moquelumnan) running around
the pole.

Lanz (Italian) a form of Lance.

Lao (Spanish) a short form of
Stanislaus.

Lap (Vietnamese) independent.

Lapidos (Hebrew) torches.

Laquan (American) a combination of
the prefix La + Quan.

Laquintin (American) a combination of
the prefix La + Quintin.

Laramie (French) tears of love.
Geography: a town in Wyoming on the
Overland Trail.

Larenzo (Italian, Spanish) a form of
Lorenzo.
Larinzo

Larkin (Irish) rough; fierce.

Larnell (American) a combination of
Larry + Darnell.

Laron (French) thief.
*Laran, La'ron, La Ron, Laronn, La
Ruan*

Larrimore (French) armorer.

Larry (Latin) a familiar form of
Lawrence.
Larrie, Lary

Lars (Scandinavian) a form of
Lawrence.
*Laris, Larris, Larse, Larsen, Larson,
Larsson, Laurans, Laurits, Lavrans,
Lorens*

LaSalle (French) hall.

Lash (Gypsy) a form of Louis.
Lashi, Lasho

Lashawn (American) a combination of
the prefix La + Shawn.

Lashon (American) a form of Lashawn.

Lasse (Finnish) a form of Nicholas.

László (Hungarian) famous ruler.

Lateef (Arabic) gentle; pleasant.

Latham (Scandinavian) barn. (English)
district.

Lathan (American) a combination of
the prefix La + Nathan.

Lathrop (English) barn, farmstead.

Latimer (English) interpreter.

Latravis (American) a combination of the prefix La + Travis.

Latrell (American) a combination of the prefix La + Kentrell.

Laudalino (Portuguese) praised.

Laughlin (Irish) servant of Saint Secundinus.
Lanty

Laurence (Latin) crowned with laurel. A form of Lawrence. See also Rance, Raulas, Raulo, Renzo.
Lauran, Laurance, Laureano, Lauren, Laurencho, Laurentij, Laurentios, Laurentiu, Laurentius, Laurentzi, Laurin, Laurits, Lauritz, Laurnet, Laurus, Lurance

Laurencio (Spanish) a form of Laurence.

Laurens (Dutch) a form of Laurence.
Laurenz

Laurent (French) a form of Laurence.

Laurie (English) a familiar form of Laurence.

Lauris (Swedish) a form of Laurence.

Lauro (Filipino) a form of Laurence.

LaValle (French) valley.

Lavan (Hebrew) white.

Lavaughan (American) a form of Lavan.

Lave (Italian) lava. (English) lord.

Lavell (French) a form of LaValle.

Lavi (Hebrew) lion.

Lavon (American) a form of Lavan.

Lavrenti (Russian) a form of Lawrence.

Lawerence (Latin) a form of Lawrence.
Lawerance

Lawford (English) ford on the hill.
Law

Lawler (Irish) soft-spoken.

Lawrence (Latin) crowned with laurel. See also Brencis, Chencho.
Laiurenty, Lanty, Larance, Laren, Larian, Larien, Laris, Larka, Larrance, Larrence, Larya, Law, Lawrance, Lawren, Lawrey, Lawrie, Lawron, Lawry, Loreca, Lourenco, Lowrance

Lawson (English) son of Lawrence.

Lawton (English) town on the hill.
Law

Layne (English) a form of Lane.

Layton (English) a form of Leighton.

Lazaro (Italian) a form of Lazarus.
Lazarillo, Lazarito, Lazzaro

Lazarus (Greek) a form of Eleazar. Bible: Lazarus was raised from the dead by Jesus.

Leander (Greek) lion-man; brave as a lion.
Ander

Leandro (Spanish) a form of Leander.

Leben (Yiddish) life.

Lebna (Ethiopian) spirit; heart.

Ledarius (American) a combination of the prefix Le + Darius.

Lee (English) a short form of Farley, Leonard, and names containing "lee."

Leggett (French) one who is sent; delegate.

Lei (Chinese) thunder. (Hawaiian) a form of Ray.

Leib (Yiddish) roaring lion.
Leibel

Leif (Scandinavian) beloved.
Laif, Lief

Leigh (English) a form of Lee.

Leighton (English) meadow farm.

Leith (Scottish) broad river.

Lek (Tai) small.

Lekeke (Hawaiian) powerful ruler.

Leks (Estonian) a familiar form of Alexander.

Lel (Gypsy) taker.

Leland (English) meadowland; protected land.
Lealand, Leeland, Leighland, Lelan, Lelann, Leyland

Lemar (French) a form of Lamar.

Lemuel (Hebrew) devoted to God.

Len (Hopi) flute. (German) a short form of Leonard.

Lenard (German) a form of Leonard.
Lennard

Lencho (Spanish) a form of Lawrence.

Lennart (Swedish) a form of Leonard.

Lenno (Native American) man.

Lennon (Irish) small cloak; cape.

Lennor (Gypsy) spring; summer.

Lennox (Scottish) with many elms.

Lenny (German) a familiar form of Leonard.
Lennie

Leo (Latin) lion. (German) a short form of Leon, Leopold.
Leão, Leibel, Léo, Léocadie, Leos, Leosko, Leosoko, Lion, Liutas, Lyon, Nardek

Leobardo (Italian) a form of Leonard.

Leon (Greek, German) a short form of Leonard, Napoleon.
Léon, Leonas, Léonce, Leoncio, Leondris, Leone, Leonek, Leonetti, Leonirez, Leonizio, Leonon, Leons, Leontes, Leontios, Leontrae, Liutas

Leonard (German) brave as a lion.
Leanard, Lena, Leno, Léonard, Leonardis, Leontes, Lynnard

Leonardo (Italian) a form of Leonard.
Leonaldo

Leonel (English) little lion. See also Lionel.

Leonhard (German) a form of Leonard.

Leonid (Russian) a form of Leonard.

Leonidas (Greek) a form of Leonard.

Leopold (German) brave people.

Leopoldo (Italian) a form of Leopold.

Leor (Hebrew) my light.

Lequinton (American) a combination of the prefix Le + Quinton.

Leron (French) round, circle. (American) a combination of the prefix Le + Ron.

Leroy (French) king. See also Delroy, Elroy.
Leeroy, Lerai, Leroi

Les (Scottish, English) a short form of Leslie, Lester.

Lesharo (Pawnee) chief.

Leshawn (American) a combination of the prefix Le + Shawn.

Leslie (Scottish) gray fortress.
Leslea, Leslee, Lesley, Lesly, Lezlie, Lezly

Lester (Latin) chosen camp. (English) from Leicester, England.
Leicester

Lev (Hebrew) heart. (Russian) a form of Leo. A short form of Leverett, Levi.

Leverett (French) young hare.

Levi (Hebrew) joined in harmony. Bible: the third son of Jacob; Levites are the priestly tribe of the Israelites.
Leavi, Leevi, Levey, Levie, Levitis, Levy, Lewi

Levin (Hebrew) a form of Levi.

Levon (American) a form of Lavon.

Lew (English) a short form of Lewis.

Lewin (English) beloved friend.

Lewis (Welsh) a form of Llewellyn. (English) a form of Louis.
Lewes, Lewie, Lewy

Lex (English) a short form of Alexander.

Lexus (Greek) a short form of Alexander.

Leyati (Moquelumnan) shape of an abalone shell.

Lí (Chinese) strong.

Liam (Irish) a form of William.

Liang (Chinese) good, excellent.

Liban (Hawaiian) a form of Laban.

Liberio (Portuguese) liberation.

Lidio (Greek, Portuguese) ancient.

Ligongo (Yao) who is this?

Likeke (Hawaiian) a form of Richard.

Liko (Chinese) protected by Buddha. (Hawaiian) bud.

Lin (Burmese) bright. (English) a short form of Lyndon.
Lyn

Linc (English) a short form of Lincoln.

Lincoln (English) settlement by the pool. History: Abraham Lincoln was the sixteenth U.S. president.
Lincon

Lindberg (German) mountain where linden grow.

Lindell (English) valley of the linden.

Linden (English) a form of Lyndon.

Lindley (English) linden field.

Lindon (English) a form of Lyndon.

Lindsay (English) a form of Lindsey.
Linsay

Lindsey (English) linden-tree island.
*Lind, Lindsee, Lindsy, Linsey,
Lyndsay, Lyndsey, Lyndsie, Lynzie*

Linford (English) linden ford.

Linfred (German) peaceful, calm.

Linley (English) flax meadow.

Linton (English) flax town.

Linu (Hindi) lily.

Linus (Greek) flaxen haired.

Linwood (English) flax wood.

Lio (Hawaiian) a form of Leo.

Lionel (French) lion cub. See also
Leonel.
*Lional, Lionell, Lionello, Lynel,
Lynell, Lyonel*

Liron (Hebrew) my song.

Lise (Moquelumnan) salmon's head
coming out of the water.

Lisimba (Yao) lion.

Lister (English) dyer.

Litton (English) town on the hill.

Liu (African) voice.

Liuz (Polish) light.

Livingston (English) Leif's town.

Liwanu (Moquelumnan) growling bear.

Llewellyn (Welsh) lionlike.

Lloyd (Welsh) gray haired; holy. See also
Floyd.
Loy, Loyd, Loyde, Loydie

Lobo (Spanish) wolf.

Lochlain (Irish, Scottish) land of lakes.

Locke (English) forest.

Loe (Hawaiian) a form of Roy.

Logan ☥ (Irish) meadow.
Logen

Lok (Chinese) happy.

Lokela (Hawaiian) a form of Roger.

Lokni (Moquelumnan) raining through
the roof.

Lomán (Irish) bare. (Slavic) sensitive.

Lombard (Latin) long bearded.

Lon (Irish) fierce. (Spanish) a short
form of Alonso, Alonzo, Leonard,
Lonnie.

Lonan (Zuni) cloud.

Lonato (Native American) flint stone.

London (English) fortress of the moon.
Geography: the capital of the United
Kingdom.

Long (Chinese) dragon. (Vietnamese)
hair.

Lonnie (German, Spanish) a familiar
form of Alonso, Alonzo.
Lonnell, Lonniel, Lonny

Lono (Hawaiian) Mythology: the god of
learning and intellect.

Lonzo (German, Spanish) a short form
of Alonso, Alonzo.

Lootah (Lakota) red.

Lopaka (Hawaiian) a form of Robert.

Loránd (Hungarian) a form of Roland.

Lóránt (Hungarian) a form of Lawrence.

Lorcan (Irish) little; fierce.

Lord (English) noble title.

Loren (Latin) a short form of Lawrence.
Lorin, Lorren, Lorrin, Loryn

Lorenzo (Italian, Spanish) a form of Lawrence.
Lerenzo, Lorenc, Lorence, Lorenco, Lorencz, Lorens, Lorentz, Lorenz, Lorenza, Lorinc, Lörinc, Lorinzo, Lorrenzo, Lorrie, Zo

Loretto (Italian) a form of Lawrence.

Lorimer (Latin) harness maker.
Lorrie

Loring (German) son of the famous warrior.
Lorrie

Loris (Dutch) clown.

Loritz (Latin, Danish) laurel.
Lauritz

Lorne (Latin) a short form of Lawrence.
Lorn, Lornie

Lorry (English) a form of Laurie.

Lot (Hebrew) hidden, covered. Bible: Lot fled from Sodom, but his wife glanced back upon its destruction and was transformed into a pillar of salt.

Lothar (German) a form of Luther.

Lou (German) a short form of Louis.

Loudon (German) low valley.

Louie (German) a familiar form of Louis.

Louis (German) famous warrior. See also Aloisio, Aloysius, Clovis, Luigi.
Lashi, Lasho, Loudovicus, Lucho, Lude, Ludek, Ludirk, Ludis, Ludko, Lughaidh, Lutek

Lourdes (French) from Lourdes, France. Religion: a place where the Virgin Mary was said to have appeared.

Louvain (English) Lou's vanity. Geography: a city in Belgium.

Lovell (English) a form of Lowell.

Lowell (French) young wolf. (English) beloved.
Lowe, Lowel

Loyal (English) faithful, loyal.
Loy

Lubomir (Polish) lover of peace.

Luboslaw (Polish) lover of glory.

Luc (French) a form of Luke.
Luce

Luca (Italian) a form of Lucius.
Luka

Lucas ♛ (German, Irish, Danish, Dutch) a form of Lucius.
Lucassie, Luckas, Lucus

Lucian (Latin) a form of Lucius.
Lukyan

Luciano (Italian) a form of Lucian.

Lucien (French) a form of Lucius.

Lucio (Italian) a form of Lucius.

Lucius (Latin) light; bringer of light.
Loukas, Luce

Lucky (American) fortunate.

Ludlow (English) prince's hill.

Ludovic (German) a form of Ludwig.

Ludwig (German) a form of Louis. Music: Ludwig van Beethoven was a famous nineteenth-century German composer.

Lui (Hawaiian) a form of Louis.

Luigi (Italian) a form of Louis. *Luigino*

Luis ♛ (Spanish) a form of Louis. *Luise*

Luiz (Spanish) forms of Louis.

Lukas, Lukus (Greek, Czech, Swedish) forms of Luke. *Loukas, Lukash, Lukasha, Lukass, Lukasz*

Luke ♛ (Latin) a form of Lucius. Bible: companion of Saint Paul and author of the third Gospel of the New Testament. *Luck, Luk, Luka, Lúkács, Lukes, Lukyan*

Lukela (Hawaiian) a form of Russel.

Luken (Basque) bringer of light. *Luk*

Luki (Basque) famous warrior.

Lukman (Arabic) prophet.

Lulani (Hawaiian) highest point in heaven.

Lumo (Ewe) born facedown.

Lundy (Scottish) grove by the island.

Lunn (Irish) warlike.

Lunt (Swedish) grove.

Lusila (Hindi) leader.

Lusio (Zuni) a form of Lucius.

Lutalo (Luganda) warrior.

Lutfi (Arabic) kind, friendly.

Luther (German) famous warrior. History: Martin Luther was one of the central figures of the Reformation. *Lutero, Luthor*

Lutherum (Gypsy) slumber.

Luyu (Moquelumnan) head shaker.

Lyall, Lyell (Scottish) loyal.

Lyle (French) island. *Lisle, Ly, Lysle*

Lyman (English) meadow.

Lynch (Irish) mariner.

Lyndal (English) valley of lime trees.

Lyndon (English) linden hill. History: Lyndon B. Johnson was the thirty-sixth U.S. president. *Lyden, Lydon, Lyn, Lynden*

Lynn (English) waterfall; brook. *Lyn, Lynell, Lynette, Lynnard, Lynoll*

Lyron (Hebrew) a form of Leron, Liron.

Lysander (Greek) liberator.

Maalik (Punjabi) a form of Málik.

Mac (Scottish) son.

Macadam (Scottish) son of Adam.

Macallister (Irish) son of Alistair.

Macario (Spanish) a form of Makarios.

Macarthur (Irish) son of Arthur.

Macaulay (Scottish) son of righteous-
ness.

Macbride (Scottish) son of a follower
of Saint Brigid.

Maccoy (Irish) son of Hugh, Coy.

Maccrea (Irish) son of grace.

Macdonald (Scottish) son of Donald.

Macdougal (Scottish) son of Dougal.

Mace (French) club. (English) a short
form of Macy, Mason.

Macgregor (Scottish) son of Gregor.

Machas (Polish) a form of Michael.

Mack (Scottish) a short form of names
beginning with "Mac" and "Mc."
*Macke, Mackey, Mackie, Macklin,
Macks*

Mackenzie (Irish) son of Kenzie.

Mackinnley (Irish) son of the learned
ruler.

Macklain (Irish) a form of Maclean.

Maclean (Irish) son of Leander.

Macmahon (Irish) son of Mahon.

Macmurray (Irish) son of Murray.

Macnair (Scottish) son of the heir.

Maco (Hungarian) a form of
Emmanuel.

Macon (German, English) maker.

Macy (French) Matthew's estate.

Maddock (Welsh) generous.

Maddox (Welsh, English) benefactor's
son.

Madhar (Hindi) full of intoxication;
relating to spring.

Madison (English) son of Maude; good
son.
Maddie, Maddison, Maddy, Madisson

Madongo (Luganda) uncircumcised.

Madu (Ibo) people.

Magar (Armenian) groom's attendant.

Magee (Irish) son of Hugh.

Magen (Hebrew) protector.

Magnar (Norwegian) strong; warrior.

Magnus (Latin) great.

Magomu (Luganda) younger of twins.

Maguire (Irish) son of the beige one.

Mahammed (Arabic) a form of
Muhammad.

Mahdi (Arabic) guided to the right path.

Mahesa (Hindi) great lord. Religion:
another name for the Hindu god Shiva.

Mahi'ai (Hawaiian) a form of George.

Mahir (Arabic, Hebrew) excellent;
industrious.

Mahkah (Lakota) earth.

Mahmoud (Arabic) a form of
Muhammad.

Mahmúd (Arabic) a form of
Muhammad.

Mahomet (Arabic) a form of
Muhammad.

Mahon (Irish) bear.

Mahpee (Lakota) sky.

Maimun (Arabic) lucky.

Mairtin (Irish) a form of Martin.

Maitias (Irish) a form of Mathias.

Maitiú (Irish) a form of Matthew.

Maitland (English) meadowland.

Majid (Arabic) great, glorious.

Major (Latin) greater; military rank.

Makaio (Hawaiian) a form of Matthew.

Makalani (Mwera) writer.

Makani (Hawaiian) wind.

Makarios (Greek) happy; blessed.

Makenzie (Irish) a form of Mackenzie.

Makin (Arabic) strong.

Makis (Greek) a form of Michael.

Makoto (Japanese) sincere.

Maks (Hungarian) a form of Max.

Maksim (Russian) a form of
Maximilian.

Maksym (Polish) a form of
Maximilian.

Makyah (Hopi) eagle hunter.

Mal (Irish) a short form of names
beginning with "Mal."

Malachi (Hebrew) angel of God. Bible:
the last canonical Hebrew prophet.
*Maeleachlainn, Malachia, Malachie,
Malchija, Malechy*

Malachy (Irish) a form of Malachi.

Malajitm (Sanskrit) garland of victory.

Malcolm (Scottish) follower of Saint
Columba who Christianized North
Scotland. (Arabic) dove.
Malcolum, Malkolm

Malcom (Scottish) a form of Malcolm.
Malcum

Malden (English) meeting place in a
pasture.

Malek (Arabic) a form of Málik.

Maleko (Hawaiian) a form of Mark.

Málik (Punjabi) lord, master. (Arabic) a
form of Malachi.
*Malak, Malik, Malikh, Maliq,
Malique, Mallik*

Malin (English) strong, little warrior.

Mallory (German) army counselor.
(French) wild duck.

Maloney (Irish) church going.

Malvern (Welsh) bare hill.

Malvin (Irish, English) a form of
Melvin.

Mamo (Hawaiian) yellow flower; yellow
bird.

Manchu (Chinese) pure.

Manco (Peruvian) supreme leader.
History: a sixteenth-century Incan king.

Mandala (Yao) flowers.

Mandeep (Punjabi) mind full of light.
Mandieep

Mandel (German) almond.

Mandek (Polish) a form of Armand,
Herman.

Mander (Gypsy) from me.

Manford (English) small ford.

Manfred (English) man of peace. See
also Fred.

Manger (French) stable.

Mango (Spanish) a familiar form of
Emmanuel, Manuel.

Manheim (German) servant's home.

Manipi (Native American) living marvel.

Manius (Scottish) a form of Magnus.

Manley (English) hero's meadow.

Mann (German) man.

Manning (English) son of the hero.

Mannix (Irish) monk.

Manny (German, Spanish) a familiar
form of Manuel.

Mano (Hawaiian) shark. (Spanish) a
short form of Manuel.

Manoj (Sanskrit) cupid.

Mansa (Swahili) king. History: a four-
teenth-century king of Mali.

Mansel (English) manse; house occu-
pied by a clergyman.

Mansfield (English) field by the river;
hero's field.

Man-Shik (Korean) deeply rooted.

Mansür (Arabic) divinely aided.

Manton (English) man's town; hero's
town.

Manu (Hindi) lawmaker. History: the
reputed writer of the Hindi compen-
dium of sacred laws and customs.
(Hawaiian) bird. (Ghanaian) second-
born son.

Manuel (Hebrew) a short form of
Emmanuel.
*Mannuel, Manolón, Manual,
Manue, Manuelli, Manuelo, Manuil,
Manyuil*

Manville (French) worker's village.
(English) hero's village.

Man-Young (Korean) ten thousand
years of prosperity.

Manzo (Japanese) third son.

Maona (Winnebago) creator, earth
maker.

Mapira (Yao) millet.

Marc (French) a form of Mark.
Marc-André, Mark-Andre

Marcel (French) a form of Marcellus.
Marcell, Marsale, Marsel

Marcelino (Italian) a form of
Marcellus.

Marcelo, Marcello (Italian) forms of
Marcellus.
Marchello, Marsello, Marselo

Marcellus (Latin) a familiar form of
Marcus.

March (English) dweller by a boundary.

Marciano (Italian) a form of Martin.
Marcio

Marcilka (Hungarian) a form of
Marcellus.

Marcin (Polish) a form of Martin.

Marco (Italian) a form of Marcus.
History: Marco Polo was a thirteenth-
century Venetian traveler who explored
Asia.
Marcko

Marcos (Spanish) a form of Marcus.
Marcous, Markos, Markose

Marcus (Latin) martial, warlike.
*Marcas, Marcio, Marckus, Marcous,
Markov*

Marek (Slavic) a form of Marcus.

Maren (Basque) sea.

Mareo (Japanese) uncommon.

Marian (Polish) a form of Mark.

Mariano (Italian) a form of Mark.

Marid (Arabic) rebellious.

Marin (French) sailor.

Marino (Italian) a form of Marin.
Marinos

Mario (Italian) a form of Marino.
Marios, Marrio

Marion (French) bitter; sea of bitterness.

Marius (Latin) a form of Marin.

Mark (Latin) a form of Marcus. Bible:
author of the second Gospel in the New
Testament. See also Maleko.
*Markee, Markey, Markos, Márkus,
Marque, Marx*

Markanthony (Italian) a combination
of Mark + Anthony.

Marke (Polish) a form of Mark.

Markel, Markell (Latin) forms of
Mark.

Markes (Portuguese) a form of
Marques.

Markese (French) a form of Marquis.

Markham (English) homestead on the
boundary.

Markis (French) a form of Marquis.

Marko (Latin) a form of Marco, Mark.
Markco

Markus (Latin) a form of Marcus.
Markas, Markcus, Markcuss, Marqus

Marland (English) lake land.

Marley (English) lake meadow.

Marlin (English) deep-sea fish.
Marlion

Marlon (French) a form of Merlin.

Marlow (English) hill by the lake.

Marmion (French) small.

Marnin (Hebrew) singer; bringer of joy.

Maro (Japanese) myself.

Marquan (American) a combination of
Mark + Quan.

Marquel (American) a form of Marcellus.

Marques (Portuguese) nobleman.
Markques, Marquest, Markqueus, Marqus

Marquez (Portuguese) a form of Marques.

Marquice (American) a form of Marquis.

Marquis, Marquise (French) nobleman.
Marcquis, Marcuis, Markuis, Marquee, Marqui, Marquie, Marquist

Marquon (American) a combination of Mark + Quon.

Marr (Spanish) divine. (Arabic) forbidden.

Mars (Latin) bold warrior. Mythology: the Roman god of war.

Marsalis (Italian) a form of Marcellus.

Marsden (English) marsh valley.

Marsh (English) swamp land. (French) a short form of Marshall.

Marshal (French) a form of Marshall.
Marschal, Marshel

Marshall (French) caretaker of the horses; military title.
Marshell

Marshawn (American) a combination of Mark + Shawn.

Marston (English) town by the marsh.

Martell (English) hammerer.
Martel

Marten (Dutch) a form of Martin.

Martez (Spanish) a form of Martin.

Marti (Spanish) a form of Martin.
Martie

Martial (French) a form of Mark.

Martin (Latin, French) a form of Martinus. History: Martin Luther King, Jr. led the Civil Rights movement and won the Nobel Peace Prize. See also Tynek.
Maartin, Marinos, Mart, Martan, Martijn, Martinas, Martine, Martiniano, Martinien, Marto, Marton, Márton, Marts, Martyn, Mattin, Mertin

Martinez (Spanish) a form of Martin.

Martinho (Portuguese) a form of Martin.

Martino (Italian) a form of Martin.

Martins (Latvian) a form of Martin.

Martinus (Latin) martial, warlike.

Marty (Latin) a familiar form of Martin.
Martey, Martie

Marut (Hindi) Religion: the Hindu god of the wind.

Marv (English) a short form of Marvin.

Marvin (English) lover of the sea.
Marvein, Marven, Marwin, Marwynn

Marwan (Arabic) history personage.

Marwood (English) forest pond.

Masaccio (Italian) twin.

Masahiro (Japanese) broad-minded.

Masamba (Yao) leaves.

Masao (Japanese) righteous.

Masato (Japanese) just.

Mashama (Shona) surprising.

Maska (Native American) powerful. (Russian) mask.

Maslin (French) little Thomas.

Mason ✤ (French) stone worker. *Maison*

Masou (Native American) fire god.

Massey (English) twin.

Massimo (Italian) greatest. *Massimiliano*

Masud (Arabic, Swahili) fortunate.

Matai (Basque, Bulgarian) a form of Matthew.

Matalino (Filipino) bright.

Mateo (Spanish) a form of Matthew.

Mateusz (Polish) a form of Matthew.

Mathe (German) a short form of Matthew.

Mather (English) powerful army.

Matheu (German) a form of Matthew.

Mathew (Hebrew) a form of Matthew.

Mathias, Matthias (German, Swedish) forms of Matthew.

Mathieu, Matthieu (French) forms of Matthew.

Matías (Spanish) a form of Mathias.

Mato (Native American) brave.

Matope (Rhodesian) our last child.

Matoskah (Lakota) white bear.

Mats (Swedish) a familiar form of Matthew.

Matson (Hebrew) son of Matt.

Matt (Hebrew) a short form of Matthew. *Mat*

Matteen (Afghan) disciplined; polite.

Matteus (Scandinavian) a form of Matthew.

Matthew ✤ (Hebrew) gift of God. Bible: author of the first Gospel of the New Testament. *Mads, Mata, Matek, Matfei, Matheson, Mathian, Mathieson, Matro, Matthaeus, Matthaios, Matthaus, Matthäus, Mattheus, Matthews, Mattmias*

Matty (Hebrew) a familiar form of Matthew.

Matus (Czech) a form of Mathias.

Matvey (Russian) a form of Matthew.

Matyas (Polish) a form of Matthew.

Mauli (Hawaiian) a form of Maurice.

Maurice (Latin) dark skinned; moor; marshland. See also Seymour. *Maur, Maurance, Maureo, Maurids, Mauriece, Maurikas, Maurin, Maurino, Maurise, Maurius, Maurrel, Maurtel, Maurycy, Morice, Morrel, Morrice, Morrill*

Mauricio (Spanish) a form of Maurice.

Mauritz (German) a form of Maurice.

Maurizio (Italian) a form of Maurice.

Mauro (Latin) a short form of Maurice.
Maur, Maurio

Maury (Latin) a familiar form of
Maurice.

Maverick (American) independent.

Mawuli (Ewe) there is a God.

Max (Latin) a short form of
Maximilian, Maxwell.
Maxe, Maxx

Maxfield (English) Mack's field.

Maxi (Czech, Hungarian, Spanish) a
familiar form of Maximilian, Máximo.

Maxim (Russian) a form of Maxime.

Maxime (French) most excellent.

Maximilian (Latin) greatest.
*Maixim, Maxamillion, Maxemilian,
Maxemilion, Maximalian, Maximili,
Maximilia, Maximilianus,
Maximilien, Maxmilian, Maxmillion,
Maxon, Maxymilian, Maxymillian*

Maximiliano (Italian) a form of
Maximilian.
Massimiliano

Maximillian (Latin) a form of
Maximilian.
Maximillion

Máximo (Spanish) a form of
Maximilian.

Maximos (Greek) a form of
Maximilian.

Maxwell (English) great spring.
Maxwel, Maxwill

Maxy (English) a familiar form of Max,
Maxwell.

Mayer (Hebrew) a form of Meir. (Latin)
a form of Magnus, Major.

Mayes (English) field.

Mayhew (English) a form of Matthew.

Maynard (English) powerful; brave. See
also Meinhard.

Mayo (Irish) yew-tree plain. (English) a
form of Mayes. Geography: a county in
Ireland.

Mayon (Indian) person of black com-
plexion. Religion: another name for
the Indian god Mal.

Mayonga (Luganda) lake sailor.

Mazi (Ibo) sir.

Mazin (Arabic) proper.

Mbita (Swahili) born on a cold night.

Mbwana (Swahili) master.

McGeorge (Scottish) son of George.

Mckade (Scottish) son of Kade.

Mckay (Scottish) son of Kay.
Mackay

McKenzie (Irish) a form of Mackenzie.

Mckinley (Irish) a form of Mackinnley.

Mead (English) meadow.

Medgar (German) a form of Edgar.

Medwin (German) faithful friend.

Mehetabel (Hebrew) who God benefits.

Mehrdad (Persian) gift of the sun.

Mehtar (Sanskrit) prince.

Meinhard (German) strong, firm. See also Maynard.

Meinrad (German) strong counsel.

Meir (Hebrew) one who brightens, shines; enlightener. History: Golda Meir was the prime minister of Israel.

Meka (Hawaiian) eyes.

Mel (English, Irish) a familiar form of Melvin.

Melbourne (English) mill stream.

Melchior (Hebrew) king.

Meldon (English) mill hill.

Melrone (Irish) servant of Saint Ruadhan.

Melvern (Native American) great chief.

Melville (French) mill town. Literature: Herman Melville was a well-known nineteenth-century American writer.

Melvin (Irish) armored chief. (English) mill friend; council friend. See also Vinny.
Melvino, Melvon, Melvyn, Melwin, Melwyn, Melwynn

Menachem (Hebrew) comforter.

Menassah (Hebrew) cause to forget.

Mendel (English) repairman.

Mengesha (Ethiopian) kingdom.

Menico (Spanish) a short form of Domenico.

Mensah (Ewe) third son.

Menz (German) a short form of Clement.

Mercer (English) storekeeper.

Mered (Hebrew) revolter.

Meredith (Welsh) guardian from the sea.

Merion (Welsh) from Merion, Wales.

Merle (French) a short form of Merlin, Merrill.
Meryl

Merlin (English) falcon. Literature: the magician who served as counselor in King Arthur's court.

Merrick (English) ruler of the sea.

Merrill (Irish) bright sea. (French) famous.
Meryl

Merritt (Latin, Irish) valuable; deserving.

Merton (English) sea town.

Merv (Irish) a short form of Mervin.

Merville (French) sea village.

Mervin (Irish) a form of Marvin.
Mervyn, Mervynn, Merwin, Merwinn, Merwyn, Murvin, Murvyn, Myrvyn, Myrvynn, Myrwyn

Meshach (Hebrew) artist. Bible: one of Daniel's three friends who emerged unharmed from the fiery furnace of Babylon.

Mesut (Turkish) happy.

Metikla (Moquelumnan) reaching a hand underwater to catch a fish.

Mette (Greek, Danish) pearl.

Meurig (Welsh) a form of Maurice.

Meyer (German) farmer.

Mhina (Swahili) delightful.

Micah (Hebrew) a form of Michael. Bible: a Hebrew prophet. *Mic, Micaiah, Michiah, Mikah, Myca, Mycah*

Micha (Hebrew) a short form of Michael.

Michael ☙ (Hebrew) who is like God? See also Micah, Miguel, Mika, Miles. *Machael, Mahail, Maichail, Maikal, Makael, Makal, Makel, Makell, Meikel, Mekal, Mekhail, Mhichael, Micael, Micahel, Mical, Michaele, Michaell, Michak, Michale, Michau, Micheil, Michelet, Michiel, Micho, Michoel, Mihalje, Mihkel, Mikell, Miquel, Mychael, Mykhas*

Michail (Russian) a form of Michael.

Michal (Polish) a form of Michael. *Michak*

Micheal (Irish) a form of Michael.

Michel (French) a form of Michael. *Michaud, Miche, Michee, Michon*

Michelangelo (Italian) a combination of Michael + Angelo. Art: Michelangelo Buonarroti was one of the greatest Renaissance painters.

Michele (Italian) a form of Michael.

Michio (Japanese) man with the strength of three thousand.

Mick (English) a short form of Michael, Mickey.

Mickael (English) a form of Michael.

Mickenzie (Irish) a form of Mackenzie.

Mickey (Irish) a familiar form of Michael. *Mickie, Micky*

Micu (Hungarian) a form of Nick.

Miguel ☙ (Portuguese, Spanish) a form of Michael. *Migeel, Migel, Miguelly, Migui*

Miguelangel (Spanish) a combination of Miguel + Angel.

Mihail (Greek, Bulgarian, Romanian) a form of Michael.

Mika (Ponca) raccoon. (Hebrew) a form of Micah. (Russian) a familiar form of Michael. *Mikah*

Mikael (Swedish) a form of Michael. *Mikaeel, Mikaele*

Mikáele (Hawaiian) a form of Michael.

Mikal (Hebrew) a form of Michael. *Mekal*

Mikasi (Omaha) coyote.

Mike (Hebrew) a short form of Michael. *Mikey, Myk*

Mikeal (Irish) a form of Michael.

Mikel (Basque) a form of Michael. *Mekel, Mekell, Mikell*

Mikelis (Latvian) a form of Michael.

Mikhail (Greek, Russian) a form of Michael. *Mekhail*

Miki (Japanese) tree.

Mikkel (Norwegian) a form of Michael.

Mikko (Finnish) a form of Michael.

Mikolaj (Polish) a form of Nicholas.

Mikolas (Greek) a form of Nicholas.

Miksa (Hungarian) a form of Max.

Milan (Italian) northerner. Geography: a city in northern Italy.

Milap (Native American) giving.

Milborough (English) middle borough.

Milek (Polish) a familiar form of Nicholas.

Miles (Greek) millstone. (Latin) soldier. (German) merciful. (English) a short form of Michael.
Milas, Milles, Milson

Milford (English) mill by the ford.

Mililani (Hawaiian) heavenly caress.

Milko (Czech) a form of Michael. (German) a familiar form of Emil.

Millard (Latin) caretaker of the mill.

Miller (English) miller; grain grinder.

Mills (English) mills.

Milo (German) a form of Miles. A familiar form of Emil.

Milos (Greek, Slavic) pleasant.

Miloslav (Czech) lover of glory.

Milt (English) a short form of Milton.

Milton (English) mill town.
Miltie, Milty, Mylton

Mimis (Greek) a familiar form of Demetrius.

Min (Burmese) king.

Mincho (Spanish) a form of Benjamin.

Minel (Spanish) a form of Manuel.

Miner (English) miner.

Mingan (Native American) gray wolf.

Mingo (Spanish) a short form of Domingo.

Minh (Vietnamese) bright.

Minkah (Akan) just, fair.

Minor (Latin) junior; younger.

Minoru (Japanese) fruitful.

Mique (Spanish) a form of Mickey.
Miquel

Miron (Polish) peace.

Miroslav (Czech) peace; glory.

Mirwais (Afghan) noble ruler.

Misael (Hebrew) a form of Michael.

Misha (Russian) a short form of Michail.

Miska (Hungarian) a form of Michael.

Mister (English) mister.

Misu (Moquelumnan) rippling water.

Mitch (English) a short form of Mitchell.

Mitchel (English) a form of Mitchell.
Mitchael, Mitchele

Mitchell (English) a form of Michael.
Mitchall, Mitchelle, Mitchem, Mytch, Mytchell

Mitsos (Greek) a familiar form of Demetrius.

Modesto (Latin) modest.

Moe (English) a short form of Moses.

Mogens (Dutch) powerful.

Mohamad (Arabic) a form of
Muhammad.
Mohamid

Mohamed (Arabic) a form of
Muhammad.

Mohamet (Arabic) a form of
Muhammad.

Mohammad (Arabic) a form of
Muhammad.
*Mahammad, Mohammadi,
Mohammd, Mohammid, Mohanad,
Mohmad*

Mohammed (Arabic) a form of
Muhammad.
Mohaned

Mohamud (Arabic) a form of
Muhammad.

Mohan (Hindi) delightful.

Moises (Portuguese, Spanish) a form
of Moses.
Moise, Moisés, Moisey, Moisis

Moishe (Yiddish) a form of Moses.

Mojag (Native American) crying baby.

Molimo (Moquelumnan) bear going
under shady trees.

Momuso (Moquelumnan) yellow jackets crowded in their nests for the winter.

Mona (Moquelumnan) gathering jim-
sonweed seed.

Monahan (Irish) monk.

Mongo (Yoruba) famous.

Monroe (Irish) Geography: the mouth
of the Roe River.

Montague (French) pointed mountain.

Montana (Spanish) mountain.
Geography: a U.S. state.

Montaro (Japanese) big boy.

Monte (Spanish) a short form of
Montgomery.
*Montae, Montaé, Montay, Montee,
Monti, Montoya*

Montel (American) a form of Montreal.

Montez (Spanish) dweller in the mountains.
Monteiz, Monteze, Montisze

Montgomery (English) rich man's
mountain.

Montre (French) show.

Montreal (French) royal mountain.
Geography: a city in Quebec.

Montrell (French) a form of Montreal.

Montsho (Tswana) black.

Monty (English) a familiar form of
Montgomery.

Moore (French) dark; moor; marshland.

Mordecai (Hebrew) martial, warlike.
Mythology: Marduk was the Babylonian
god of war. Bible: wise counselor to
Queen Esther.

Mordred (Latin) painful. Literature: the
bastard son of King Arthur.

Morel (French) an edible mushroom.
Morrel

Moreland (English) moor; marshland.

Morell (French) dark; from Morocco.
Morrill

Morey (Greek) a familiar form of Moris.
(Latin) a form of Morrie.
Morry

Morgan (Scottish) sea warrior.
Morgen, Morgun, Morrgan

Morio (Japanese) forest.

Moris (Greek) son of the dark one.
(English) a form of Morris.

Moritz (German) a form of Maurice,
Morris.

Morley (English) meadow by the moor.

Morrie (Latin) a familiar form of
Maurice, Morse.
Morry

Morris (Latin) dark skinned; moor;
marshland. (English) a form of
Maurice.
Moriss, Morriss, Morry

Morse (English) son of Maurice.

Mort (French, English) a short form of
Morten, Mortimer, Morton.

Morten (Norwegian) a form of Martin.

Mortimer (French) still water.

Morton (English) town near the moor.

Morven (Scottish) mariner.

Mose (Hebrew) a short form of Moses.

Moses (Hebrew) drawn out of the water.
(Egyptian) son, child. Bible: the Hebrew
lawgiver who brought the Ten Com-
mandments down from Mount Sinai.
*Moise, Moïse, Moisei, Mosese, Mosiah,
Mosie, Mosya, Mosze, Moszek, Moyses*

Moshe (Hebrew, Polish) a form of Moses.
Mosheh

Mosi (Swahili) first-born.

Moss (Irish) a short form of Maurice,
Morris. (English) a short form of Moses.

Moswen (African) light in color.

Motega (Native American) new arrow.

Mouhamed (Arabic) a form of
Muhammad.

Mousa (Arabic) a form of Moses.

Moze (Lithuanian) a form of Moses.

Mpasa (Nguni) mat.

Mposi (Nyakyusa) blacksmith.

Mpoza (Luganda) tax collector.

Msrah (Akan) sixth-born.

Mtima (Nguni) heart.

Muata (Moquelumnan) yellow jackets
in their nest.

Mugamba (Runyoro) talks too much.

Mugisa (Rutooro) lucky.

Muhammad (Arabic) praised. History:
the founder of the Islamic religion. See
also Ahmad, Hamid, Yasin.
*Muhamad, Muhamet,
Muhammadali, Muhammed*

Muhannad (Arabic) sword.

Muhsin (Arabic) beneficent; charitable.

Muhtadi (Arabic) rightly guided.

Muir (Scottish) moor; marshland.

Mujahid (Arabic) fighter in the way of Allah.

Mukasa (Luganda) God's chief administrator.

Mukhtar (Arabic) chosen.

Mukul (Sanskrit) bud, blossom; soul.

Mulogo (Musoga) wizard.

Mundan (Rhodesian) garden.

Mundo (Spanish) a short form of Edmundo.

Mundy (Irish) from Reamonn.

Mungo (Scottish) amiable.

Mun-Hee (Korean) literate; shiny.

Munir (Arabic) brilliant; shining.

Munny (Cambodian) wise.

Muraco (Native American) white moon.

Murali (Hindi) flute. Religion: the instrument the Hindu god Krishna is usually depicted as playing.

Murat (Turkish) wish come true.

Murdock (Scottish) wealthy sailor.

Murphy (Irish) sea warrior.

Murray (Scottish) sailor.
Moray, Murrey, Murry

Murtagh (Irish) a form of Murdock.

Musa (Swahili) child.

Musád (Arabic) untied camel.

Musoke (Rukonjo) born while a rainbow was in the sky.

Mustafa (Arabic) chosen; royal.
Mostafa, Mostaffa, Moustafa, Mustafah

Mustapha (Arabic) a form of Mustafa.

Muti (Arabic) obedient.

Mwaka (Luganda) born on New Year's Eve.

Mwamba (Nyakyusa) strong.

Mwanje (Luganda) leopard.

Mwinyi (Swahili) king.

Mwita (Swahili) summoner.

Mychajlo (Latvian) a form of Michael.
Mykhas

Mychal (American) a form of Michael.

Myer (English) a form of Meir.

Mykal, Mykel (American) forms of Michael.

Myles (Latin) soldier. (German) a form of Miles.

Mynor (Latin) a form of Minor.

Myo (Burmese) city.

Myron (Greek) fragrant ointment.
Mehran, Mehrayan, My, Myran, Myrone

Myung-Dae (Korean) right; great.

Mzuzi (Swahili) inventive.

N

Naaman (Hebrew) pleasant.

Nabiha (Arabic) intelligent.

Nabil (Arabic) noble.

Nachman (Hebrew) a short form of Menachem.

Nada (Arabic) generous.

Nadav (Hebrew) generous; noble.

Nadidah (Arabic) equal to anyone else.

Nadim (Arabic) friend.

Nadir (Afghan, Arabic) dear, rare.

Nadisu (Hindi) beautiful river.

Naeem (Arabic) benevolent.

Naftali (Hebrew) wreath.

Nagid (Hebrew) ruler; prince.

Nahele (Hawaiian) forest.

Nahma (Native American) sturgeon.

Nailah (Arabic) successful.

Nairn (Scottish) river with alder trees.

Najee (Arabic) a form of Naji.

Naji (Arabic) safe.

Najíb (Arabic) born to nobility.

Najji (Muganda) second child.

Nakia (Arabic) pure.

Nakos (Arapaho) sage, wise.

Naldo (Spanish) a familiar form of Reginald.

Nalren (Dene) thawed out.

Nam (Vietnamese) scrape off.

Namaka (Hawaiian) eyes.

Namid (Ojibwa) star dancer.

Namir (Hebrew) leopard.

Nandin (Hindi) Religion: a servant of the Hindu god Shiva.

Nando (German) a familiar form of Ferdinand.

Nangila (Abaluhya) born while parents traveled.

Nangwaya (Mwera) don't mess with me.

Nansen (Swedish) son of Nancy.

Nantai (Navajo) chief.

Nantan (Apache) spokesman.

Naoko (Japanese) straight, honest.

Napayshni (Lakota) he does not flee; courageous.

Napier (Spanish) new city.

Napoleon (Greek) lion of the woodland. (Italian) from Naples, Italy. History: Napoleon Bonaparte was a famous nineteenth-century French emperor.

Naquan (American) a combination of the prefix Na + Quan.

Narain (Hindi) protector. Religion: another name for the Hindu god Vishnu.

Narcisse (French) a form of Narcissus.

Narcissus (Greek) daffodil. Mythology: the youth who fell in love with his own reflection.

Nard (Persian) chess player.

Nardo (German) strong, hardy. (Spanish) a short form of Bernardo.

Narve (Dutch) healthy, strong.

Nashashuk (Fox, Sauk) loud thunder.

Nashoba (Choctaw) wolf.

Nasim (Persian) breeze; fresh air.

Nasser (Arabic) victorious.

Nat (English) a short form of Nathan, Nathaniel.

Natal (Spanish) a form of Noël.

Natan (Hebrew, Hungarian, Polish, Russian, Spanish) God has given.

Natanael (Hebrew) a form of Nathaniel.
Nataniel

Nate (Hebrew) a short form of Nathan, Nathaniel.

Natesh (Hindi) destroyer. Religion: another name for the Hindu god Shiva.

Nathan ✴ (Hebrew) a short form of Nathaniel. Bible: a prophet during the reigns of David and Solomon.
Naethan, Nathann, Nathean, Nathian, Nathin, Nathon, Natthan, Naythan

Nathanael (Hebrew) gift of God. Bible: one of the Twelve Apostles. Also known as Bartholomew.
Nathanae, Nathanal, Nathaneal, Nathaneil, Nathanel, Nathaneol

Nathanial (Hebrew) a form of Nathaniel.
Nathanyal

Nathanie (Hebrew) a familiar form of Nathaniel.
Nathania, Nathanni

Nathaniel ✴ (Hebrew) gift of God.
Nathanielle, Nathanuel, Nathanyel, Natheal, Nathel, Nathinel

Nathen (Hebrew) a form of Nathan.

Nav (Gypsy) name.

Navarro (Spanish) plains.

Navdeep (Sikh) new light.

Navin (Hindi) new, novel.

Nawat (Native American) left-handed.

Nawkaw (Winnebago) wood.

Nayati (Native American) wrestler.

Nayland (English) island dweller.

Nazareth (Hebrew) born in Nazareth, Israel.

Nazih (Arabic) pure, chaste.

Ndale (Nguni) trick.

Neal (Irish) a form of Neil.
Neale, Neall, Nealle, Nealon, Nealy

Neci (Latin) a familiar form of Ignatius.

Nectarios (Greek) saint. Religion: a saint in the Greek Orthodox Church.

Ned (English) a familiar form of Edward, Edwin.

Nehemiah (Hebrew) compassion of Jehovah. Bible: a Jewish leader.

Nehru (Hindi) canal.

Neil (Irish) champion.
Neel, Neibl, Neile, Neill, Neille, Niele

Neka (Native American) wild goose.

Nelek (Polish) a form of Cornelius.

Nellie (English) a familiar form of Cornelius, Cornell, Nelson.

Nelius (Latin) a short form of Cornelius.

Nelo (Spanish) a form of Daniel.

Nels (Scandinavian) a form of Neil, Nelson.

Nelson (English) son of Neil.

Nemesio (Spanish) just.

Nemo (Greek) glen, glade. (Hebrew) a short form of Nehemiah.

Nen (Egyptian) ancient waters.

Neptune (Latin) sea ruler. Mythology: the Roman god of the sea.

Nero (Latin, Spanish) stern. History: a cruel Roman emperor.

Nesbit (English) nose-shaped bend in a river.

Nestor (Greek) traveler; wise.

Nethaniel (Hebrew) a form of Nathaniel.

Neto (Spanish) a short form of Ernesto.

Nevada (Spanish) covered in snow. Geography: a U.S. state.

Nevan (Irish) holy.

Neville (French) new town.
Nev

Nevin (Irish) worshiper of the saint. (English) middle; herb.
Nefen, Nev, Neven, Nevins, Niven

Newbold (English) new tree.

Newell (English) new hall.

Newland (English) new land.

Newlin (Welsh) new lake.

Newman (English) newcomer.

Newton (English) new town.

Ngai (Vietnamese) herb.

Nghia (Vietnamese) forever.

Ngozi (Ibo) blessing.

Ngu (Vietnamese) sleep.

Nguyen (Vietnamese) a form of Ngu.

Nhean (Cambodian) self-knowledge.

Niall (Irish) a form of Neil. History: Niall of the Nine Hostages was a famous Irish king.
Nial, Nialle

Nibal (Arabic) arrows.

Nibaw (Native American) standing tall.

Nicabar (Gypsy) stealthy.

Nicho (Spanish) a form of Dennis.

Nicholas ※ (Greek) victorious people.
Religion: Nicholas of Myra is a patron
saint of children. See also Caelan,
Claus, Cola, Colar, Cole, Colin, Colson,
Klaus, Lasse, Mikolaj, Mikolas, Milek.
*Niccolas, Nichalas, Nichelas, Nichele,
Nichlas, Nichlos, Nichola, Nichole,
Nicholl, Niclas, Niclasse, Nicoles,
Nicolis, Nicoll, Nikhil, Nikili, Nioclás,
Niocol, Nycholas*

Nicholaus (Greek) a form of Nicholas.

Nichols, Nicholson (English) son of
Nicholas.

Nick (English) a short form of Dominic,
Nicholas. See also Micu.
Nic, Nik

Nickalus (Greek) a form of Nicholas.

Nicklaus, Nicklas (Greek) forms of
Nicholas.
*Nickolau, Nickolaus, Nicolaus,
Niklaus*

Nickolas (Greek) a form of Nicholas.
Nickolaos, Nickolus

Nicky (Greek) a familiar form of
Nicholas.

Nico (Greek) a short form of Nicholas.

Nicodemus (Greek) conqueror of the
people.

Nicola (Italian) a form of Nicholas. See
also Cola.

Nicolai (Norwegian, Russian) a form of
Nicholas.

Nicolas (Italian) a form of Nicholas.
*Nicolaas, Nicolás, Nicolaus, Nicoles,
Nicolis*

Nicolo (Italian) a form of Nicholas.
Nicol, Nicolao

Niels (Danish) a form of Neil.

Nien (Vietnamese) year.

Nigan (Native American) ahead.

Nigel (Latin) dark night.
*Niegel, Nigal, Nigiel, Nigil, Nigle,
Nijel, Nygel*

Nika (Yoruba) ferocious.

Nike (Greek) victorious.

Niki (Hungarian) a familiar form of
Nicholas.

Nikita (Russian) a form of Nicholas.

Nikiti (Native American) round and
smooth like an abalone shell.

Nikko, Niko (Hungarian) forms of
Nicholas.

Niklas (Latvian, Swedish) a form of
Nicholas.
Niklaus

Nikola (Greek) a short form of
Nicholas.
Nikolao

Nikolai (Estonian, Russian) a form of
Nicholas.

Nikolas (Greek) a form of Nicholas.
*Nicanor, Nikalus, Nikolaas, Nikolaos,
Nikolis, Nikos, Nilos, Nykolas*

Nikolaus (Greek) a form of Nicholas.
Nikolaos

Nikolos (Greek) a form of Nicholas. See
also Kolya.
Nikolaos, Nikos, Nilos

Nil (Russian) a form of Neil.

Nila (Hindi) blue.

Niles (English) son of Neil.

Nilo (Finnish) a form of Neil.

Nils (Swedish) a short form of Nicholas.

Nimrod (Hebrew) rebel. Bible: a great-grandson of Noah.

Niño (Spanish) young child.

Niran (Tai) eternal.

Nishan (Armenian) cross, sign, mark.

Nissan (Hebrew) sign, omen; miracle.

Nitis (Native American) friend.

Nixon (English) son of Nick.

Nizam (Arabic) leader.

Nkunda (Runyankore) loves those who hate him.

N'namdi (Ibo) his father's name lives on.

Noach (Hebrew) a form of Noah.

Noah ☀ (Hebrew) peaceful, restful. Bible: the patriarch who built the ark to survive the Flood.
Noak, Noi

Noam (Hebrew) sweet; friend.

Noble (Latin) born to nobility.

Nodin (Native American) wind.

Noe (Czech, French) a form of Noah.

Noé (Hebrew, Spanish) quiet, peaceful. See also Noah.

Noël (French) day of Christ's birth. See also Natal.
Noel, Noël, Nole, Noli, Nowel, Nowell

Nohea (Hawaiian) handsome.

Nokonyu (Native American) katydid's nose.

Nolan (Irish) famous; noble.
Noland, Nolen, Nolin, Nollan, Nolyn

Nollie (Latin, Scandinavian) a familiar form of Oliver.

Norbert (Scandinavian) brilliant hero.

Norberto (Spanish) a form of Norbert.

Norman (French) Norseman. History: a name for the Scandinavians who settled in northern France in the tenth century, and who later conquered England in 1066.
Norm, Normand, Normen, Normie, Normy

Norris (French) northerner. (English) Norman's horse.

Northcliff (English) northern cliff.

Northrop (English) north farm.

Norton (English) northern town.

Norville (French, English) northern town.

Norvin (English) northern friend.

Norward (English) protector of the north.

Norwood (English) northern woods.

Notaku (Moquelumnan) growing bear.

Nowles (English) a short form of Knowles.

Nsoah (Akan) seventh-born.

Numa (Arabic) pleasant.

Numair (Arabic) panther.

Nuncio (Italian) messenger.

Nuri (Hebrew, Arabic) my fire.

Nuriel (Hebrew, Arabic) fire of the Lord.

Nuru (Swahili) born in daylight.

Nusair (Arabic) bird of prey.

Nwa (Nigerian) son.

Nwake (Nigerian) born on market day.

Nye (English) a familiar form of Aneurin, Nigel.

Nyle (English) island. (Irish) a form of Neil.

Oakes (English) oak trees.

Oakley (English) oak-tree field.

Oalo (Spanish) a form of Paul.

Oba (Yoruba) king.

Obadele (Yoruba) king arrives at the house.

Obadiah (Hebrew) servant of God.

Obed (English) a short form of Obadiah.

Oberon (German) noble; bearlike. Literature: the king of the fairies in the Shakespearean play *A Midsummer Night's Dream*. See also Auberon, Aubrey.

Obert (German) wealthy; bright.

Obie (English) a familiar form of Obadiah.

Ocan (Luo) hard times.

Octavio (Latin) eighth. See also Tavey, Tavian.

Octavious, Octavius (Latin) forms of Octavio.

Odakota (Lakota) friendly.

Odd (Norwegian) point.

Ode (Benin) born along the road. (Irish, English) a short form of Odell.

Oded (Hebrew) encouraging.

Odell (Greek) ode, melody. (Irish) otter. (English) forested hill.

Odin (Scandinavian) ruler. Mythology: the Norse god of wisdom and war.

Odion (Benin) first of twins.

Odo (Norwegian) a form of Otto.

Odolf (German) prosperous wolf.

Odom (Ghanaian) oak tree.

Odon (Hungarian) wealthy protector.

Odran (Irish) pale green.
Orin, Orren

Odysseus (Greek) wrathful. Literature: the hero of Homer's epic poem *Odyssey*.

Ofer (Hebrew) young deer.

Og (Aramaic) king. Bible: the king of Basham.

Ogaleesha (Lakota) red shirt.

Ogbay (Ethiopian) don't take him from me.

Ogbonna (Ibo) image of his father.

Ogden (English) oak valley. Literature: Ogden Nash was a twentieth-century American writer of light verse.

Ogima (Chippewa) chief.

Ogun (Nigerian) Mythology: the god of war.

Ohanko (Native American) restless.

Ohannes (Turkish) a form of John.

Ohanzee (Lakota) comforting shadow.

Ohin (African) chief.

Ohitekah (Lakota) brave.

Oistin (Irish) a form of Austin.

OJ (American) a combination of the initials O. + J.

Ojo (Yoruba) difficult delivery.

Okapi (Swahili) an African animal related to the giraffe but having a short neck.

Oke (Hawaiian) a form of Oscar.

Okechuku (Ibo) God's gift.

Okeke (Ibo) born on market day.

Okie (American) from Oklahoma.

Oko (Ghanaian) older twin. (Yoruba) god of war.

Okorie (Ibo) a form of Okeke.

Okpara (Ibo) first son.

Okuth (Luo) born in a rain shower.

Ola (Yoruba) wealthy, rich.

Olaf (Scandinavian) ancestor. History: a patron saint and king of Norway.

Olajuwon (Yoruba) wealth and honor are God's gifts.

Olamina (Yoruba) this is my wealth.

Olatunji (Yoruba) honor reawakens.

Olav (Scandinavian) a form of Olaf.

Ole (Scandinavian) a familiar form of Olaf, Olav.

Oleg (Latvian, Russian) holy.

Oleksandr (Russian) a form of Alexander.

Olés (Polish) a familiar form of Alexander.

Olin (English) holly.

Olindo (Italian) from Olinthos, Greece.

Oliver (Latin) olive tree. (Scandinavian) kind; affectionate.
Oilibhéar, Oliverio, Oliverios, Olivero, Oliviero, Olliver, Ollivor, Olvan

Olivier (French) a form of Oliver.

Oliwa (Hawaiian) a form of Oliver.

Ollie (English) a familiar form of Oliver.

Olo (Spanish) a short form of Orlando, Rolando.

Olubayo (Yoruba) highest joy.

Olufemi (Yoruba) wealth and honor favors me.

Olujimi (Yoruba) God gave me this.

Olushola (Yoruba) God has blessed me.

Omar (Arabic) highest; follower of the Prophet. (Hebrew) reverent.
Omair, Omarr

Omari (Swahili) a form of Omar.

Omer (Arabic) a form of Omar.

Omolara (Benin) child born at the right time.

On (Burmese) coconut. (Chinese) peace.

Onan (Turkish) prosperous.

Onaona (Hawaiian) pleasant fragrance.

Ondro (Czech) a form of Andrew.

O'neil (Irish) son of Neil.

Onkar (Hindi) God in his entirety.

Onofrio (German) a form of Humphrey.

Onslow (English) enthusiast's hill.

Onufry (Polish) a form of Humphrey.

Onur (Turkish) honor.

Ophir (Hebrew) faithful. Bible: an Old Testament people and country.

Opio (Ateso) first of twin boys.

Oral (Latin) verbal; speaker.

Oran (Irish) green.

Oratio (Latin) a form of Horatio.

Orbán (Hungarian) born in the city.

Ordell (Latin) beginning.

Oren (Hebrew) pine tree. (Irish) light skinned, white.
Orin, Oris, Orren

Orestes (Greek) mountain man. Mythology: the son of the Greek leader Agamemnon.

Ori (Hebrew) my light.

Orien (Latin) visitor from the east.
Orin, Oris

Orion (Greek) son of fire. Mythology: a giant hunter who was killed by Artemis. See also Zorion.

Orji (Ibo) mighty tree.

Orlando (German) famous throughout the land. (Spanish) a form of Roland.
Olando, Orlan, Orland, Orlanda, Orlandus, Orlo, Orlondo, Orlondon

Orleans (Latin) golden.

Orman (German) mariner, seaman. (Scandinavian) serpent, worm.

Ormond (English) bear mountain; spear protector.

Oro (Spanish) golden.

Orono (Latin) a form of Oren.

Orrick (English) old oak tree.

Orrin (English) river.
Orin

Orris (Latin) a form of Horatio.
Oris

Orry (Latin) from the Orient.
Oarrie, Orrey, Orrie

Orsino (Italian) a form of Orson.

Orson (Latin) bearlike.

Orton (English) shore town.

Ortzi (Basque) sky.

Orunjan (Yoruba) born under the midday sun.

Orval (English) a form of Orville.

Orville (French) golden village. History: Orville Wright and his brother Wilbur were the first men to fly an airplane.

Orvin (English) spear friend.

Osahar (Benin) God hears.

Osayaba (Benin) God forgives.

Osaze (Benin) whom God likes.

Osbert (English) divine; bright.

Osborn (Scandinavian) divine bear. (English) warrior of God.

Oscar (Scandinavian) divine spearman.
Osker, Oszkar

Osei (Fante) noble.

Osgood (English) divinely good.

O'Shea (Irish) son of Shea.

Osip (Russian, Ukrainian) a form of Joseph, Yosef. See also Osya.

Oskar (Scandinavian) a form of Oscar.
Osker

Osman (Turkish) ruler. (English) servant of God.

Osmar (English) divine; wonderful.

Osmond (English) divine protector.

Osric (English) divine ruler.

Ostin (Latin) a form of Austin.

Osvaldo (Spanish) a form of Oswald.
Osvald, Osvalda

Oswald (English) God's power; God's crest. See also Waldo.
Oswold

Oswaldo (Spanish) a form of Oswald.

Oswin (English) divine friend.

Osya (Russian) a familiar form of Osip.

Ota (Czech) prosperous.
Otik

Otadan (Native American) plentiful.

Otaktay (Lakota) kills many; strikes many.

Otek (Polish) a form of Otto.

Otello (Italian) a form of Othello.

Otem (Luo) born away from home.

Othello (Spanish) a form of Otto. Literature: the title character in the Shakespearean tragedy *Othello*.

Othman (German) wealthy.

Otis (Greek) keen of hearing. (German) son of Otto.
Oates, Odis, Otes, Otess, Ottis, Otys

Ottah (Nigerian) thin baby.

Ottar (Norwegian) point warrior; fright warrior.

Ottmar (Turkish) a form of Osman.

Otto (German) rich.
Otfried, Otho, Othon, Otik, Otilio, Otman, Oto, Otón, Otton, Ottone

Ottokar (German) happy warrior.

Otu (Native American) collecting seashells in a basket.

Ouray (Ute) arrow. Astrology: born under the sign of Sagittarius.

Oved (Hebrew) worshiper, follower.

Owen ☝ (Irish) born to nobility; young warrior. (Welsh) a form of Evan. *Owain, Owens, Owin*

Owney (Irish) elderly.

Oxford (English) place where oxen cross the river.

Oya (Moquelumnan) speaking of the jacksnipe.

Oystein (Norwegian) rock of happiness.

Oz (Hebrew) a short form of Osborn, Oswald.

Ozturk (Turkish) pure; genuine Turk.

Ozzie (English) a familiar form of Osborn, Oswald.

P

Paavo (Finnish) a form of Paul.

Pablo (Spanish) a form of Paul. *Pable, Paublo*

Pace (English) a form of Pascal.

Pacifico (Filipino) peaceful.

Paco (Italian) pack. (Spanish) a familiar form of Francisco. (Native American) bald eagle. See also Quico.

Paddy (Irish) a familiar form of Padraic, Patrick.

Paden (English) a form of Patton.

Padget (English) a form of Page.

Padraic (Irish) a form of Patrick.

Page (French) youthful assistant.

Paige (English) a form of Page.

Pakelika (Hawaiian) a form of Patrick.

Paki (African) witness.

Pal (Swedish) a form of Paul.

Pál (Hungarian) a form of Paul.

Palaina (Hawaiian) a form of Brian.

Palani (Hawaiian) a form of Frank.

Palash (Hindi) flowery tree.

Palben (Basque) blond.

Palladin (Native American) fighter.

Palmer (English) palm-bearing pilgrim.

Palti (Hebrew) God liberates.

Panas (Russian) immortal.

Panayiotis (Greek) a form of Peter.

Pancho (Spanish) a familiar form of Francisco, Frank.

Panos (Greek) a form of Peter.

Paolo (Italian) a form of Paul.

Paquito (Spanish) a familiar form of Paco.

Paramesh (Hindi) greatest. Religion: another name for the Hindu god Shiva.

Pardeep (Sikh) mystic light.

Paris (Greek) lover. Geography: the capital of France. Mythology: the prince of Troy who started the Trojan War by abducting Helen.
Paras, Paree, Parris

Park (Chinese) cypress tree. (English) a short form of Parker.

Parker (English) park keeper.

Parkin (English) little Peter.

Parlan (Scottish) a form of Bartholomew. See also Parthalán.

Parnell (French) little Peter. History: Charles Stewart Parnell was a famous Irish politician.

Parr (English) cattle enclosure, barn.

Parrish (English) church district.

Parry (Welsh) son of Harry.

Parth (Irish) a short form of Parthalán.

Parthalán (Irish) plowman. See also Bartholomew.

Parthenios (Greek) virgin. Religion: a Greek Orthodox saint.

Pascal (French) born on Easter or Passover.
Pascale, Pascalle, Paschal, Paschalis, Pascoe, Pascow

Pascual (Spanish) a form of Pascal.

Pasha (Russian) a form of Paul.

Pasquale (Italian) a form of Pascal.
Pascuale, Pasquel

Pastor (Latin) spiritual leader.

Pat (Native American) fish. (English) a short form of Patrick.

Patakusu (Moquelumnan) ant biting a person.

Patamon (Native American) raging.

Patek (Polish) a form of Patrick.

Patric (Latin) a form of Patrick.

Patrice (French) a form of Patrick.

Patricio (Spanish) a form of Patrick.

Patrick (Latin) nobleman. Religion: the patron saint of Ireland. See also Fitzpatrick, Ticho.
Patrik, Patrique, Patrizius, Pats, Patsy

Patrin (Gypsy) leaf trail.

Patryk (Latin) a form of Patrick.
Patryck

Patterson (Irish) son of Pat.

Pattin (Gypsy) leaf.

Patton (English) warrior's town.
Paton

Patwin (Native American) man.

Patxi (Basque, Teutonic) free.

Paul (Latin) small. Bible: Saul, later renamed Paul, was the first to bring the teachings of Christ to the Gentiles.
Pall, Pasko, Paulia, Paulis, Pauls, Paulus, Pavlos

Pauli (Latin) a familiar form of Paul.

Paulin (German, Polish) a form of Paul.

Paulino (Spanish) a form of Paul.

Paulo (Portuguese, Swedish, Hawaiian) a form of Paul.

Pavel (Russian) a form of Paul.

Pavit (Hindi) pious, pure.

Pawel (Polish) a form of Paul.

Pax (Latin) peaceful.

Paxton (Latin) peaceful town.

Payat (Native American) he is on his way.

Payden (English) a form of Payton.
Paydon

Payne (Latin) from the country.

Paytah (Lakota) fire.

Payton (English) a form of Patton.
Paiton, Pate

Paz (Spanish) a form of Pax.

Pearce (English) a form of Pierce.
Pears

Pearson (English) son of Peter. See also Pierson.
Pearsson

Peder (Scandinavian) a form of Peter.

Pedro (Spanish) a form of Peter.
Pedrín, Pedrín, Petronio

Peers (English) a form of Peter.

Peeter (Estonian) a form of Peter.
Peet

Peirce (English) a form of Peter.

Pekelo (Hawaiian) a form of Peter.

Peleke (Hawaiian) a form of Frederick.

Pelham (English) tannery town.

Pelí (Latin, Basque) happy.

Pell (English) parchment.
Pall

Pello (Greek, Basque) stone.

Pelton (English) town by a pool.

Pembroke (Welsh) headland. (French) wine dealer. (English) broken fence.

Peniamina (Hawaiian) a form of Benjamin.

Penley (English) enclosed meadow.

Penn (Latin) pen, quill. (English) enclosure. (German) a short form of Penrod.

Penrod (German) famous commander.

Pepa (Czech) a familiar form of Joseph.

Pepe (Spanish) a familiar form of José.

Pepin (German) determined; petitioner. History: Pepin the Short was an eighth-century king of the Franks.

Peppe (Italian) a familiar form of Joseph.

Per (Swedish) a form of Peter.

Perben (Greek, Danish) stone.

Percival (French) pierce the valley. Literature: a knight of the Round Table who first appears in Chrétien de Troyes's poem about the quest for the Holy Grail.

Percy (French) a familiar form of Percival.
Pearcey, Pearcy, Percey, Percie, Piercey, Piercy

Peregrine (Latin) traveler; pilgrim; falcon.

Pericles (Greek) just leader. History: an Athenian statesman.

Perico (Spanish) a form of Peter.

Perine (Latin) a short form of Peregrine.
Perion

Perkin (English) little Peter.

Pernell (French) a form of Parnell.
Perren

Perry (English) a familiar form of Peregrine, Peter.
Perrie

Perth (Scottish) thorn-bush thicket. Geography: a burgh in Scotland; a city in Australia.

Pervis (Latin) passage.

Pesach (Hebrew) spared. Religion: another name for Passover.

Petar (Greek) a form of Peter.

Pete (English) a short form of Peter.
Peat, Peet, Petey, Peti, Petie, Piet, Pit

Peter (Greek, Latin) small rock. Bible: Simon, renamed Peter, was the leader of the Twelve Apostles. See also Boutros, Ferris, Takis.
Panayiotos, Peadair, Perion, Péter, Peterke, Peterus, Petruno, Piaras, Pietrek, Piter, Pjeter

Peterson (English) son of Peter.
Peteris

Petiri (Shona) where we are.

Petr (Bulgarian) a form of Peter.

Petras (Lithuanian) a form of Peter.

Petros (Greek) a form of Peter.

Petru (Romanian) a form of Peter.

Petter (Norwegian) a form of Peter.

Peverell (French) piper.

Peyo (Spanish) a form of Peter.

Peyton (English) a form of Patton, Payton.

Pharaoh (Latin) ruler. History: a title for the ancient kings of Egypt.

Phelan (Irish) wolf.

Phelipe (Spanish) a form of Philip.

Phelix (Latin) a form of Felix.

Phelps (English) son of Phillip.

Phil (Greek) a short form of Philip, Phillip.

Philander (Greek) lover of mankind.

Philbert (English) a form of Filbert.

Philemon (Greek) kiss.

Philip (Greek) lover of horses. Bible: one of the Twelve Apostles. See also Felipe, Felippo, Filip, Fillippo, Filya, Fischel, Flip.
Philippo, Philly, Philp, Pilib, Pippo

Philipp (German) a form of Philip.
Phillipp

Philippe (French) a form of Philip.
Philipe, Phillepe

Phillip (Greek) a form of Philip.
Phillipp, Phillips

Phillipos (Greek) a form of Phillip.

Philly (American) a familiar form of Philip, Phillip.

Philo (Greek) love.

Phinean (Irish) a form of Finian.

Phineas (English) a form of Pinchas.

Phirun (Cambodian) rain.

Phoenix (Latin) phoenix, a legendary bird.

Phuok (Vietnamese) good.

Pias (Gypsy) fun.

Pickford (English) ford at the peak.

Pickworth (English) wood cutter's estate.

Pierce (English) a form of Peter.
Peerce, Piercy

Piero (Italian) a form of Peter.

Pierre (French) a form of Peter.
Peirre, Piere, Pierrot

Pierre-Luc (French) a combination of Pierre + Luc.
Piere

Piers (English) a form of Philip.

Pierson (English) son of Peter. See also Pearson.
Piersson

Pieter (Dutch) a form of Peter.

Pietro (Italian) a form of Peter.

Pilar (Spanish) pillar.

Pili (Swahili) second born.

Pilipo (Hawaiian) a form of Philip.

Pillan (Native American) supreme essence.

Pin (Vietnamese) faithful boy.

Pinchas (Hebrew) oracle. (Egyptian) dark skinned.

Pinky (American) a familiar form of Pinchas.

Pino (Italian) a form of Joseph.

Piñon (Tupi-Guarani) Mythology: the hunter who became the constellation Orion.

Pio (Latin) pious.

Piotr (Bulgarian) a form of Peter.

Pippin (German) father.

Piran (Irish) prayer. Religion: the patron saint of miners.

Pirro (Greek, Spanish) flaming hair.

Pista (Hungarian) a familiar form of István.

Piti (Spanish) a form of Peter.

Pitin (Spanish) a form of Felix.

Pitney (English) island of the strong-willed man.

Pitt (English) pit, ditch.

Placido (Spanish) serene.

Plato (Greek) broad shouldered. History: a famous Greek philosopher.

Platt (French) flatland.

Pol (Swedish) a form of Paul.

Poldi (German) a familiar form of Leopold.

Pollard (German) close-cropped head.

Pollock (English) a form of Pollux. Art: American artist Jackson Pollock was a leader of abstract expressionism.

Pollux (Greek) crown. Astronomy: one of the stars in the constellation Gemini.

Polo (Tibetan) brave wanderer. (Greek) a short form of Apollo. Culture: a game played on horseback. History: Marco Polo was a thirteenth-century Venetian explorer who traveled throughout Asia.

Pomeroy (French) apple orchard.

Ponce (Spanish) fifth. History: Juan Ponce de León of Spain searched for the Fountain of Youth in Florida.

Pony (Scottish) small horse.

Porfirio (Greek, Spanish) purple stone.

Porter (Latin) gatekeeper.

Poshita (Sanskrit) cherished.

Po Sin (Chinese) grandfather elephant.

Poul (Danish) a form of Paul.

Pov (Gypsy) earth.

Powa (Native American) wealthy.

Powell (English) alert.

Pramad (Hindi) rejoicing.

Pravat (Tai) history.

Prem (Hindi) love.

Prentice (English) apprentice.

Prescott (English) priest's cottage. See also Scott.

Presley (English) priest's meadow. Music: Elvis Presley was an influential American rock 'n' roll singer.

Preston (English) priest's estate.
Prestin

Prewitt (French) brave little one.

Price (Welsh) son of the ardent one.

Pricha (Tai) clever.

Primo (Italian) first; premier quality.

Prince (Latin) chief; prince.
Prence, Prinz, Prinze

Princeton (English) princely town.

Proctor (Latin) official, administrator.

Prokopios (Greek) declared leader.

Prosper (Latin) fortunate.

Pryor (Latin) head of the monastery; prior.

Pumeet (Sanskrit) pure.

Purdy (Hindi) recluse.

Purvis (French, English) providing food.

Putnam (English) dweller by the pond.

Pyotr (Russian) a form of Peter.

Q

Qabil (Arabic) able.

Qadim (Arabic) ancient.

Qadir (Arabic) powerful.

Qamar (Arabic) moon.

Qasim (Arabic) divider.

Qimat (Hindi) valuable.

Quaashie (Ewe) born on Sunday.

Quadarius (American) a combination of Quan + Darius.

Quade (Latin) fourth.

Quamaine (American) a combination of Quan + Jermaine.

Quan (Comanche) a short form of Quanah.

Quanah (Comanche) fragrant.

Quandre (American) a combination of Quan + Andre.

Quant (Greek) how much?

Quantavius (American) a combination of Quan + Octavius.

Quashawn (American) a combination of Quan + Shawn.

Qudamah (Arabic) courage.

Quenby (Scandinavian) a form of Quimby.

Quennell (French) small oak.

Quenten (Latin) a form of Quentin.

Quentin (Latin) fifth. (English) queen's town.
Qeuntin, Quantin, Quent, Quientin, Qwentin

Quenton (Latin) a form of Quentin.
Quienton

Quico (Spanish) a familiar form of many names.

Quigley (Irish) maternal side.

Quillan (Irish) cub.

Quimby (Scandinavian) woman's estate.

Quincy (French) fifth son's estate.
Quincey, Quinnsy, Quinsey

Quindarius (American) a combination of Quinn + Darius.

Quinlan (Irish) strong; well shaped.

Quinn (Irish) a short form of Quincy, Quinlan, Quinton.

Quintavius (American) a combination of Quinn + Octavius.

Quinten (Latin) a form of Quentin.

Quintin (Latin) a form of Quentin.

Quinton (Latin) a form of Quentin.
Quinneton, Quint, Quintan, Quintann, Quintus, Quiton, Qunton, Qwinton

Quiqui (Spanish) a familiar form of Enrique.

Quitin (Latin) a short form of Quinton.
Quiton

Quito (Spanish) a short form of Quinton.

Quon (Chinese) bright.

R

Raanan (Hebrew) fresh; luxuriant.

Rabi (Arabic) breeze.

Race (English) race.

Racham (Hebrew) compassionate.

Rad (English) advisor. (Slavic) happy.

Radbert (English) brilliant advisor.

Radburn (English) red brook; brook with reeds.

Radcliff (English) red cliff; cliff with reeds.

Radford (English) red ford; ford with reeds.

Radley (English) red meadow; meadow of reeds.

Radman (Slavic) joyful.

Radnor (English) red shore; shore with reeds.

Radomil (Slavic) happy peace.

Radoslaw (Polish) happy glory.

Raekwon (American) a form of Raquan.

Raequan (American) a form of Raquan.

Raeshawn (American) a form of Rashawn.

Rafael (Spanish) a form of Raphael. See also Falito.
Rafaelle, Rafaello, Rafaelo, Rafeal, Rafeé, Rafel, Rafello, Raffael, Raffaelo, Raffeal

Rafaele (Italian) a form of Raphael.

Rafal (Polish) a form of Raphael.

Rafe (English) a short form of Rafferty, Ralph.

Rafer (Irish) a short form of Rafferty.

Rafferty (Irish) rich, prosperous.

Rafi (Arabic) exalted. (Hebrew) a familiar form of Raphael.

Rafiq (Arabic) friend.

Raghib (Arabic) desirous.

Raghnall (Irish) wise power.

Ragnar (Norwegian) powerful army.

Rago (Hausa) ram.

Raheem (Punjabi) compassionate God.

Rahim (Arabic) merciful.
Raheim, Rahiem, Rahiim

Rahman (Arabic) compassionate.

Rahul (Arabic) traveler.

Raíd (Arabic) leader.

Raiden (Japanese) Mythology: the thunder god.

Raimondo (Italian) a form of Raymond.

Raimund (German) a form of Raymond.

Raimundo (Portuguese, Spanish) a form of Raymond.

Raine (English) lord; wise.

Rainer (German) counselor.

Rainey (German) a familiar form of Rainer.

Raini (Tupi-Guarani) Religion: the god who created the world.

Raishawn (American) a form of Rashawn.

Rajabu (Swahili) born in the seventh month of the Islamic calendar.

Rajah (Hindi) prince; chief.

Rajak (Hindi) cleansing.

Rajan (Hindi) a form of Rajah.

Rakeem (Punjabi) a form of Raheem.

Rakim (Arabic) a form of Rahim.

Rakin (Arabic) respectable.

Raktim (Hindi) bright red.

Raleigh (English) a form of Rawleigh.

Ralph (English) wolf counselor.
Radolphus, Ralf, Ralpheal, Ralphel

Ralphie (English) a familiar form of Ralph.

Ralston (English) Ralph's settlement.

Ram (Hindi) god; godlike. Religion: another name for the Hindu god Rama. (English) male sheep. A short form of Ramsey.

Ramadan (Arabic) ninth month of the Arabic year in the Islamic calendar.

Ramanan (Hindi) god; godlike.

Rami (Hindi, English) a form of Ram. (Spanish) a short form of Ramiro.

Ramiro (Portuguese, Spanish) supreme judge.

Ramón (Spanish) a form of Raymond.
Ramon, Remone, Romone

Ramone (Dutch) a form of Raymond.
Ramond, Remone

Ramsden (English) valley of rams.

Ramsey (English) ram's island.
Ramsay, Ramsy, Ramzee, Ramzi

Rance (English) a short form of Laurence. (American) a familiar form of Laurence.

Rand (English) shield; warrior.

Randal (English) a form of Randall.
Randale, Randel, Randle

Randall (English) a form of Randolph.
Randell

Randolph (English) shield wolf.
Randol, Randolf, Randolfo, Randolpho, Ranolph

Randy (English) a familiar form of Rand, Randall, Randolph.
Randey, Randi, Randie, Ranndy

Ranger (French) forest keeper.

Rangle (American) cowboy.

Rangsey (Cambodian) seven kinds of colors.

Rani (Hebrew) my song; my joy.

Ranieri (Italian) a form of Ragnar.

Ranjan (Hindi) delighted; gladdened.

Rankin (English) small shield.

Ransford (English) raven's ford.

Ransley (English) raven's field.

Ransom (Latin) redeemer. (English) son of the shield.

Raoul (French) a form of Ralph, Rudolph.

Raphael (Hebrew) God has healed.
Bible: one of the archangels. Art: a
prominent painter of the Renaissance.
See also Falito, Rafi.
*Rafel, Raphaél, Raphale, Raphaello,
Raphel, Raphello, Rephael*

Rapheal (Hebrew) a form of Raphael.
Rafel

Rapier (French) blade-sharp.

Raquan (American) a combination of
the prefix Ra + Quan.

Rashaad (Arabic) a form of Rashad.

Rashaan (American) a form of
Rashawn.
Rashann

Rashad (Arabic) wise counselor.
*Raashad, Rachad, Rachard, Raeshad,
Raishard, Rhashad*

Rashard (American) a form of Richard.

Rashaud (Arabic) a form of Rashad.
Rachaud, Rashaude

Rashaun (American) a form of
Rashawn.

Rashawn (American) a combination of
the prefix Ra + Shawn.
*Rashaw, Rashun, Raushan,
Raushawn, Rhashan, Rhashaun,
Rhashawn*

Rashean (American) a combination of
the prefix Ra + Sean.
Rashane, Rasheen, Rashien, Rashiena

Rasheed (Arabic) a form of Rashad.

Rashid (Arabic) a form of Rashad.

Rashida (Swahili) righteous.

Rashidi (Swahili) wise counselor.

Rashod (Arabic) a form of Rashad.
Rashoda, Rashodd, Rhashod

Rashon (American) a form of Rashawn.
Rashun

Rasmus (Greek, Danish) a short form of
Erasmus.

Raul (French) a form of Ralph.

Raulas (Lithuanian) a form of
Laurence.

Raulo (Lithuanian) a form of Laurence.

Raven (English) a short form of
Ravenel.

Ravenel (English) raven.

Ravi (Hindi) sun.
Ravee, Ravijot

Ravid (Hebrew) a form of Arvid.

Raviv (Hebrew) rain, dew.

Ravon (English) a form of Raven.

Rawdon (English) rough hill.

Rawleigh (English) deer meadow.

Rawlins (French) a form of Roland.

Ray (French) kingly, royal. (English) a
short form of Rayburn, Raymond. See
also Lei.
Rae, Raye

Rayan (Irish) a form of Ryan.

Rayburn (English) deer brook.

Rayce (English) a form of Race.

Rayden (Japanese) a form of Raiden.

Rayhan (Arabic) favored by God.

Rayi (Hebrew) my friend, my companion.

Raymon (English) a form of Raymond.
Rayman, Reamonn

Raymond (English) mighty; wise protector. See also Aymon.
Radmond, Raemond, Ramond, Ramonde, Raymand, Rayment, Raymont, Raymund, Raymunde

Raymundo (Spanish) a form of Raymond.
Raemondo

Raynaldo (Spanish) a form of Reynold.

Raynard (French) a form of Renard, Reynard.

Rayne (English) a form of Raine.

Raynor (Scandinavian) a form of Ragnar.

Rayshawn (American) a combination of Ray + Shawn.

Rayshod (American) a form of Rashad.

Rayvon (American) a form of Ravon.

Razi (Aramaic) my secret.

Read (English) a form of Reed, Reid.
Raeed

Reading (English) son of the red wanderer.

Reagan (Irish) little king. History: Ronald Wilson Reagan was the fortieth U.S. president.

Rebel (American) rebel.

Red (American) red, redhead.

Reda (Arabic) satisfied.

Redford (English) red river crossing.

Redley (English) red meadow; meadow with reeds.

Redmond (German) protecting counselor. (English) a form of Raymond.
Radmond

Redpath (English) red path.

Reece (Welsh) enthusiastic; stream.
Reice

Reed (English) a form of Reid.
Raeed

Reese (Welsh) a form of Reece.
Rees, Reis, Riess

Reeve (English) steward.

Reg (English) a short form of Reginald.

Regan (Irish) a form of Reagan.

Reggie (English) a familiar form of Reginald.

Reginal (English) a form of Reginald.
Reginale, Reginel

Reginald (English) king's advisor. A form of Reynold. See also Naldo.
Reggis, Reginaldo, Reginalt, Reginauld, Reginault, Regnauld

Regis (Latin) regal.

Rehema (Swahili) second-born.

Rei (Japanese) rule, law.

Reid (English) redhead.
Reide, Ried

Reidar (Norwegian) nest warrior.

Reilly (Irish) a form of Riley.

Reinaldo (Spanish) a form of Reynold.

Reinhart (German) a form of Reynard.

Reinhold (Swedish) a form of Ragnar.

Reku (Finnish) a form of Richard.

Remi, Rémi (French) forms of Remy.
Remie, Remmie

Remington (English) raven estate.

Remus (Latin) speedy, quick.
Mythology: Remus and his twin
brother, Romulus, founded Rome.

Remy (French) from Rheims, France.

Renaldo (Spanish) a form of Reynold.

Renard (French) a form of Reynard.

Renardo (Italian) a form of Reynard.

Renato (Italian) reborn.

Renaud (French) a form of Reynard,
Reynold.
Renault

Rendor (Hungarian) policeman.

René (French) reborn.
*Renat, Renatus, Renault, Rene,
Renee*

Renfred (English) lasting peace.

Renfrew (Welsh) raven woods.

Renjiro (Japanese) virtuous.

Renny (Irish) small but strong.
(French) a familiar form of René.

Reno (American) gambler. Geography: a
city in Nevada known for gambling.

Renshaw (English) raven woods.

Renton (English) settlement of the roe
deer.

Renzo (Latin) a familiar form of
Laurence. (Italian) a short form of
Lorenzo.

Reshad (American) a form of Rashad.

Reshawn (American) a combination of
the prefix Re + Shawn.

Reshean (American) a combination of
the prefix Re + Sean.

Reuben (Hebrew) behold a son.
*Reuban, Reubin, Rheuben, Rube,
Rubey, Rubin*

Reuven (Hebrew) a form of Reuben.

Rex (Latin) king.

Rexford (English) king's ford.

Rexton (English) king's town.

Rey (Spanish) a short form of Reynaldo,
Reynard, Reynold.

Reyes (English) a form of Reece.

Reyhan (Arabic) favored by God.

Reymond (English) a form of
Raymond.

Reymundo (Spanish) a form of
Raymond.

Reynaldo (Spanish) a form of Reynold.

Reynard (French) wise; bold, courageous.

Reynold (English) king's advisor. See
also Reginald.
Ranald

Réz (Hungarian) copper; redhead.

Rhett (Welsh) a form of Rhys. Literature: Rhett Butler was the hero of Margaret Mitchell's novel *Gone with the Wind.*

Rhodes (Greek) where roses grow. Geography: an island of southeast Greece.

Rhyan (Irish) a form of Rian.

Rhys (Welsh) a form of Reece, Reese.

Rian (Irish) little king.

Ric (Italian, Spanish) a short form of Rico.
Ricci

Ricardo (Portuguese, Spanish) a form of Richard.
Racardo, Recard, Ricaldo, Ricard, Ricardos, Riccardo, Ricciardo, Richardo

Rice (English) rich, noble. (Welsh) a form of Reece.

Rich (English) a short form of Richard.

Richard ☙ (English) a form of Richart. See also Aric, Dick, Juku, Likeke.
Richar, Richards, Richardson, Richer, Richerd, Richshard, Rickert, Rihardos, Rihards, Riocard, Riócard, Risa, Risardas, Rishard, Ristéard, Rostik, Rysio, Ryszard

Richart (German) rich and powerful ruler.

Richie (English) a familiar form of Richard.

Richman (English) powerful.

Richmond (German) powerful protector.

Rick (German, English) a short form of Cedric, Frederick, Richard.
Ricke, Ricks, Rik, Rykk

Rickard (Swedish) a form of Richard.

Ricker (English) powerful army.

Rickey (English) a familiar form of Richard, Rick, Riqui.

Rickie (English) a form of Ricky.
Ricki

Rickward (English) mighty guardian.

Ricky (English) a familiar form of Richard, Rick.
Ricci, Riczi, Rikki, Rikky

Rico (Spanish) a familiar form of Richard. (Italian) a short form of Enrico.

Rida (Arabic) favor.

Riddock (Irish) smooth field.

Rider (English) horseman.

Ridge (English) ridge of a cliff.

Ridgeley (English) meadow near the ridge.

Ridgeway (English) path along the ridge.

Ridley (English) meadow of reeds.

Riel (Spanish) a short form of Gabriel.

Rigby (English) ruler's valley.

Rigel (Arabic) foot. Astronomy: one of the stars in the constellation Orion.

Rigg (English) ridge.

Rigoberto (German) splendid; wealthy.

Rikard (Scandinavian) a form of
Richard.

Riki (Estonian) a form of Rick.
Rikki

Riley (Irish) valiant.
Rilley, Rilye

Rinaldo (Italian) a form of Reynold.

Ring (English) ring.

Ringo (Japanese) apple. (English) a
familiar form of Ring.

Rio (Spanish) river. Geography: Rio de
Janeiro is a city in Brazil.

Riordan (Irish) bard, royal poet.

Rip (Dutch) ripe; full grown. (English) a
short form of Ripley.

Ripley (English) meadow near the river.

Riqui (Spanish) a form of Rickey.

Rishad (American) a form of Rashad.

Rishawn (American) a combination of
the prefix Ri + Shawn.

Rishi (Hindi) sage.

Risley (English) meadow with shrubs.

Risto (Finnish) a short form of
Christopher.

Riston (English) settlement near the
shrubs.

Ritchard (English) a form of Richard.

Ritchie (English) a form of Richie.

Rithisak (Cambodian) powerful.

Ritter (German) knight; chivalrous.

River (English) river; riverbank.

Riyad (Arabic) gardens.

Roald (Norwegian) famous ruler.

Roan (English) a short form of Rowan.

Roar (Norwegian) praised warrior.

Roarke (Irish) famous ruler.

Rob (English) a short form of Robert.

Robbie (English) a familiar form of
Robert.
Robie, Robbi

Robby (English) a familiar form of
Robert.
Robbey, Robhy, Roby

Robert ☀ (English) famous brilliance.
See also Bobek, Dob, Lopaka.
*Rab, Rabbie, Raby, Riobard, Riobart,
Robars, Robart, Rober, Roberd,
Robers, Roibeárd, Rosertas, Ruberto,
Rudbert*

Roberto (Italian, Portuguese, Spanish)
a form of Robert.

Roberts, Robertson (English) son of
Robert.

Robin (English) a short form of Robert.
*Robben, Robbin, Robbyn, Roben,
Robinet, Robinn, Robins, Roibín*

Robinson (English) a form of Roberts.

Robyn (English) a form of Robin.

Rocco (Italian) rock.
Rocca, Roko, Roque

Rochester (English) rocky fortress.

Rock (English) a short form of
Rockwell.

Rockford (English) rocky ford.

Rockland (English) rocky land.

Rockledge (English) rocky ledge.

Rockley (English) rocky field.

Rockwell (English) rocky spring. Art: Norman Rockwell was a well-known twentieth-century American illustrator.

Rocky (American) a familiar form of Rocco, Rock.
Rockey, Rockie

Rod (English) a short form of Penrod, Roderick, Rodney.

Rodas (Greek, Spanish) a form of Rhodes.

Roddy (English) a familiar form of Roderick.

Roden (English) red valley. Art: Auguste Rodin was an innovative French sculptor.

Roderich (German) a form of Roderick.

Roderick (German) famous ruler. See also Broderick.
Rhoderick, Rodderick, Roderic, Roderigo, Roderik, Roderyck, Rodgrick, Rodricki, Rodrigue, Rodrugue, Roodney, Rurik

Rodger (German) a form of Roger.
Rodge, Rodgy

Rodman (German) famous man, hero.

Rodney (English) island clearing.
Rhodney, Rodnee, Rodni, Rodnie, Rodnne

Rodolfo (Spanish) a form of Rudolph.
Rodolpho, Rodulfo

Rodrick (German) a form of Roderick.
Roddrick, Rodric, Rodrich, Rodrique, Rodryck, Rodryk

Rodrigo (Italian, Spanish) a form of Roderick.

Rodriguez (Spanish) son of Rodrigo.

Rodrik (German) famous ruler.

Rodriquez (Spanish) a form of Rodriguez.

Roe (English) roe deer.
Rowe

Rogan (Irish) redhead.

Rogelio (Spanish) famous warrior.
Rojelio

Roger (German) famous spearman. See also Lokela.
Rog, Rogerick, Rogers, Rogiero, Rojelio, Rüdiger

Rogerio (Portuguese, Spanish) a form of Roger.

Rohan (Hindi) sandalwood.

Rohin (Hindi) upward path.

Rohit (Hindi) big and beautiful fish.

Roi (French) a form of Roy.

Roja (Spanish) red.

Roland (German) famous throughout the land.
Rolan, Rolanda, Rolek, Rolland, Rowe

Rolando (Portuguese, Spanish) a form of Roland.
Roldan, Roldán

Rolf (German) a form of Ralph. A short form of Rudolph.

Rolle (Swedish) a familiar form of Roland, Rolf.

Rollie (English) a familiar form of Roland.

Rollin (English) a form of Roland.

Rollo (English) a familiar form of Roland.

Rolon (Spanish) famous wolf.

Romain (French) a form of Roman.

Roman (Latin) from Rome, Italy.
Roma, Romman

Romanos (Greek) a form of Roman.

Romario (Italian) a form of Romeo.

Romel (Latin) a short form of Romulus.

Romello (Italian) of Romel.

Romeo (Italian) pilgrim to Rome; Roman. Literature: the title character of the Shakespearean play *Romeo and Juliet*.

Romero (Latin) a form of Romeo.

Romney (Welsh) winding river.

Romulus (Latin) citizen of Rome. Mythology: Romulus and his twin brother, Remus, founded Rome.

Romy (Italian) a familiar form of Roman.

Ron (Hebrew) a short form of Aaron, Ronald.
Ronn

Ronald (Scottish) a form of Reginald.
Ranald, Ronal, Ronney, Ronnold, Ronoldo

Ronaldo (Portuguese) a form of Ronald.

Rónán (Irish) seal.

Rondel (French) short poem.

Ronel (American) a form of Rondel.

Roni (Hebrew) my song; my joy.

Ronnie (Scottish) a familiar form of Ronald.
Ronie

Ronny (Scottish) a form of Ronnie.
Ronney

Ronson (Scottish) son of Ronald.

Ronté (American) a combination of Ron + the suffix Te.

Rooney (Irish) redhead.

Roosevelt (Dutch) rose field. History: Theodore and Franklin D. Roosevelt were the twenty-sixth and thirty-second U.S. presidents, respectively.
Rosevelt

Roper (English) rope maker.

Rory (German) a familiar form of Roderick. (Irish) red king.
Rorey

Rosalio (Spanish) rose.

Rosario (Portuguese) rosary.

Roscoe (Scandinavian) deer forest.
Rosco

Roshad (American) a form of Rashad.

Roshean (American) a combination of the prefix Ro + Sean.

Rosito (Filipino) rose.

Ross (Latin) rose. (Scottish) peninsula. (French) red.
Rosse, Rossell, Rossi, Rossie, Rossy

Rosswell (English) springtime of roses.

Rostislav (Czech) growing glory.

Roswald (English) field of roses.

Roth (German) redhead.

Rothwell (Scandinavian) red spring.

Rover (English) traveler.

Rowan (English) tree with red berries.
Rowe

Rowell (English) roe-deer well.

Rowland (English) rough land. (German) a form of Roland.

Rowley (English) rough meadow.

Rowson (English) son of the redhead.

Roxbury (English) rook's town or fortress.

Roy (French) king. A short form of Royal, Royce. See also Conroy, Delroy, Fitzroy, Leroy, Loe.

Royal (French) kingly, royal.

Royce (English) son of Roy.
Roice

Royden (English) rye hill.

Ruben (Hebrew) a form of Reuben.
Rube, Rubin

Rubert (Czech) a form of Robert.

Ruby (Hebrew) a familiar form of Reuben, Ruben.

Rudd (English) a short form of Rudyard.

Ruda (Czech) a form of Rudolph.
Rudek

Rudi (Spanish) a familiar form of Rudolph.

Rudo (Shona) love.

Rudolf (German) a form of Rudolph.

Rudolph (German) famous wolf. See also Dolf.
Rezsó, Rodolph, Rodolphe, Rudek, Rudolphus

Rudolpho (Italian) a form of Rudolph.

Rudy (English) a familiar form of Rudolph.
Ruddy, Ruddie, Rudey

Rudyard (English) red enclosure.

Rueben (Hebrew) a form of Reuben.

Ruff (French) redhead.

Rufin (Polish) redhead.
Rufino

Ruford (English) red ford; ford with reeds.

Rufus (Latin) redhead.
Rayfus, Rufe, Ruffis, Ruffus, Rufino, Rufo, Rufous

Rugby (English) rook fortress. History: a famous British school after which the sport of Rugby was named.

Ruggerio (Italian) a form of Roger.

Ruhakana (Rukiga) argumentative.

Ruland (German) a form of Roland.

Rumford (English) wide river crossing.

Runako (Shona) handsome.

Rune (German, Swedish) secret.

Runrot (Tai) prosperous.

Rupert (German) a form of Robert.

Ruperto (Italian) a form of Rupert.

Ruprecht (German) a form of Rupert.

Rush (French) redhead. (English) a
short form of Russell.

Rushford (English) ford with rushes.

Rusk (Spanish) twisted bread.

Ruskin (French) redhead.

Russ (French) a short form of Russell.

Russel (French) a form of Russell.

Russell (French) redhead; fox colored.
See also Lukela.
Roussell, Russelle

Rusty (French) a familiar form of Russell.
Rustie, Rustin, Rustyn

Rutger (Scandinavian) a form of Roger.

Rutherford (English) cattle ford.

Rutland (Scandinavian) red land.

Rutledge (English) red ledge.

Rutley (English) red meadow.

Ruy (Spanish) a short form of Roderick.

Ryan ☀ (Irish) little king.
*Rhyne, Ryane, Ryann, Ryin, Ryuan,
Ryun*

Rycroft (English) rye field.

Ryder (English) a form of Rider.

Rye (English) a short form of Ryder. A
grain used in cereal and whiskey.
(Gypsy) gentleman.

Ryen (Irish) a form of Ryan.

Ryerson (English) son of Rider, Ryder.

Ryese (English) a form of Reece.

Ryker (American) a surname used as a
first name.

Rylan (English) land where rye is
grown.
Rylin

Ryland (English) a form of Rylan.
Ryeland, Rylund

Ryle (English) rye hill.

Rylee (Irish) a form of Riley.
Rylie

Ryley (Irish) a form of Riley.

Ryman (English) rye seller.

Ryne (Irish) a form of Ryan.

Ryon (Irish) a form of Ryan.

S

Sabastian (Greek) a form of Sebastian.
Sabastien

Saber (French) sword.

Sabin (Basque) ancient tribe of central
Italy.

Sabiti (Rutooro) born on Sunday.

Sabola (Nguni) pepper.

Saburo (Japanese) third-born son.

Sacha (Russian) a form of Sasha.
Sascha

Sachar (Russian) a form of Zachary.

Saddam (Arabic) powerful ruler.

Sadiki (Swahili) faithful.

Sadler (English) saddle maker.

Safari (Swahili) born while traveling.

Safford (English) willow river crossing.

Sage (English) wise. Botany: an herb.

Sahale (Native American) falcon.

Sahen (Hindi) above.

Sahil (Native American) a form of Sahale.

Sahir (Hindi) friend.

Sa'id (Arabic) happy.

Sajag (Hindi) watchful.

Saka (Swahili) hunter.

Sakeri (Danish) a form of Zachary.

Sakima (Native American) king.

Sakuruta (Pawnee) coming sun.

Sal (Italian) a short form of Salvatore.

Salam (Arabic) lamb.

Salamon (Spanish) a form of Solomon.

Salaun (French) a form of Solomon.

Sálih (Arabic) right, good.

Salim (Swahili) peaceful.

Salím (Arabic) peaceful, safe.

Salmalin (Hindi) taloned.

Salman (Czech) a form of Salím, Solomon.

Salomon (French) a form of Solomon.

Salton (English) manor town; willow town.

Salvador (Spanish) savior.
Salvadore

Salvatore (Italian) savior. See also Xavier.
Salbatore, Sallie, Sally, Salvator, Salvidor, Sauveur

Sam (Hebrew) a short form of Samuel.
Samm, Sem

Sambo (American) a familiar form of Samuel.

Sameer (Arabic) a form of Samír.

Sami, Samy (Hebrew) forms of Sammy.
Sameeh, Sameh, Samie

Samír (Arabic) entertaining companion.

Samman (Arabic) grocer.

Sammy (Hebrew) a familiar form of Samuel.
Saamy, Samey, Sammee, Sammey, Sammie

Samo (Czech) a form of Samuel.

Samson (Hebrew) like the sun. Bible: a judge and powerful warrior betrayed by Delilah.
Sampson, Sansao, Sansom

Samual (Hebrew) a form of Samuel.

Samuel ☼ (Hebrew) heard God; asked of God. Bible: a famous Old Testament prophet and judge. See also Kamuela, Zamiel, Zanvil.
Samael, Samaru, Samauel, Samaul, Sameul, Samiel, Sammail, Sammel, Sammuel, Samouel, Samu, Samuelis, Samuello, Samuil, Samuka, Samule, Samvel, Sanko, Saumel, Schmuel, Simuel, Sombhairle, Zamuel

Samuele (Italian) a form of Samuel.

Samuru (Japanese) a form of Samuel.

Sanat (Hindi) ancient.

Sanborn (English) sandy brook.

Sanchez (Latin) a form of Sancho.

Sancho (Latin) sanctified; sincere. Literature: Sancho Panza was Don Quixote's squire.

Sandeep (Punjabi) enlightened.

Sander (English) a short form of Alexander, Lysander.

Sanders (English) son of Sander.

Sándor (Hungarian) a short form of Alexander.

Sandro (Greek, Italian) a short form of Alexander.

Sandy (English) a familiar form of Alexander.
Sande, Sandey, Sandie

Sanford (English) sandy river crossing.

Sani (Hindi) the planet Saturn. (Navajo) old.

Sanjay (American) a combination of Sanford + Jay.

Sanjiv (Hindi) long lived.

Sankar (Hindi) a form of Shankara, another name for the Hindu god Shiva.

Sansón (Spanish) a form of Samson.

Santana (Spanish) History: Antonio López de Santa Anna was a Mexican general and political leader.

Santiago (Spanish) a form of James.

Santino (Spanish) a form of Santonio.

Santo (Italian, Spanish) holy.

Santon (English) sandy town.

Santonio (Spanish) Geography: a short form of San Antonio, a city in Texas.

Santos (Spanish) saint.

Santosh (Hindi) satisfied.

Sanyu (Luganda) happy.

Saqr (Arabic) falcon.

Saquan (American) a combination of the prefix Sa + Quan.

Sarad (Hindi) born in the autumn.

Sargent (French) army officer.

Sarito (Spanish) a form of Caesar.

Sariyah (Arabic) clouds at night.

Sarngin (Hindi) archer; protector.

Sarojin (Hindi) like a lotus.

Sasha (Russian) a short form of Alexander.
Sausha

Sasson (Hebrew) joyful.

Satchel (French) small bag.

Satordi (French) Saturn.

Saul (Hebrew) asked for, borrowed.
Bible: in the Old Testament, a king of
Israel and the father of Jonathan; in
the New Testament, Saint Paul's origi-
nal name was Saul.
Saül, Shaul

Saverio (Italian) a form of Xavier.

Saville (French) willow town.

Savon (Spanish) a treeless plain.

Saw (Burmese) early.

Sawyer (English) wood worker.

Sax (English) a short form of Saxon.

Saxon (English) swordsman. History:
the Roman name for the Teutonic
raiders who ravaged the Roman British
coasts.

Sayer (Welsh) carpenter.

Sayyid (Arabic) master.

Scanlon (Irish) little trapper.

Schafer (German) shepherd.

Schmidt (German) blacksmith.

Schneider (German) tailor.

Schön (German) handsome.

Schuyler (Dutch) sheltering.
Schuylar, Scoy, Scy, Skuyler, Sky

Schyler (Dutch) a form of Schuyler.
Schylar

Scorpio (Latin) dangerous, deadly.
Astronomy: a southern constellation
near Libra and Sagittarius. Astrology:
the eighth sign of the zodiac.

Scott (English) from Scotland. A familiar form of Prescott.
Scot, Scotto

Scottie (English) a familiar form of
Scott.
Scotie, Scotti

Scotty (English) a familiar form of
Scott.

Scoville (French) Scott's town.

Scully (Irish) town crier.

Seabert (English) shining sea.

Seabrook (English) brook near the sea.

Seamus (Irish) a form of James.
Seamas

Sean ☀ (Irish) a form of John.
*Seaghan, Séan, Seán, Seanán, Seane,
Seann, Shaan, Siôn*

Searlas (Irish, French) a form of
Charles.

Searle (English) armor.

Seasar (Latin) a form of Caesar.

Seaton (English) town near the sea.

Sebastian ☀ (Greek) venerable.
(Latin) revered.
*Bastian, Sabastien, Sebastiano,
Sebastin, Sebbie, Sebestyén, Sebo,
Sepasetiano*

Sebastien, Sébastien (French) forms
of Sebastian.
Sebasten

Sebastion (Greek) a form of Sebastian.

Sedgely (English) sword meadow.

Sedric (Irish) a form of Cedric.

Seeley (English) blessed.

Sef (Egyptian) yesterday. Mythology: one of the two lions that make up the Akeru, guardian of the gates of morning and night.

Sefton (English) village of rushes.

Sefu (Swahili) sword.

Seger (English) sea spear; sea warrior.

Segun (Yoruba) conqueror.

Segundo (Spanish) second.

Seibert (English) bright sea.

Seif (Arabic) religion's sword.

Seifert (German) a form of Siegfried.

Sein (Basque) innocent.

Sekaye (Shona) laughter.

Selby (English) village by the mansion.

Seldon (English) willow tree valley.

Selig (German) a form of Seeley.

Selwyn (English) friend from the palace.

Semanda (Luganda) cow clan.

Semer (Ethiopian) a form of George.

Semon (Greek) a form of Simon.

Sempala (Luganda) born in prosperous times.

Sen (Japanese) wood fairy.

Sener (Turkish) bringer of joy.

Senior (French) lord.

Sennett (French) elderly.

Senon (Spanish) living.

Senwe (African) dry as a grain stalk.

Sepp (German) a form of Joseph.

Septimus (Latin) seventh.

Serafino (Portuguese) a form of Seraphim.

Seraphim (Hebrew) fiery, burning. Bible: the highest order of angels, known for their zeal and love.

Sereno (Latin) calm, tranquil.

Serge (Latin) attendant.
Seargeob, Serg, Sergios, Sergius, Sergiusz, Serguel, Sirgio, Sirgios

Sergei (Russian) a form of Serge.

Sergio (Italian) a form of Serge.
Serginio, Serigo, Serjio

Servando (Spanish) to serve.

Seth ☙ (Hebrew) appointed. Bible: the third son of Adam.
Set, Sethan, Sethe, Shet

Setimba (Luganda) river dweller. Geography: a river in Uganda.

Seumas (Scottish) a form of James.

Severiano (Italian) a form of Séverin.

Séverin (French) severe.

Severn (English) boundary.

Sevilen (Turkish) beloved.

Seward (English) sea guardian.

Sewati (Moquelumnan) curved bear claws.

Sexton (English) church official; sexton.

Sextus (Latin) sixth.

Seymour (French) prayer. Religion: name honoring Saint Maur. See also Maurice.

Shabouh (Armenian) king, noble. History: a fourth-century Persian king.

Shad (Punjabi) happy-go-lucky. *Shadd*

Shadi (Arabic) singer.

Shadrach (Babylonian) god; godlike. Bible: one of three companions who emerged unharmed from the fiery furnace of Babylon.

Shadwell (English) shed by a well.

Shah (Persian) king. History: a title for rulers of Iran.

Shaheem (American) a combination of Shah + Raheem.

Shahid (Arabic) a form of Sa'id.

Shai (Hebrew) a short form of Yeshaya.

Shaiming (Chinese) life; sunshine.

Shaine (Irish) a form of Sean.

Shaka (Zulu) founder, first. History: Shaka Zulu was the founder of the Zulu empire.

Shakeel (Arabic) a form of Shaquille.

Shakir (Arabic) thankful.

Shakur (Arabic) a form of Shakir.

Shalom (Hebrew) peace.

Shalya (Hindi) throne.

Shaman (Sanskrit) holy man, mystic, medicine man.

Shamar (Hebrew) a form of Shamir.

Shamir (Hebrew) precious stone.

Shamus (American) slang for detective.

Shan (Irish) a form of Shane.

Shanahan (Irish) wise, clever.

Shandy (English) rambunctious.

Shane (Irish) a form of Sean. *Shayn*

Shangobunni (Yoruba) gift from Shango.

Shanley (Irish) small; ancient.

Shannon (Irish) small and wise. *Shanan, Shannan, Shannen, Shanon*

Shantae (French) a form of Chante.

Shap (English) a form of Shep.

Shaquan (American) a combination of the prefix Sha + Quan.

Shaquell (American) a form of Shaquille.

Shaquille (Arabic) handsome.

Shaquon (American) a combination of the prefix Sha + Quon.

Sharad (Pakistani) autumn.

Sharíf (Arabic) honest; noble.
*Shareef, Sharef, Shareff, Sharif, Shariff,
Shariyf, Sharyif*

Sharod (Pakistani) a form of Sharad.

Sharron (Hebrew) flat area, plain.

Shattuck (English) little shad fish.

Shaun (Irish) a form of Sean.
*Shaughan, Shaughn, Shauna,
Shaunahan, Shaune, Shaunn*

Shavar (Hebrew) comet.
Shavit

Shavon (American) a combination of
the prefix Sha + Yvon.
Shawon

Shaw (English) grove.

Shawn (Irish) a form of Sean.
*Shawen, Shawne, Shawnee, Shawnn,
Shawon*

Shawnta (American) a combination of
Shawn + the suffix Ta.

Shay (Irish) a form of Shea.
Shae, Shaye, Shey

Shayan (Cheyenne) a form of
Cheyenne.

Shayne (Hebrew) a form of Sean.
Shayn

Shea (Irish) courteous.

Shedrick (Babylonian) a form of
Shadrach.

Sheehan (Irish) little; peaceful.

Sheffield (English) crooked field.

Shel (English) a short form of Shelby,
Sheldon, Shelton.

Shelby (English) ledge estate.
Shelbey, Shelbie, Shell, Shelly

Sheldon (English) farm on the ledge.
Shelden, Sheldin, Shell, Shelly

Shelley (English) a familiar form of
Shelby, Sheldon, Shelton. Literature:
Percy Bysshe Shelley was a nineteenth-
century British poet.
Shell, Shelly

Shelton (English) town on a ledge.

Shem (Hebrew) name; reputation.
(English) a short form of Samuel.
Bible: Noah's oldest son.

Shen (Egyptian) sacred amulet.
(Chinese) meditation.

Shep (English) a short form of
Shepherd.

Shepherd (English) shepherd.

Shepley (English) sheep meadow.

Sherborn (English) clear brook.

Sheridan (Irish) wild.

Sherill (English) shire on a hill.

Sherlock (English) light haired.
Literature: Sherlock Holmes is a
famous British detective character,
created by Sir Arthur Conan Doyle.

Sherman (English) sheep shearer;
resident of a shire.
*Scherman, Schermann, Sherm,
Shermann, Shermie, Shermy*

Sherrod (English) clearer of the land.

Sherwin (English) swift runner, one
who cuts the wind.

Sherwood (English) bright forest.

Shihab (Arabic) blaze.

Shilín (Chinese) intellectual.

Shiloh (Hebrew) God's gift.

Shimon (Hebrew) a form of Simon.

Shimshon (Hebrew) a form of Samson.

Shing (Chinese) victory.

Shipton (English) sheep village; ship village.

Shiquan (American) a combination of the prefix Shi + Quan.

Shiro (Japanese) fourth-born son.

Shiva (Hindi) life and death. Religion: the most common name for the Hindu god of destruction and reproduction.

Shlomo (Hebrew) a form of Solomon.

Shmuel (Hebrew) a form of Samuel.

Shneur (Yiddish) senior.

Shon (German) a form of Schön. (American) a form of Sean.

Shunnar (Arabic) pheasant.

Si (Hebrew) a short form of Silas, Simon.

Sid (French) a short form of Sidney.

Siddel (English) wide valley.

Siddhartha (Hindi) History: Siddhartha Gautama was the original name of Buddha, the founder of Buddhism.

Sidney (French) from Saint-Denis, France.
Cydney, Sidnee, Sidon, Sydny

Sidonio (Spanish) a form of Sidney.

Sidwell (English) wide stream.

Siegfried (German) victorious peace. See also Zigfrid, Ziggy.

Sierra (Irish) black. (Spanish) saw-toothed.

Sig (German) a short form of Siegfried, Sigmund.

Sigifredo (German) a form of Siegfried.

Siggy (German) a familiar form of Siegfried, Sigmund.

Sigmund (German) victorious protector. See also Ziggy, Zsigmond, Zygmunt.

Sigurd (German, Scandinavian) victorious guardian.

Sigwald (German) victorious leader.

Silas (Latin) a short form of Silvan.
Sias

Silvan (Latin) forest dweller.

Silvano (Italian) a form of Silvan.

Silvester (Latin) a form of Sylvester.

Silvestro (Italian) a form of Sylvester.

Silvio (Italian) a form of Silvan.

Simão (Portuguese) a form of Samuel.

Simba (Swahili) lion. (Yao) a short form of Lisimba.
Sim

Simcha (Hebrew) joyful.

Simeon (French) a form of Simon.
Simone

Simms (Hebrew) son of Simon.
Simm

Simmy (Hebrew) a familiar form of Simcha, Simon.

Simon (Hebrew) he heard. Bible: one of the Twelve Disciples. See also Symington, Ximenes.
Saimon, Samien, Sim, Simao, Simen, Simion, Simm, Simmon, Simmonds, Simmons, Simonas, Simone, Simson, Simyon, Síomón

Simpson (Hebrew) son of Simon.
Simson

Sinclair (French) prayer. Religion: name honoring Saint Clair.

Singh (Hindi) lion.

Sinjon (English) saint, holy man. Religion: name honoring Saint John.

Sipatu (Moquelumnan) pulled out.

Sipho (Zulu) present.

Siraj (Arabic) lamp, light.

Siseal (Irish) a form of Cecil.

Sisi (Fante) born on Sunday.

Siva (Hindi) a form of Shiva.

Sivan (Hebrew) ninth month of the Jewish year.

Siwatu (Swahili) born during a time of conflict.

Siwili (Native American) long fox's tail.

Skah (Lakota) white.

Skee (Scandinavian) projectile.

Skeeter (English) swift.

Skelly (Irish) storyteller.
Shell

Skelton (Dutch) shell town.

Skerry (Scandinavian) stony island.

Skip (Scandinavian) a short form of Skipper.

Skipper (Scandinavian) shipmaster.

Skiriki (Pawnee) coyote.

Skule (Norwegian) hidden.

Skye (Dutch) a short form of Skylar, Skyler, Skylor.
Sky

Skylar (Dutch) a form of Schuyler.
Skyelar

Skyler (Dutch) a form of Schuyler.
Skyeler, Skylee

Skylor (Dutch) a form of Schuyler.

Slade (English) child of the valley.

Slane (Czech) salty.

Slater (English) roof slater.

Slava (Russian) a short form of Stanislav, Vladislav, Vyacheslav.

Slawek (Polish) a short form of Radoslaw.

Slevin (Irish) mountaineer.

Sloan (Irish) warrior.

Smedley (English) flat meadow.

Smith (English) blacksmith.

Snowden (English) snowy hill.

Socrates (Greek) wise, learned. History: a famous ancient Greek philosopher.

Sofian (Arabic) devoted.

Sohrab (Persian) ancient hero.

Soja (Yoruba) soldier.

Sol (Hebrew) a short form of Saul, Solomon.

Solly (Hebrew) a familiar form of Saul, Solomon.

Solomon (Hebrew) peaceful. Bible: a king of Israel famous for his wisdom. See also Zalman.
Salamen, Salamun, Salomo, Selim, Shelomah, Solamb, Solaman, Solmon, Soloman, Solomonas

Solon (Greek) wise. History: a noted ancient Athenian lawmaker.

Somerset (English) place of the summer settlers. Literature: William Somerset Maugham was a well-known British writer.

Somerville (English) summer village.

Son (Vietnamese) mountain. (Native American) star. (English) son, boy. A short form of Madison, Orson.

Songan (Native American) strong.

Sonny (English) a familiar form of Grayson, Madison, Orson, Son.
Sonnie

Sono (Akan) elephant.

Sören (Danish) thunder; war.

Sorrel (French) reddish brown.

Soroush (Persian) happy.

Soterios (Greek) savior.

Southwell (English) south well.

Sovann (Cambodian) gold.

Sowande (Yoruba) wise healer sought me out.

Spalding (English) divided field.

Spangler (German) tinsmith.

Spark (English) happy.

Spear (English) spear carrier.

Speedy (English) quick; successful.

Spence (English) a short form of Spencer.
Spense

Spencer (English) dispenser of provisions.
Spencre

Spenser (English) a form of Spencer. Literature: Edmund Spenser was the British poet who wrote *The Faerie Queen*.
Spanser, Spense

Spike (English) ear of grain; long nail.

Spiro (Greek) round basket; breath.

Spoor (English) spur maker.

Sproule (English) energetic.

Spurgeon (English) shrub.

Spyros (Greek) a form of Spiro.

Squire (English) knight's assistant; large landholder.

Stacey, Stacy (English) familiar forms of Eustace.
Stace, Stacee

Stafford (English) riverbank landing.

Stamford (English) a form of Stanford.

Stamos (Greek) a form of Stephen.

Stan (Latin, English) a short form of
   Stanley.

Stanbury (English) stone fortification.

Stancio (Spanish) a form of
   Constantine.

Stancliff (English) stony cliff.

Standish (English) stony parkland.
   History: Miles Standish was a leader in
   colonial America.

Stane (Slavic) a short form of
   Stanislaus.

Stanfield (English) stony field.

Stanford (English) rocky ford.

Stanislaus (Latin) stand of glory. See
   also Lao, Tano.

Stanislav (Slavic) a form of Stanislaus.
   See also Slava.

Stanley (English) stony meadow.
   Sianlea, Stanlee, Stanleigh, Stanly

Stanmore (English) stony lake.

Stannard (English) hard as stone.

Stanton (English) stony farm.

Stanway (English) stony road.

Stanwick (English) stony village.

Stanwood (English) stony woods.

Starbuck (English) challenger of fate.
   Literature: a character in Herman
   Melville's novel *Moby-Dick*.

Stark (German) strong, vigorous.

Starling (English) bird.

Starr (English) star.

Stasik (Russian) a familiar form of
   Stanislaus.

Stasio (Polish) a form of Stanislaus.

Stavros (Greek) a form of Stephen.

Steadman (English) owner of a farmstead.

Steel (English) like steel.

Steen (German, Danish) stone.

Steeve (Greek) a short form of Steeven.

Steeven (Greek) a form of Steven.
   Steevan

Stefan (German, Polish, Swedish) a
   form of Stephen.
   *Steafeán, Stefane, Stefanson, Stefaun,
   Stefawn*

Stefano (Italian) a form of Stephen.

Stefanos (Greek) a form of Stephen.
   Stephano, Stephanos

Stefen (Norwegian) a form of Stephen.
   Steffen, Steffin, Stefin

Steffan (Swedish) a form of Stefan.
   Staffan

Stefon (Polish) a form of Stephon.
   Staffon, Steffon, Stefone

Stein (German) a form of Steen.

Steinar (Norwegian) rock warrior.

Stepan (Russian) a form of Stephen.

Steph (English) a short form of
   Stephen.

Stephan (Greek) a form of Stephen.
   *Stephanas, Stephano, Stephanos,
   Stephanus*

Stéphane (French) a form of Stephen.
Stefane, Stephane, Stepháne

Stephen (Greek) crowned. See also
Estében, Estebe, Estevan, Estevao,
Étienne, István, Szczepan, Tapani, Teb,
Teppo, Tiennot.
*Stenya, Stepanos, Stephanas, Stephens,
Stephenson, Stephfan, Stephin, Stepven*

Stephon (Greek) a form of Stephen.
Stepfon, Stephone

Sterling (English) valuable; silver
penny. A form of Starling.

Stern (German) star.

Sterne (English) austere.

Stetson (Danish) stepson.

Stevan (Greek) a form of Steven.

Steve (Greek) a short form of Stephen,
Steven.
Steave, Stevy

Steven ☙ (Greek) a form of Stephen.
Steiven

Stevens (English) son of Steven.

Stevie (English) a familiar form of
Stephen, Steven.
Stevey, Stevy

Stevin, Stevon (Greek) forms of
Steven.

Stewart (English) a form of Stuart.
Steward

Stian (Norwegian) quick on his feet.

Stig (Swedish) mount.

Stiggur (Gypsy) gate.

Stillman (English) quiet.

Sting (English) spike of grain.

Stockman (English) tree-stump remover.

Stockton (English) tree-stump town.

Stockwell (English) tree-stump well.

Stoddard (English) horse keeper.

Stoffel (German) a short form of
Christopher.

Stoker (English) furnace tender.

Stone (English) stone.

Storm (English) tempest, storm.

Storr (Norwegian) great.

Stover (English) stove tender.

Stowe (English) hidden; packed away.

Strahan (Irish) minstrel.

Stratford (English) bridge over the river.
Literature: Stratford-upon-Avon was
Shakespeare's birthplace.

Stratton (Scottish) river valley town.

Strephon (Greek) one who turns.

Strom (Greek) bed, mattress. (German)
stream.

Strong (English) powerful.

Stroud (English) thicket.

Struthers (Irish) brook.

Stu (English) a short form of Stewart,
Stuart.

Stuart (English) caretaker, steward.
History: a Scottish and English royal
family.
Stuarrt

Studs (English) rounded nail heads; shirt ornaments; male horses used for breeding. History: Louis "Studs" Terkel is a famous American journalist.

Styles (English) stairs put over a wall to help cross it.

Subhi (Arabic) early morning.

Suck Chin (Korean) unshakable rock.

Sudi (Swahili) lucky.

Sued (Arabic) master, chief.

Suffield (English) southern field.

Sugden (English) valley of sows.

Suhail (Arabic) gentle.

Suhuba (Swahili) friend.

Sukru (Turkish) grateful.

Sulaiman (Arabic) a form of Solomon.

Sullivan (Irish) black eyed.

Sully (Irish) a familiar form of Sullivan. (French) stain, tarnish. (English) south.

Sultan (Swahili) ruler.

Sum (Tai) appropriate.

Summit (English) peak, top.

Sumner (English) church officer; summoner.

Sundeep (Punjabi) light; enlightened. *Sundip*

Sunny (English) sunny, sunshine.

Sunreep (Hindi) pure.

Sutcliff (English) southern cliff.

Sutherland (Scandinavian) southern land.

Sutton (English) southern town.

Sven (Scandinavian) youth.

Swaggart (English) one who sways and staggers.

Swain (English) herdsman; knight's attendant.

Swaley (English) winding stream.

Sweeney (Irish) small hero.

Swinbourne (English) stream used by swine.

Swindel (English) valley of the swine.

Swinfen (English) swine's mud.

Swinford (English) swine's crossing.

Swinton (English) swine town.

Sy (Latin) a short form of Sylas, Symon.

Sydney (French) a form of Sidney.

Syed (Arabic) happy.

Sying (Chinese) star.

Sylas (Latin) a form of Silas.

Sylvain (French) a form of Silvan, Sylvester.

Sylvester (Latin) forest dweller. *Sly, Syl, Sylverster, Sylvestre*

Symington (English) Simon's town, Simon's estate.

Symon (Greek) a form of Simon.

Szczepan (Polish) a form of Stephen.

Szygfrid (Hungarian) a form of Siegfried.

Szymon (Polish) a form of Simon.

T

Taaveti (Finnish) a form of David.

Tab (German) shining, brilliant. (English) drummer.

Tabari (Arabic) he remembers.

Tabib (Turkish) physician.

Tabo (Spanish) a short form of Gustave.

Tabor (Persian) drummer. (Hungarian) encampment.

Tad (Welsh) father. (Greek, Latin) a short form of Thaddeus.
Tadd, Taddy, Tade, Tadek, Tadey

Tadan (Native American) plentiful.

Tadarius (American) a combination of the prefix Ta + Darius.

Taddeo (Italian) a form of Thaddeus.

Taddeus (Greek, Latin) a form of Thaddeus.

Tadi (Omaha) wind.

Tadzi (Carrier) loon.

Tadzio (Polish, Spanish) a form of Thaddeus.

Taffy (Welsh) a form of David. (English) a familiar form of Taft.

Taft (English) river.

Tage (Danish) day.

Taggart (Irish) son of the priest.

Tahír (Arabic) innocent, pure.

Tai (Vietnamese) weather; prosperous; talented.

Taima (Native American) born during a storm.

Taishawn (American) a combination of Tai + Shawn.

Tait (Scandinavian) a form of Tate.

Taiwan (Chinese) island; island dweller. Geography: a country off the coast of China.

Taiwo (Yoruba) first-born of twins.

Taj (Urdu) crown.

Tajo (Spanish) day.

Tajuan (American) a combination of the prefix Ta + Juan.

Takeo (Japanese) strong as bamboo.

Takis (Greek) a familiar form of Peter.

Takoda (Lakota) friend to everyone.

Tal (Hebrew) dew; rain.

Talbert (German) bright valley.

Talbot (French) boot maker.

Talcott (English) cottage near the lake.

Tale (Tswana) green.

Talen (English) a form of Talon.

Talib (Arabic) seeker.

Taliesin (Welsh) radiant brow.

Taliki (Hausa) fellow.

Talli (Delaware) legendary hero.

Talmadge (English) lake between two towns.

Talmai (Aramaic) mound; furrow.

Talman (Aramaic) injured; oppressed.

Talon (French, English) claw, nail.
Tallin, Tallon

Talor (English) a form of Tal, Taylor.

Tam (Vietnamese) number eight. (Hebrew) honest. (English) a short form of Thomas.

Taman (Slavic) dark, black.

Tamar (Hebrew) date; palm tree.

Tambo (Swahili) vigorous.

Tamir (Arabic) tall as a palm tree.

Tammy (English) a familiar form of Thomas.

Tamson (Scandinavian) son of Thomas.

Tan (Burmese) million. (Vietnamese) new.

Tanek (Greek) immortal. See also Atek.

Taneli (Finnish) God is my judge.

Taner (English) a form of Tanner.

Tanguy (French) warrior.

Tani (Japanese) valley.

Tanmay (Sanskrit) engrossed.

Tanner (English) leather worker; tanner.
Tanery, Tann, Tannor

Tannin (English) tan colored; dark.

Tanny (English) a familiar form of Tanner.

Tano (Spanish) camp glory. (Ghanaian) Geography: a river in Ghana. (Russian) a short form of Stanislaus.

Tanton (English) town by the still river.

Tapan (Sanskrit) sun; summer.

Tapani (Finnish) a form of Stephen.

Täpko (Kiowa) antelope.

Taquan (American) a combination of the prefix Ta + Quan.

Tarak (Sanskrit) star; protector.

Taran (Sanskrit) heaven.

Tarek (Arabic) a form of Táriq.
Tareek

Tarell (German) a form of Terrell.

Taren (American) a form of Taron.

Tarif (Arabic) uncommon.

Tarik (Arabic) a form of Táriq.
Tarick

Táriq (Arabic) conqueror. History: Tariq bin Ziyad was the Muslim general who conquered Spain.
Tareck, Tarreq, Tereik

Tarleton (English) Thor's settlement.

Taro (Japanese) first-born male.

Taron (American) a combination of Tad + Ron.

Tarrant (Welsh) thunder.

Tarun (Sanskrit) young, youth.

Tarver (English) tower; hill; leader.

Taryn (American) a form of Taron.

Tas (Gypsy) bird's nest.

Tashawn (American) a combination of the prefix Ta + Shawn.

Tass (Hungarian) ancient mythology name.

Tasunke (Dakota) horse.

Tate (Scandinavian, English) cheerful. (Native American) long-winded talker. *Tayte*

Tatius (Latin) king, ruler. History: a Sabine king.

Tatum (English) cheerful.

Tau (Tswana) lion.

Tauno (Finnish) a form of Donald.

Taurean (Latin) strong; forceful. Astrology: born under the sign of Taurus.

Taurus (Latin) Astrology: the second sign of the zodiac. *Tauris*

Tavares (Aramaic) a form of Tavor. *Tarvarres, Tavarres, Taveress*

Tavaris (Aramaic) a form of Tavor. *Tarvaris, Tavar, Tavaras, Tavari, Tavarian, Tavarius, Tavarri, Tavarris, Tavars, Tavarse, Tavarus, Tevaris, Tevarus*

Tavey (Latin) a familiar form of Octavio.

Tavi (Aramaic) good.

Tavian (Latin) a form of Octavio.

Tavish (Scottish) a form of Thomas.

Tavo (Slavic) a short form of Gustave.

Tavon (American) a form of Tavian.

Tavor (Aramaic) misfortune.

Tawno (Gypsy) little one.

Tayib (Hindi) good; delicate.

Tayler (English) a form of Taylor. *Tailer, Teyler*

Taylor (English) tailor. *Tailor, Taylour*

Tayshawn (American) a combination of Taylor + Shawn.

Tayvon (American) a form of Tavian.

Taz (Arabic) shallow ornamental cup.

Tazio (Italian) a form of Tatius.

Teagan (Irish) a form of Teague.

Teague (Irish) bard, poet.

Tearence (Latin) a form of Terrence. *Tearance, Tearrance*

Tearlach (Scottish) a form of Charles.

Tearle (English) stern, severe.

Teasdale (English) river dweller. Geography: a river in England.

Teb (Spanish) a short form of Stephen.

Ted (English) a short form of Edward, Edwin, Theodore. *Tedd, Tedek, Tedik, Tedson*

Teddy (English) a familiar form of Edward, Theodore. *Teddey, Teddie*

Tedmund (English) protector of the land.

Tedorik (Polish) a form of Theodore.

Tedrick (American) a combination of Ted + Rick.

Teetonka (Lakota) big lodge.

Tefere (Ethiopian) seed.

Tegan (Irish) a form of Teague.

Tej (Sanskrit) light; lustrous.

Tejas (Sanskrit) sharp.

Tekle (Ethiopian) plant.

Telek (Polish) a form of Telford.

Telem (Hebrew) mound; furrow.

Telford (French) iron cutter.

Teller (English) storyteller.

Telly (Greek) a familiar form of Teller, Theodore.

Telmo (English) tiller, cultivator.

Telutci (Moquelumnan) bear making dust as it runs.

Telvin (American) a combination of the prefix Te + Melvin.

Tem (Gypsy) country.

Teman (Hebrew) on the right side; southward.

Tembo (Swahili) elephant.

Tempest (French) storm.

Temple (Latin) sanctuary.

Templeton (English) town near the temple.

Tennant (English) tenant, renter.

Tennessee (Cherokee) mighty warrior. Geography: a southern U.S. state.

Tennyson (English) a form of Dennison. Literature: Alfred, Lord Tennyson was a nineteenth-century British poet.

Teo (Vietnamese) a form of Tom.

Teobaldo (Italian, Spanish) a form of Theobald.

Teodoro (Italian, Spanish) a form of Theodore.

Teppo (French) a familiar form of Stephen.

Tequan (American) a combination of the prefix Te + Quan.

Terance (Latin) a form of Terrence.

Terell (German) a form of Terrell.

Teremun (Tiv) father's acceptance.

Terence (Latin) a form of Terrence. *Teren, Teryn*

Terencio (Spanish) a form of Terrence.

Terran (Latin) a short form of Terrance. *Teren, Terren*

Terrance (Latin) a form of Terrence. *Tarrance*

Terrell (German) thunder ruler. *Terrail, Terral, Terrale, Terrall, Terreal, Terrel, Terrelle, Terryal, Terryel, Tirel, Tirrell, Turrell*

Terrence (Latin) smooth.
Tarrance, Terren

Terrick (American) a combination of the prefix Te + Derrick.

Terrill (German) a form of Terrell.

Terrin (Latin) a short form of Terrence. *Teryn*

Terris (Latin) son of Terry.

Terron (American) a form of Tyrone.

Terry (English) a familiar form of Terrence. See also Keli. *Tarry, Terrey, Terri, Terrie*

Tertius (Latin) third.

Teshawn (American) a combination of the prefix Te + Shawn.

Teva (Hebrew) nature.

Tevan (American) a form of Tevin.

Tevel (Yiddish) a form of David.

Tevin (American) a combination of the prefix Te + Kevin.

Tevis (Scottish) a form of Thomas.

Tevon (American) a form of Tevin.

Tewdor (German) a form of Theodore.

Tex (American) from Texas.

Thabit (Arabic) firm, strong.

Thad (Greek, Latin) a short form of Thaddeus.

Thaddeus (Greek) courageous. (Latin) praiser. Bible: one of the Twelve Apostles. See also Fadey. *Thaddaeus, Thaddaus, Thaddeau, Thaddeaus, Thaddeo, Thaddiaus,* *Thaddius, Thadeaou, Thadeous, Thadeus, Thadieus, Thadious, Thadius, Thadus*

Thady (Irish) praise.

Thai (Vietnamese) many, multiple.

Thaman (Hindi) god; godlike.

Than (Burma) million.

Thane (English) attendant warrior.

Thang (Vietnamese) victorious.

Thanh (Vietnamese) finished.

Thaniel (Hebrew) a short form of Nathaniel.

Thanos (Greek) nobleman; bear-man.

Thatcher (English) roof thatcher, repairer of roofs.

Thaw (English) melting ice.

Thayer (French) nation's army.

Thel (English) upper story.

Thenga (Yao) bring him.

Theo (English) a short form of Theodore.

Theobald (German) people's prince. See also Dietbald.

Theodore (Greek) gift of God. See also Feodor, Fyodor. *Téadóir, Teador, Tedor, Tedorek, Teodomiro, Teodus, Teos, Theodor, Theódor, Theodors, Theodorus, Theodosios, Theodrekr, Tivadar, Tolek*

Theodoric (German) ruler of the people. See also Dedrick, Derek, Dirk.

Theophilus (Greek) loved by God.

Theron (Greek) hunter.
Theran, Theren, Therin, Therron

Thian (Vietnamese) smooth.

Thibault (French) a form of Theobald.

Thierry (French) a form of Theodoric.

Thom (English) a short form of Thomas.

Thoma (German) a form of Thomas.

Thomas ✺ (Greek, Aramaic) twin. Bible: one of the Twelve Apostles. See also Chuma, Foma, Maslin.
Thomason, Thomeson, Thomison, Thomson, Tomcy

Thompson (English) son of Thomas.
Thomason, Thomison, Thomson

Thor (Scandinavian) thunder. Mythology: the Norse god of thunder.

Thorald (Scandinavian) Thor's follower.

Thorbert (Scandinavian) Thor's brightness.

Thorbjorn (Scandinavian) Thor's bear.

Thorgood (English) Thor is good.

Thorleif (Scandinavian) Thor's beloved.

Thorley (English) Thor's meadow.

Thorndike (English) thorny embankment.

Thorne (English) a short form of names beginning with "Thorn."

Thornley (English) thorny meadow.

Thornton (English) thorny town.

Thorpe (English) village.

Thorwald (Scandinavian) Thor's forest.

Thuc (Vietnamese) aware.

Thurlow (English) Thor's hill.

Thurmond (English) defended by Thor.

Thurston (Scandinavian) Thor's stone.

Tiago (Spanish) a form of Jacob.

Tiberio (Italian) from the Tiber River region.

Tibor (Hungarian) holy place.

Tichawanna (Shona) we shall see.

Ticho (Spanish) a short form of Patrick.

Tieler (English) a form of Tyler.

Tiennot (French) a form of Stephen.

Tiernan (Irish) lord.

Tierney (Irish) lordly.

Tige (English) a short form of Tiger.

Tiger (American) tiger; powerful and energetic.

Tiimu (Moquelumnan) caterpillar coming out of the ground.

Tilden (English) tilled valley.

Tiktu (Moquelumnan) bird digging up potatoes.

Tilford (English) prosperous ford.

Till (German) a short form of Theodoric.

Tilton (English) prosperous town.

Tim (Greek) a short form of Timothy.
Timmie

Timin (Arabic) born near the sea.

Timmothy (Greek) a form of Timothy.
Timmathy, Timmoty, Timmthy

Timmy (Greek) a familiar form of
Timothy.
Timmie

Timo (Finnish) a form of Timothy.

Timofey (Russian) a form of Timothy.

Timon (Greek) honorable.

Timoteo (Portuguese, Spanish) a form
of Timothy.

Timothy ✵ (Greek) honoring God. See
also Kimokeo.
*Tadhg, Taidgh, Tiege, Tima, Timithy,
Timkin, Timok, Timontheo, Timonthy,
Timót, Timote, Timotei, Timoteus,
Timothé, Timothée, Timotheo,
Timotheos, Timotheus, Timothey,
Timthie, Tiomóid, Tomothy*

Timur (Hebrew) a form of Tamar.
(Russian) conqueror.

Tin (Vietnamese) thinker.

Tino (Spanish) venerable, majestic.
(Italian) small. A familiar form of
Antonio. (Greek) a short form of
Augustine.

Tinsley (English) fortified field.

Tiquan (American) a combination of
the prefix Ti + Quan.

Tisha (Russian) a form of Timothy.

Tishawn (American) a combination of
the prefix Ti + Shawn.

Tito (Italian) a form of Titus.

Titus (Greek) giant. (Latin) hero. A form
of Tatius. History: a Roman emperor.
Tite, Titek

Tivon (Hebrew) nature lover.

TJ (American) a combination of the
initials T. + J.

Tobal (Spanish) a short form of
Christopher.

Tobar (Gypsy) road.

Tobi (Yoruba) great.

Tobias (Hebrew) God is good.
Tobia, Tobiah, Tobiás, Tobit

Tobin (Hebrew) a form of Tobias.
Tobyn, Tovin

Toby (Hebrew) a familiar form of
Tobias.
Tobby, Tobe, Tobey, Tobie

Todd (English) fox.
Tod, Toddie, Toddy

Todor (Basque, Russian) a form of
Theodore.

Toft (English) small farm.

Tohon (Native American) cougar.

Tokala (Dakota) fox.

Toland (English) owner of taxed land.

Tolbert (English) bright tax collector.

Toller (English) tax collector.

Tom (English) a short form of Tomas,
Thomas.
Tommey

Toma (Romanian) a form of Thomas.

Tomas (German) a form of Thomas.
*Tomaisin, Tomaz, Tomcio, Tome,
Tomek, Tomelis, Tomico, Tomik,
Tomislaw, Tomo, Tomson*

Tomás (Irish, Spanish) a form of
Thomas.

Tomasso (Italian) a form of Thomas.

Tombe (Kakwa) northerners.

Tomey (Irish) a familiar form of
Thomas.
Tome

Tomi (Japanese) rich. (Hungarian) a
form of Thomas.

Tomlin (English) little Tom.

Tommie (Hebrew) a form of Tommy.
Tommi

Tommy (Hebrew) a familiar form of
Thomas.

Tonda (Czech) a form of Tony.
Tonek

Tong (Vietnamese) fragrant.

Toni (Greek, German, Slavic) a form of
Tony.

Tonio (Portuguese) a form of Tony.
(Italian) a short form of Antonio.

Tony (Greek) flourishing. (Latin) praise-
worthy. (English) a short form of
Anthony. A familiar form of
Remington.
Tonek, Toney, Tonik

Tooantuh (Cherokee) spring frog.

Toomas (Estonian) a form of Thomas.

Topher (Greek) a short form of
Christopher, Kristopher.

Topo (Spanish) gopher.

Topper (English) hill.

Tor (Norwegian) thunder. (Tiv) royalty,
king.

Torian (Irish) a form of Torin.

Torin (Irish) chief.
Torrin

Torkel (Swedish) Thor's cauldron.

Tormey (Irish) thunder spirit.

Tormod (Scottish) north.

Torn (Irish) a short form of Torrence.

Torquil (Danish) Thor's kettle.

Torr (English) tower.

Torrance (Irish) a form of Torrence.
Torance

Torren (Irish) a short form of Torrence.
Toren

Torrence (Irish) knolls. (Latin) a form
of Terrence.
*Taurence, Toreence, Torreon, Torrin,
Torry, Tuarence, Turance*

Torrey (English) a form of Tory.
Toreey, Torre, Torri, Torrie, Torry

Toru (Japanese) sea.

Tory (English) familiar form of Torr,
Torrence.
Tori

Toshi-Shita (Japanese) junior.

Tovi (Hebrew) good.

Townley (English) town meadow.

Townsend (English) town's end.

Trace (Irish) a form of Tracy.

Tracey (Irish) a form of Tracy.

Tracy (Greek) harvester. (Latin) courageous. (Irish) battler.
Tracie, Treacy

Trader (English) well-trodden path; skilled worker.

Trae (English) a form of Trey.
Trai

Trahern (Welsh) strong as iron.

Tramaine (Scottish) a form of Tremaine, Tremayne.

Traquan (American) a combination of Travis + Quan.

Trashawn (American) a combination of Travis + Shawn.

Traugott (German) God's truth.

Travaris (French) a form of Travers.

Travell (English) traveler.

Traven (American) a form of Trevon.

Travers (French) crossroads.

Travion (American) a form of Trevon.

Travis (English) a form of Travers.
Travais, Traves, Traveus, Travious, Traviss, Travus, Travys, Trevais

Travon (American) a form of Trevon.

Tray (English) a form of Trey.

Trayton (English) town full of trees.

Trayvon (American) a combination of Tray + Von.

Treavon (American) a form of Trevon.

Tredway (English) well-worn road.

Tremaine, Tremayne (Scottish) house of stone.
Tremain, Treymaine, Trimaine

Trent (Latin) torrent, rapid stream. (French) thirty. Geography: a city in northern Italy.
Trente, Trentino, Trento, Trentonio

Trenton (Latin) town by the rapid stream. Geography: the capital of New Jersey.
Trendon, Trendun, Trenten, Trentin, Trinton

Trequan (American) a combination of Trey + Quan.

Treshawn (American) a combination of Trey + Shawn.

Treston (Welsh) a form of Tristan.
Trestan

Trev (Irish, Welsh) a short form of Trevor.

Trevaughn (American) a combination of Trey + Vaughn.

Trevelyan (English) Elian's homestead.

Trevin (American) a form of Trevon.

Trevion (American) a form of Trevon.

Trevis (English) a form of Travis.

Trevon (American) a combination of Trey + Von.

Trevor ☀ (Irish) prudent. (Welsh) homestead.
Trefor, Trevar, Trever, Treyvor

Trey (English) three; third.
Trai

Treyvon (American) a form of Trevon.

Trigg (Scandinavian) trusty.

Trini (Latin) a short form of Trinity.

Trinity (Latin) holy trinity.

Trip, Tripp (English) traveler.

Tristan (Welsh) bold. Literature: a knight in the Arthurian legends who fell in love with his uncle's wife. *Tris, Trisan, Tristian*

Tristano (Italian) a form of Tristan.

Tristen (Welsh) a form of Tristan.

Tristin (Welsh) a form of Tristan. *Tristian*

Triston (Welsh) a form of Tristan.

Tristram (Welsh) sorrowful. Literature: the title character in Laurence Sterne's eighteenth-century novel *Tristram Shandy*.

Tristyn (Welsh) a form of Tristan.

Trot (English) trickling stream.

Trowbridge (English) bridge by the tree.

Troy (Irish) foot soldier. (French) curly haired. (English) water. See also Koi. *Troi, Troye, Troyton*

True (English) faithful, loyal.

Truesdale (English) faithful one's homestead.

Truitt (English) little and honest.

Truman (English) honest. History: Harry S. Truman was the thirty-third U.S. president.

Trumble (English) strong; bold.

Trustin (English) trustworthy.

Trygve (Norwegian) brave victor.

Trystan (Welsh) a form of Tristan.

Tsalani (Nguni) good-bye.

Tse (Ewe) younger of twins.

Tu (Vietnamese) tree.

Tuaco (Ghanaian) eleventh-born.

Tuan (Vietnamese) goes smoothly.

Tucker (English) fuller, tucker of cloth. *Tuck, Tuckie, Tucky*

Tudor (Welsh) a form of Theodore. History: an English ruling dynasty.

Tug (Scandinavian) draw, pull.

Tuketu (Moquelumnan) bear making dust as it runs.

Tukuli (Moquelumnan) caterpillar crawling down a tree.

Tulio (Italian, Spanish) lively.

Tullis (Latin) title, rank.

Tully (Irish) at peace with God. (Latin) a familiar form of Tullis.

Tumaini (Mwera) hope.

Tumu (Moquelumnan) deer thinking about eating wild onions.

Tung (Vietnamese) stately, dignified. (Chinese) everyone.

Tungar (Sanskrit) high; lofty.

Tupi (Moquelumnan) pulled up.

Tupper (English) ram raiser.

Turi (Spanish) a short form of Arthur.

Turk (English) from Turkey.

Turner (Latin) lathe worker; wood worker.

Turpin (Scandinavian) Finn named after Thor.

Tut (Arabic) strong and courageous. History: a short form of Tutankhamen, an Egyptian king.

Tutu (Spanish) a familiar form of Justin.

Tuvya (Hebrew) a form of Tobias.

Tuwile (Mwera) death is inevitable.

Tuyen (Vietnamese) angel.

Twain (English) divided in two. Literature: Mark Twain (whose real name was Samuel Langhorne Clemens) was one of the most prominent nineteenth-century American writers.

Twia (Fante) born after twins.

Twitchell (English) narrow passage.

Twyford (English) double river crossing.

Txomin (Basque) like the Lord.

Ty (English) a short form of Tyler, Tyrone, Tyrus.
Tye

Tyee (Native American) chief.

Tyger (English) a form of Tiger.

Tylar (English) a form of Tyler.

Tyler ☿ (English) tile maker.
Tiler, Tyel, Tyle, Tylee, Tylere, Tyller

Tylor (English) a form of Tyler.

Tymon (Polish) a form of Timothy. (Greek) a form of Timon.

Tymothy (English) a form of Timothy.

Tynan (Irish) dark.

Tynek (Czech) a form of Martin.

Tyquan (American) a combination of Ty + Quan.

Tyran (American) a form of Tyrone.

Tyree (Scottish) island dweller. Geography: Tiree is an island off the west coast of Scotland.
Tyra, Tyrae, Tyrai, Tyray, Tyre, Tyrea, Tyrée

Tyreese (American) a form of Terrence.

Tyrel, Tyrell (American) forms of Terrell.

Tyrick (American) a combination of Ty + Rick.

Tyrin (American) a form of Tyrone.

Tyron (American) a form of Tyrone.
Tyronn, Tyronna, Tyronne

Tyrone (Greek) sovereign. (Irish) land of Owen.
Teirone, Tyerone, Tyroney, Tyronne, Tyroon, Tyroun

Tyrus (English) a form of Thor.

Tyshawn (American) a combination of Ty + Shawn.

Tyson (French) son of Ty.
Tison, Tiszon, Tyce, Tyesn, Tyeson, Tysen, Tysie, Tysne, Tysone

Tytus (Polish) a form of Titus.

Tyvon (American) a combination of Ty + Von.

Tywan (Chinese) a form of Taiwan.

Tzadok (Hebrew) righteous.

Tzion (Hebrew) sign from God.

Tzuriel (Hebrew) God is my rock.

Tzvi (Hebrew) deer.

U

Uaine (Irish) a form of Owen.

Ubadah (Arabic) serves God.

Ubaid (Arabic) faithful.

Uberto (Italian) a form of Hubert.

Uche (Ibo) thought.

Uday (Sanskrit) to rise.

Udell (English) yew-tree valley.

Udit (Sanskrit) grown; shining.

Udo (Japanese) ginseng plant. (German) a short form of Udolf.

Udolf (English) prosperous wolf.

Ugo (Italian) a form of Hugh, Hugo.

Ugutz (Basque) a form of John.

Uilliam (Irish) a form of William.
Ulick

Uinseann (Irish) a form of Vincent.

Uistean (Irish) intelligent.

Uja (Sanskrit) growing.

Uku (Hawaiian) flea, insect; skilled ukulele player.

Ulan (African) first-born twin.

Ulbrecht (German) a form of Albert.

Ulf (German) wolf.

Ulfred (German) peaceful wolf.

Ulger (German) warring wolf.

Ulises (Latin) a form of Ulysses.
Ulishes, Ulisse, Ulisses

Ullock (German) sporting wolf.

Ulmer (English) famous wolf.

Ulmo (German) from Ulm, Germany.

Ulric (German) a form of Ulrich.

Ulrich (German) wolf ruler; ruler of all. See also Alaric.

Ultman (Hindi) god; godlike.

Ulyses (Latin) a form of Ulysses.

Ulysses (Latin) wrathful. A form of Odysseus.
Ulick, Ulysse

Umang (Sanskrit) enthusiastic.

Umar (Arabic) a form of Omar.

Umberto (Italian) a form of Humbert.

Umi (Yao) life.

Umit (Turkish) hope.

Unai (Basque) shepherd.

Uner (Turkish) famous.

Unika (Lomwe) brighten.

Unique (Latin) only, unique.

Unwin (English) nonfriend.

Upshaw (English) upper wooded area.

Upton (English) upper town.

Upwood (English) upper forest.

Urban (Latin) city dweller; courteous.

Urbane (English) a form of Urban.

Urbano (Italian) a form of Urban.

Uri (Hebrew) a short form of Uriah.

Uriah (Hebrew) my light. Bible: a soldier and the husband of Bathsheba. See also Yuri.
Uria, Urias, Urijah

Urian (Greek) heaven.

Uriel (Hebrew) God is my light.

Urson (French) a form of Orson.

Urtzi (Basque) sky.

Usamah (Arabic) like a lion.

Useni (Yao) tell me.

Usi (Yao) smoke.

Ustin (Russian) a form of Justin.

Utatci (Moquelumnan) bear scratching itself.

Uthman (Arabic) companion of the Prophet.

Uttam (Sanskrit) best.

Uwe (German) a familiar form of Ulrich.

Uzi (Hebrew) my strength.

Uziel (Hebrew) God is my strength; mighty force.

Uzoma (Nigerian) born during a journey.

Uzumati (Moquelumnan) grizzly bear.

V

Vachel (French) small cow.

Vaclav (Czech) wreath of glory.

Vadin (Hindi) speaker.

Vail (English) valley.

Val (Latin) a short form of Valentin.

Valborg (Swedish) mighty mountain.

Valdemar (Swedish) famous ruler.

Valentin (Latin) strong; healthy.

Valentino (Italian) a form of Valentin.

Valerian (Latin) strong; healthy.

Valerii (Russian) a form of Valerian.

Valfrid (Swedish) strong peace.

Valin (Hindi) a form of Balin. Mythology: a tyrannical monkey king.

Vallis (French) from Wales.

Valter (Lithuanian, Swedish) a form of Walter.

Van (Dutch) a short form of Vandyke.
Vander, Vane, Vann, Vanno

Vance (English) thresher.

Vanda (Lithuanian) a form of Walter.
Vander

Vandyke (Dutch) dyke.

Vanya (Russian) a familiar form of
Ivan.

Vardon (French) green knoll.

Varian (Latin) variable.

Varick (German) protecting ruler.

Vartan (Armenian) rose producer; rose
giver.

Varun (Hindi) rain god.

Vasant (Sanskrit) spring.

Vashawn (American) a combination of
the prefix Va + Shawn.

Vasilis (Greek) a form of Basil.

Vasily (Russian) a form of Vasilis.

Vasin (Hindi) ruler, lord.

Vasu (Sanskrit) wealth.

Vasyl (German, Slavic) a form of
William.

Vaughn (Welsh) small.
Vaughan, Vaughen, Vaun, Voughn

Veasna (Cambodian) lucky.

Ved (Sanskrit) sacred knowledge.

Vedie (Latin) sight.

Veer (Sanskrit) brave.

Vegard (Norwegian) sanctuary; protec-
tion.

Velvel (Yiddish) wolf.

Vencel (Hungarian) a short form of
Wenceslaus.

Venedictos (Greek) a form of Benedict.

Veniamin (Bulgarian) a form of
Benjamin.

Venkat (Hindi) god; godlike. Religion:
another name for the Hindu god
Vishnu.

Venya (Russian) a familiar form of
Benedict.

Vere (Latin, French) true.

Vered (Hebrew) rose.

Vergil (Latin) a form of Virgil. Literature:
a Roman poet best known for his epic
poem *Aeneid*.

Vern (Latin) a short form of Vernon.

Vernados (German) courage of the
bear.

Verner (German) defending army.

Verney (French) alder grove.

Vernon (Latin) springlike; youthful.
Vernen, Vernin

Verrill (German) masculine. (French)
loyal.

Vian (English) full of life.

Vic (Latin) a short form of Victor.

Vicente (Spanish) a form of Vincent.
Vicent, Visente

Vicenzo (Italian) a form of Vincent.

Victoir (French) a form of Victor.

Victor ☼ (Latin) victor, conqueror.
*Victa, Victer, Victoriano, Victorien,
Victorin, Vitin*

Victorio (Spanish) a form of Victor.

Vidal (Spanish) a form of Vitas.

Vidar (Norwegian) tree warrior.

Vidor (Hungarian) cheerful.

Vidur (Hindi) wise.

Viho (Cheyenne) chief.

Vijay (Hindi) victorious.

Vikas (Hindi) growing.

Vikram (Hindi) valorous.

Vikrant (Hindi) powerful.

Viktor (German, Hungarian, Russian) a
form of Victor.

Vilhelm (German) a form of William.

Vili (Hungarian) a short form of
William.

Viliam (Czech) a form of William.

Viljo (Finnish) a form of William.

Ville (Swedish) a short form of William.

Vimal (Hindi) pure.

Vin (Latin) a short form of Vincent.

Vinay (Hindi) polite.

Vince (English) a short form of Vincent.
Vence, Vint

Vincent (Latin) victor, conqueror. See
also Binkentios, Binky.
*Vencent, Vikent, Vikenti, Vikesha,
Vincence, Vincens, Vincentius,*

*Vincents, Vincenty, Vincien, Vincient,
Vinciente*

Vincente (Spanish) a form of Vincent.

Vincenzo (Italian) a form of Vincent.
Vincenz, Vincenzio, Vinzenz

Vinci (Hungarian, Italian) a familiar
form of Vincent.

Vinny (English) a familiar form of
Calvin, Melvin, Vincent.

Vinod (Hindi) happy, joyful.

Vinson (English) son of Vincent.

Vipul (Hindi) plentiful.

Viraj (Hindi) resplendent.

Virat (Hindi) very big.

Virgil (Latin) rod bearer, staff bearer.
Virge, Virgial, Virgie

Virgilio (Spanish) a form of Virgil.

Virote (Tai) strong, powerful.

Vishal (Hindi) huge; great.

Vishnu (Hindi) protector.

Vitas (Latin) alive, vital.
Vitus

Vito (Latin) a short form of Vittorio.
*Veit, Vital, Vitale, Vitalis, Vitin, Vitis,
Vitus, Vytas*

Vittorio (Italian) a form of Victor.

Vitya (Russian) a form of Victor.

Vivek (Hindi) wisdom.

Vladimir (Russian) famous prince. See
also Dima, Waldemar, Walter.
Vimka, Vlad, Vladamir, Vladik,

Vladimar, Vladimeer, Vladimire,
Vladjimir, Vladka, Vladko, Vladlen,
Volodya, Volya, Wladimir

Vladislav (Slavic) glorious ruler. See
also Slava.
Vladik

Vlas (Russian) a short form of Vladislav.

Volker (German) people's guard.

Volney (German) national spirit.

Von (German) a short form of many
German names.

Vova (Russian) a form of Walter.

Vuai (Swahili) savior.

Vyacheslav (Russian) a form of
Vladislav. See also Slava.

W

Waban (Ojibwa) white.

Wade (English) ford; river crossing.
Wadesworth, Wadie, Waide, Wayde,
Waydell

Wadley (English) ford meadow.

Wadsworth (English) village near the
ford.

Wagner (German) wagoner, wagon
maker. Music: Richard Wagner was a
famous nineteenth-century German
composer.

Wahid (Arabic) single; exclusively
unequaled.

Wahkan (Lakota) sacred.

Wahkoowah (Lakota) charging.

Wain (English) a short form of
Wainwright. A form of Wayne.

Wainwright (English) wagon maker.

Waite (English) watchman.

Wakefield (English) wet field.

Wakely (English) wet meadow.

Wakeman (English) watchman.

Wakiza (Native American) determined
warrior.

Walcott (English) cottage by the wall.

Waldemar (German) powerful;
famous. See also Vladimir.

Walden (English) wooded valley.
Literature: Henry David Thoreau made
Walden Pond famous with his book
Walden.

Waldo (German) a familiar form of
Oswald, Waldemar, Walden.

Waldron (English) ruler.

Waleed (Arabic) newborn.

Walerian (Polish) strong; brave.

Wales (English) from Wales.

Walford (English) Welshman's ford.

Walfred (German) peaceful ruler.

Wali (Arabic) all-governing.

Walker (English) cloth walker; cloth
cleaner.
Wallie

Wallace (English) from Wales.
Wallas, Wallie, Wallis

Wallach (German) a form of Wallace.

Waller (German) powerful. (English) wall maker.

Wally (English) a familiar form of Walter.
Wallie

Walmond (German) mighty ruler.

Walsh (English) a form of Wallace.

Walt (English) a short form of Walter, Walton.
Waltti

Walter (German) army ruler, general. (English) woodsman. See also Gautier, Gualberto, Gualtiero, Gutierre, Ladislav, Vladimir.
Walaer, Waltti, Wat

Walther (German) a form of Walter.

Walton (English) walled town.

Waltr (Czech) a form of Walter.

Walworth (English) fenced-in farm.

Walwyn (English) Welsh friend.

Wamblee (Lakota) eagle.

Wang (Chinese) hope; wish.

Wanikiya (Lakota) savior.

Wanya (Russian) a form of Vanya.

Wapi (Native American) lucky.

Warburton (English) fortified town.

Ward (English) watchman, guardian.

Wardell (English) watchman's hill.

Wardley (English) watchman's meadow.

Ware (English) wary, cautious.

Warfield (English) field near the weir or fish trap.

Warford (English) ford near the weir or fish trap.

Warley (English) meadow near the weir or fish trap.

Warner (German) armed defender. (French) park keeper.

Warren (German) general; warden; rabbit hutch.
Waring, Warrenson, Warrin, Warriner, Worrin

Warton (English) town near the weir or fish trap.

Warwick (English) buildings near the weir or fish trap.

Washburn (English) overflowing river.

Washington (English) town near water. History: George Washington was the first U.S. president.

Wasili (Russian) a form of Basil.

Wasim (Arabic) graceful; good-looking.

Watende (Nyakyusa) there will be revenge.

Waterio (Spanish) a form of Walter.

Watford (English) wattle ford; dam made of twigs and sticks.

Watkins (English) son of Walter.

Watson (English) son of Walter.

Waverly (English) quaking aspen-tree meadow.

Wayland (English) a form of Waylon.

Waylon (English) land by the road.
Wallen, Walon, Way, Waylan,
Waylen, Waylin

Wayman (English) road man; traveler.

Wayne (English) wagon maker. A short
form of Wainwright.
Wanye, Wayn, Waynell

Wazir (Arabic) minister.

Webb (English) weaver.

Weber (German) weaver.

Webley (English) weaver's meadow.

Webster (English) weaver.

Weddel (English) valley near the ford.

Wei-Quo (Chinese) ruler of the country.

Welborne (English) spring-fed stream.

Welby (German) farm near the well.

Weldon (English) hill near the well.

Welfel (Yiddish) a form of William.

Welford (English) ford near the well.

Wells (English) springs.

Welsh (English) a form of Wallace,
Walsh.

Welton (English) town near the well.

Wemilat (Native American) all give to
him.

Wemilo (Native American) all speak to
him.

Wen (Gypsy) born in winter.

Wenceslaus (Slavic) wreath of honor.

Wendell (German) wanderer. (English)
good dale, good valley.
Wandale, Wendall, Wendel, Wendle,
Wendy

Wene (Hawaiian) a form of Wayne.

Wenford (English) white ford.

Wentworth (English) pale man's settlement.

Wenutu (Native American) clear sky.

Werner (English) a form of Warner.

Wes (English) a short form of Wesley.

Wesh (Gypsy) woods.

Wesley (English) western meadow.
Weslee, Wesleyan, Weslie, Wesly,
Wessley, Westleigh

West (English) west.

Westbrook (English) western brook.

Westby (English) western farmstead.

Westcott (English) western cottage.

Westley (English) a form of Wesley.

Weston (English) western town.
Westen, Westin

Wetherby (English) wether-sheep farm.

Wetherell (English) wether-sheep
corner.

Wetherly (English) wether-sheep
meadow.

Weylin (English) a form of Waylon.

Whalley (English) woods near a hill.

Wharton (English) town on the bank of a lake.

Wheatley (English) wheat field.

Wheaton (English) wheat town.

Wheeler (English) wheel maker; wagon driver.

Whistler (English) whistler, piper.

Whit (English) a short form of Whitman, Whitney.

Whitby (English) white house.

Whitcomb (English) white valley.

Whitelaw (English) small hill.

Whitey (English) white skinned; white haired.

Whitfield (English) white field.

Whitford (English) white ford.

Whitley (English) white meadow.

Whitman (English) white-haired man.

Whitmore (English) white moor.

Whitney (English) white island; white water.
Whittney, Widney, Widny

Whittaker (English) white field.

Wicasa (Dakota) man.

Wicent (Polish) a form of Vincent.

Wichado (Native American) willing.

Wickham (English) village enclosure.

Wickley (English) village meadow.

Wid (English) wide.

Wies (German) renowned warrior.

Wikoli (Hawaiian) a form of Victor.

Wiktor (Polish) a form of Victor.

Wilanu (Moquelumnan) pouring water on flour.

Wilbert (German) brilliant; resolute.
Wilberto, Wilburt

Wilbur (English) wall fortification; bright willows.
Wilburt

Wilder (English) wilderness, wild.

Wildon (English) wooded hill.

Wile (Hawaiian) a form of Willie.

Wiley (English) willow meadow; Will's meadow.
Willey

Wilford (English) willow-tree ford.
Wilferd

Wilfred (German) determined peace-maker.
Wilferd, Wilfrid, Wilfride, Wilfried, Wilfryd, Willfred, Willfried

Wilfredo (Spanish) a form of Wilfred.
Wifredo, Willfredo

Wilhelm (German) determined guardian.

Wiliama (Hawaiian) a form of William.

Wilkie (English) a familiar form of Wilkins.

Wilkins (English) William's kin.

Wilkinson (English) son of little William.

Will (English) a short form of William.
Wilm, Wim

Willard (German) determined and brave.

Willem (German) a form of William.

William ☀ (English) a form of Wilhelm. See also Gilamu, Guglielmo, Guilherme, Guillaume, Guillermo, Gwilym, Liam, Uilliam, Wilhelm.
Villiam, Wilek, Wiliame, Willaim, Willam, Willeam, Willil, Williw, Willyam, Wim

Williams (German) son of William.

Willie (German) a familiar form of William.
Wille, Willi, Willia

Willis (German) son of Willie.
Willice, Willus

Willoughby (English) willow farm.

Wills (English) son of Will.

Willy (German) a form of Willie.
Willey, Wily

Wilmer (German) determined and famous.
Wilm

Wilmot (Teutonic) resolute spirit.
Wilm

Wilny (Native American) eagle singing while flying.

Wilson (English) son of Will.
Willson

Wilt (English) a short form of Wilton.

Wilton (English) farm by the spring.

Wilu (Moquelumnan) chicken hawk squawking.

Win (Cambodian) bright. (English) a short form of Winston and names ending in "win."

Wincent (Polish) a form of Vincent.

Winchell (English) bend in the road; bend in the land.

Windsor (English) riverbank with a winch. History: the surname of the British royal family.

Winfield (English) friendly field.

Winfried (German) friend of peace.

Wing (Chinese) glory.

Wingate (English) winding gate.

Wingi (Native American) willing.

Winslow (English) friend's hill.

Winston (English) friendly town; victory town.
Winsten, Winstonn, Wynstan, Wynston

Winter (English) born in winter.

Winthrop (English) victory at the crossroads.

Winton (English) a form of Winston.

Winward (English) friend's guardian; friend's forest.

Wit (Polish) life. (English) a form of Whit. (Flemish) a short form of DeWitt.

Witek (Polish) a form of Victor.

Witha (Arabic) handsome.

Witter (English) wise warrior.

Witton (English) wise man's estate.

Wladislav (Polish) a form of Vladislav.

Wolcott (English) cottage in the woods.

Wolf (German, English) a short form of Wolfe, Wolfgang.

Wolfe (English) wolf.

Wolfgang (German) wolf quarrel. Music: Wolfgang Amadeus Mozart was a famous eighteenth-century Austrian composer.

Wood (English) a short form of Elwood, Garwood, Woodrow.

Woodfield (English) forest meadow.

Woodford (English) ford through the forest.

Woodrow (English) passage in the woods. History: Thomas Woodrow Wilson was the twenty-eighth U.S. president.

Woodruff (English) forest ranger.

Woodson (English) son of Wood.

Woodward (English) forest warden.

Woodville (English) town at the edge of the woods.

Woody (American) a familiar form of Elwood, Garwood, Woodrow.

Woolsey (English) victorious wolf.

Worcester (English) forest army camp.

Wordsworth (English) wolf-guardian's farm. Literature: William Wordsworth was a famous British poet.

Worie (Ibo) born on market day.

Worth (English) a short form of Wordsworth.

Worton (English) farm town.

Wouter (German) powerful warrior.

Wrangle (American) a form of Rangle.

Wray (Scandinavian) corner property. (English) crooked.

Wren (Welsh) chief, ruler. (English) wren.

Wright (English) a short form of Wainwright.

Wrisley (English) a form of Risley.

Wriston (English) a form of Riston.

Wuliton (Native American) will do well.

Wunand (Native American) God is good.

Wuyi (Moquelumnan) turkey vulture flying.

Wyatt (French) little warrior. *Wiatt, Wyat, Wyatte, Wye, Wyeth*

Wybert (English) battle bright.

Wyborn (Scandinavian) war bear.

Wyck (Scandinavian) village.

Wycliff (English) white cliff; village near the cliff.

Wylie (English) charming. *Wye*

Wyman (English) fighter, warrior.

Wymer (English) famous in battle.

Wyn (Welsh) light skinned; white. (English) friend. A short form of Selwyn.

Wyndham (Scottish) village near the winding road.

Wynono (Native American) first-born son.

Wythe (English) willow tree.

X

Xabat (Basque) savior.

Xaiver (Basque) a form of Xavier. *Xzaiver*

Xan (Greek) a short form of Alexander.

Xander (Greek) a short form of Alexander.

Xanthus (Latin) golden haired.

Xarles (Basque) a form of Charles.

Xavier (Arabic) bright. (Basque) owner of the new house. See also Exavier, Javier, Salvatore, Saverio. *Xabier, Xaver, Xavian, Xavon, Xever, Xizavier*

Xenophon (Greek) strange voice.

Xenos (Greek) stranger; guest.

Xerxes (Persian) ruler. History: a king of Persia.

Ximenes (Spanish) a form of Simon.

Xylon (Greek) forest.

Xzavier (Basque) a form of Xavier. *Xzavaier, Xzaver, Xzavion*

Y

Yadid (Hebrew) friend; beloved.

Yadon (Hebrew) he will judge.

Yael (Hebrew) a form of Jael.

Yafeu (Ibo) bold.

Yagil (Hebrew) he will rejoice.

Yago (Spanish) a form of James.

Yahto (Lakota) blue.

Yahya (Arabic) living.

Yair (Hebrew) he will enlighten.

Yakecen (Dene) sky song.

Yakez (Carrier) heaven.

Yakov (Russian) a form of Jacob. *Yaacob, Yaacov, Yaakov, Yachov, Yacov, Yakob*

Yale (German) productive. (English) old.

Yan, Yann (Russian) forms of John.

Yana (Native American) bear.

Yancy (Native American) Englishman, Yankee.

Yanick, Yannick (Russian) familiar forms of Yan.

Yanka (Russian) a familiar form of John.

Yanni (Greek) a form of John.

Yanton (Hebrew) a form of Johnathon, Jonathon.

Yao (Ewe) born on Thursday.

Yaphet (Hebrew) a form of Japheth.

Yarb (Gypsy) herb.

Yardan (Arabic) king.

Yarden (Hebrew) a form of Jordan.

Yardley (English) enclosed meadow.

Yarom (Hebrew) he will raise up.

Yaron (Hebrew) he will sing; he will cry out.

Yasashiku (Japanese) gentle; polite.

Yash (Hindi) victorious; glory.

Yasha (Russian) a form of Jacob, James.

Yashwant (Hindi) glorious.

Yasin (Arabic) prophet.

Yasir (Afghan) humble; takes it easy. (Arabic) wealthy.

Yasuo (Japanese) restful.

Yates (English) gates.

Yatin (Hindi) ascetic.

Yavin (Hebrew) he will understand.

Yawo (Akan) born on Thursday.

Yazid (Arabic) his power will increase.

Yechiel (Hebrew) God lives.

Yedidya (Hebrew) a form of Jedidiah. See also Didi.

Yegor (Russian) a form of George. See also Egor, Igor.

Yehoshua (Hebrew) a form of Joshua.

Yehoyakem (Hebrew) a form of Joachim, Joaquín.

Yehudi (Hebrew) a form of Judah.

Yelutci (Moquelumnan) bear walking silently.

Yeoman (English) attendant; retainer.

Yeremey (Russian) a form of Jeremiah.

Yervant (Armenian) king, ruler. History: an Armenian king.

Yeshaya (Hebrew) gift. See also Shai.

Yeshurun (Hebrew) right way.

Yeska (Russian) a form of Joseph.

Yestin (Welsh) just.

Yevgenyi (Russian) a form of Eugene. *Yevgeni, Yevgenij*

Yigal (Hebrew) he will redeem.

Yirmaya (Hebrew) a form of Jeremiah.

Yishai (Hebrew) a form of Jesse.

Yisrael (Hebrew) a form of Israel.

Yitro (Hebrew) a form of Jethro.

Yitzchak (Hebrew) a form of Isaac. See also Itzak.

Yngve (Swedish) ancestor; lord, master.

Yo (Cambodian) honest.

Yoakim (Slavic) a form of Jacob.

Yoan (German) a form of Johan, Johann.

Yoav (Hebrew) a form of Joab.

Yochanan (Hebrew) a form of John.

Yoel (Hebrew) a form of Joel.

Yogesh (Hindi) ascetic. Religion: another name for the Hindu god Shiva.

Yohance (Hausa) a form of John.

Yohan, Yohann (German) forms of Johan, Johann.

Yonah (Hebrew) a form of Jonah.

Yonatan (Hebrew) a form of Jonathan.

Yong (Chinese) courageous.

Yong-Sun (Korean) dragon in the first position; courageous.

Yoni (Greek) a form of Yanni.

Yoofi (Akan) born on Friday.

Yooku (Fante) born on Wednesday.

Yoram (Hebrew) God is high.

Yorgos (Greek) a form of George.

York (English) boar estate; yew-tree estate.

Yorkoo (Fante) born on Thursday.

Yosef (Hebrew) a form of Joseph. See also Osip.

Yóshi (Japanese) adopted son.

Yoshiyahu (Hebrew) a form of Josiah.

Yoskolo (Moquelumnan) breaking off pine cones.

Yosu (Hebrew) a form of Jesus.

Yotimo (Moquelumnan) yellow jacket carrying food to its hive.

Yottoko (Native American) mud at the water's edge.

Young (English) young.

Young-Jae (Korean) pile of prosperity.

Young-Soo (Korean) keeping the prosperity.

Youri (Russian) a form of Yuri.

Yousef (Yiddish) a form of Joseph.

Youssel (Yiddish) a familiar form of Joseph.

Yov (Russian) a short form of Yoakim.

Yovani (Slavic) a form of Jovan. *Yovan*

Yoyi (Hebrew) a form of George.

Yrjo (Finnish) a form of George.

Ysidro (Greek) a short form of Isidore.

Yu (Chinese) universe.

Yudell (English) a form of Udell.

Yuki (Japanese) snow.

Yul (Mongolian) beyond the horizon.

Yule (English) born at Christmas.

Yuli (Basque) youthful.

Yuma (Native American) son of a chief.

Yunus (Turkish) a form of Jonah.

Yurcel (Turkish) sublime.

Yuri (Russian, Ukrainian) a form of George. (Hebrew) a familiar form of Uriah.

Yusif (Russian) a form of Joseph.

Yustyn (Russian) a form of Justin.

Yusuf (Arabic, Swahili) a form of Joseph.
Yusef, Yusuff

Yutu (Moquelumnan) coyote out hunting.

Yuval (Hebrew) rejoicing.

Yves (French) a form of Ivar, Ives.
Yvens

Yvon (French) a form of Ivar, Yves.

Z

Zac (Hebrew) a short form of Zachariah, Zachary.

Zacarias (Portuguese, Spanish) a form of Zachariah.
Zacaria

Zacary (Hebrew) a form of Zachary.

Zaccary (Hebrew) a form of Zachary.

Zaccheus (Hebrew) innocent, pure.

Zach (Hebrew) a short form of Zachariah, Zachary.

Zachari (Hebrew) a form of Zachary.

Zacharia (Hebrew) a form of Zachary.

Zachariah (Hebrew) God remembered.
Zacarius, Zachury, Zaquero, Zecharia, Zecharya, Zeggery, Zhachory

Zacharias (German) a form of Zachariah.
Zekarias

Zacharie (Hebrew) a form of Zachary.
Zachare, Zacharee

Zachary ☙ (Hebrew) a familiar form of Zachariah. History: Zachary Taylor was the twelfth U.S. president. See also Sachar, Sakeri.
Zacha, Zachaios, Zacharey, Zachaury, Zachury

Zachery (Hebrew) a form of Zachary.
Zacherey, Zacheria, Zacherias, Zacheriah, Zacherie, Zacherius

Zachory (Hebrew) a form of Zachary.

Zachry (Hebrew) a form of Zachary.

Zack (Hebrew) a short form of Zachariah, Zachary.

Zackary (Hebrew) a form of Zachary.
Zackari, Zackariah, Zackarie, Zackie, Zackree, Zackrey, Zackry

Zackery (Hebrew) a form of Zachery.

Zackory (Hebrew) a form of Zachary.
Zackorie

Zadok (Hebrew) a short form of Tzadok.

Zadornin (Basque) Saturn.

Zafir (Arabic) victorious.

Zahid (Arabic) self-denying, ascetic.

Zahir (Arabic) shining, bright.

Zahur (Swahili) flower.

Zaid (Arabic) increase, growth.

Zaide (Hebrew) older.

Zaim (Arabic) brigadier general.

Zain (English) a form of Zane.

Zakaria (Hebrew) a form of Zachariah.

Zakariyya (Arabic) prophet. Religion: an Islamic prophet.

Zakary (Hebrew) a form of Zachery.

Zakery (Hebrew) a form of Zachary.

Zaki (Arabic) bright; pure. (Hausa) lion.

Zakia (Swahili) intelligent.

Zakkary (Hebrew) a form of Zachary.

Zako (Hungarian) a form of Zachariah.

Zale (Greek) sea strength.

Zalmai (Afghan) young.

Zalman (Yiddish) a form of Solomon.

Zamiel (German) a form of Samuel.
Zamuel

Zamir (Hebrew) song; bird.

Zan (Italian) clown.

Zander (Greek) a short form of
Alexander.

Zane (English) a form of John.

Zanis (Latvian) a form of Janis.

Zanvil (Hebrew) a form of Samuel.

Zaquan (American) a combination of
the prefix Za + Quan.

Zareb (African) protector.

Zared (Hebrew) ambush.

Zarek (Polish) may God protect the
king.

Zavier (Arabic) a form of Xavier.

Zayit (Hebrew) olive.

Zayne (English) a form of Zane.

Zdenek (Czech) follower of Saint Denis.

Zeb (Hebrew) a short form of Zebediah,
Zebulon.

Zebediah (Hebrew) God's gift.

Zebedee (Hebrew) a familiar form of
Zebediah.

Zebulon (Hebrew) exalted, honored;
lofty house.

Zechariah (Hebrew) a form of
Zachariah.
Zecharia, Zekarias, Zekeriah

Zed (Hebrew) a short form of Zedekiah.

Zedekiah (Hebrew) God is mighty and
just.

Zedidiah (Hebrew) a form of Zebediah.

Zeeman (Dutch) seaman.

Zeév (Hebrew) wolf.

Zeheb (Turkish) gold.

Zeke (Hebrew) a short form of Ezekiel,
Zachariah, Zachary, Zechariah.

Zeki (Turkish) clever, intelligent.

Zelgai (Afghan) heart.

Zelig (Yiddish) a form of Selig.

Zelimir (Slavic) wishes for peace.

Zemar (Afghan) lion.

Zen (Japanese) religious. Religion: a
form of Buddhism.

Zenda (Czech) a form of Eugene.

Zeno (Greek) cart; harness. History: a
Greek philosopher.

Zephaniah (Hebrew) treasured by God.

Zephyr (Greek) west wind.

Zero (Arabic) empty, void.

Zeroun (Armenian) wise and respected.

Zeshawn (American) a combination of the prefix Ze + Shawn.

Zesiro (Luganda) older of twins.

Zeus (Greek) living. Mythology: chief god of the Greek pantheon.

Zeusef (Portuguese) a form of Joseph.

Zev (Hebrew) a short form of Zebulon.

Zevi (Hebrew) a form of Tzvi.

Zhek (Russian) a short form of Evgeny.

Zhìxin (Chinese) ambitious.

Zhuàng (Chinese) strong.

Zhora (Russian) a form of George.

Zia (Hebrew) trembling; moving. (Arabic) light.

Zigfrid (Latvian, Russian) a form of Siegfried.

Ziggy (American) a familiar form of Siegfried, Sigmund.

Zigor (Basque) punishment.

Zikomo (Nguni) thank-you.

Zilaba (Luganda) born while sick.

Zimra (Hebrew) song of praise.

Zimraan (Arabic) praise.

Zinan (Japanese) second son.

Zindel (Yiddish) a form of Alexander.

Zion (Hebrew) sign, omen; excellent. Bible: the name used to refer to Israel and to the Jewish people.

Ziskind (Yiddish) sweet child.

Ziv (Hebrew) shining brightly. (Slavic) a short form of Ziven.

Ziven (Slavic) vigorous, lively.

Ziyad (Arabic) increase.

Zlatan (Czech) gold.

Zohar (Hebrew) bright light.

Zollie, Zolly (Hebrew) forms of Solly.

Zoltán (Hungarian) life.

Zorba (Greek) live each day.

Zorion (Basque) a form of Orion.

Zorya (Slavic) star; dawn.

Zotikos (Greek) saintly, holy. Religion: a saint in the Eastern Orthodox Church.

Zotom (Kiowa) a biter.

Zsigmond (Hungarian) a form of Sigmund.

Zuberi (Swahili) strong.

Zubin (Hebrew) a short form of Zebulon.

Zuhayr (Arabic) brilliant, shining.

Zuka (Shona) sixpence.

Zuriel (Hebrew) God is my rock.

Zygmunt (Polish) a form of Sigmund.

Also from Meadowbrook Press

✦ *The Best Baby Shower Book*
The number one baby shower planner has been updated for the new millennium. This contemporary guide for planning baby showers is full of helpful hints, recipes, decorating ideas, and activities that are fun without being juvenile.

✦ *Pregnancy, Childbirth, and the Newborn*
More complete and up-to-date than any other pregnancy guide, this remarkable book is the "bible" for childbirth educators. Now revised with a greatly expanded treatment of pregnancy tests, complications, and infections; an expanded list of drugs and medications (plus advice for uses); and a brand-new chapter on creating a detailed birth plan.

✦ *First-Year Baby Care*
This leading baby-care book is now totally revised with the most up-to-date medical facts and new illustrations. It contains complete information on the basics of baby care, including bathing, diapering, medical facts, and feeding your baby. Includes step-by-step illustrated instructions to make finding information easy, newborn screening and immunization schedules, breastfeeding information for working mothers, expanded information on child care options, reference guides to common illnesses, and environmental and safety tips.